T0263096

Oral Cavity and Oropharyngeal Cancer

Editors

JEFFREY N. MYERS
ERICH M. STURGIS

OTOLARYNGOLOGIC CLINICS OF NORTH AMERICA

www.oto.theclinics.com

August 2013 • Volume 46 • Number 4

ELSEVIER

1600 John F. Kennedy Boulevard • Suite 1800 • Philadelphia, Pennsylvania, 19103-2899

http://www.oto.theclinics.com

OTOLARYNGOLOGIC CLINICS OF NORTH AMERICA Volume 46, Number 4
August 2013 ISSN 0030-6665, ISBN-13: 978-0-323-18613-1

Editor: Joanne Husovski
Development Editor: Donald Mumford

Otolaryngologic Clinics of North America (ISSN 0030-6665) is published bimonthly by Elsevier, Inc., 360 Park Avenue South, New York, NY 10010-1710. Months of issue are February, April, June, August, October, and December. Business and Editorial Offices: 1600 John F. Kennedy Blvd., Suite 1800, Philadelphia, PA 19103-2899. Customer Service Office: 6277 Sea Harbor Drive, Orlando, FL 32887-4800. Periodicals postage paid at New York, NY and additional mailing offices. Subscription prices is $348.00 per year (US individuals), $653.00 per year (US institutions), $167.00 per year (US student/resident), $460.00 per year (Canadian individuals), $819.00 per year (Canadian institutions), $516.00 per year (international individuals), $819.00 per year (international institutions), $258.00 per year (international & Canadian student/resident). Foreign air speed delivery is included in all *Clinics*' subscription prices. All prices are subject to change without notice. **POSTMASTER:** Send address changes to *Otolaryngologic Clinics of North America*, Elsevier Health Sciences Division, Subscription Customer Service, 3251 Riverport Lane, Maryland Heights, MO 63043. **Telephone: 1-800-654-2452 (U.S. and Canada); 314-447-8871 (outside U.S. and Canada). Fax: 314-447-8029. E-mail: journalscustomerservice-usa@elsevier.com (for print support); journalsonlinesupport-usa@elsevier.com (for online support).**

Reprints. For copies of 100 or more of articles in this publication, please contact the Commercial Reprints Department, Elsevier Inc., 360 Park Avenue South, New York, NY 10010-1710. Tel.: 212-633-3812; Fax: 212-462-1935; E-mail: reprints@elsevier.com.

Otolaryngologic Clinics of North America is also published in Spanish by McGraw-Hill Interamericana Editores S.A., P.O. Box 5-237, 06500 Mexico D.F., Mexico.

Otolaryngologic Clinics of North America is covered in *MEDLINE/PubMed (Index Medicus), Current Contents/Clinical Medicine, Excerpta Medica, BIOSIS, Science Citation Index,* and *ISI/BIOMED.*

Printed and bound by CPI Group (UK) Ltd, Croydon, CR0 4YY
Transferred to digital print 2013

Contributors

EDITORS

JEFFREY N. MYERS, MD, PhD
Professor, Department of Head and Neck Surgery, The University of Texas MD Anderson Cancer Center, Houston, Texas

ERICH M. STURGIS, MD, MPH
Professor, Department of Head and Neck Surgery; Department of Epidemiology, The University of Texas MD Anderson Cancer Center, Houston, Texas

AUTHORS

NISHANT AGRAWAL, MD
Associate Professor, Department of Otolaryngology-Head and Neck Surgery, Johns Hopkins University School of Medicine, Baltimore, Maryland

CHLOÉ BERTOLUS, MD, PhD
Associate Professor, Department of Maxillofacial Surgery, Pitié-Salpêtrière Hospital, Paris, France

JULIANA BONILLA-VELEZ, MD
Postdoctoral Research Fellow, Department of Otolaryngology, Massachusetts Eye and Ear Infirmary, Harvard Medical School, Boston, Massachusetts

DANIEL R. CLAYBURGH, MD, PhD
Resident, Department of Otolaryngology-Head and Neck Surgery, Oregon Health and Science University, Portland, Oregon

JEAN-PHILIPPE FOY, MD
Fellow, Department of Maxillofacial Surgery, Pitié-Salpêtrière Hospital, Paris, France

STEVEN J. FRANK, MD
Associate Professor, Director of Advanced Technologies, Department of Radiation Oncology, The University of Texas MD Anderson Cancer Center, Houston, Texas

IAN GANLY, MD, PhD
Head and Neck Service, Department of Surgery, Memorial Sloan Kettering Cancer Center, New York, New York

KATHRYN A. GOLD, MD
Assistant Professor, Department of Thoracic/Head and Neck Medical Oncology, The University of Texas MD Anderson Cancer Center, Houston, Texas

NEIL GROSS, MD, FACS
Associate Professor, Head and Neck Surgery and Oncology, Department of Otolaryngology-Head and Neck Surgery, Knight Cancer Institute, Oregon Health and Science University, Portland, Oregon

G. BRANDON GUNN, MD
Assistant Professor, Department of Radiation Oncology, The University of Texas MD Anderson Cancer Center, Houston, Texas

REBECCA J. HAMMON, MD
Clinical Research Fellow, Department of Otolaryngology, Massachusetts Eye and Ear Infirmary, Harvard Medical School, Boston, Massachusetts

MIA HASHIBE, PhD
Associate Professor, Division of Public Health, Department of Family and Preventive Medicine, Huntsman Cancer Institute, University of Utah School of Medicine, Salt Lake City, Utah

KATHERINE A. HUTCHESON, PhD
Assistant Professor, Department of Head and Neck Surgery, Section of Speech Pathology & Audiology, The University of Texas MD Anderson Cancer Center, Houston, Texas

DAVID I. KUTLER, MD, FACS
Associate Professor, Division of Head and Neck Surgery, Department of Otolaryngology-Head and Neck Surgery, Weill Cornell Medical Center, New York Presbyterian Hospital, New York, New York

JAN S. LEWIN, PhD
Section Chief, Speech Pathology and Audiology, Professor, Department of Head and Neck Surgery, The University of Texas MD Anderson Cancer Center, Houston, Texas

CAROL M. LEWIS, MD, MPH
Assistant Professor, Department of Head and Neck Surgery, The University of Texas MD Anderson Cancer Center, Houston, Texas

JIAHUI LIN
Medical Student, Weill Cornell Medical College, New York, New York

PABLO H. MONTERO-MIRANDA, MD
Head and Neck Service, Department of Surgery, Memorial Sloan Kettering Cancer Center, New York, New York

EDMUND A. MROZ, PhD
Research Scientist, Center for Cancer Research, Department of Surgery, Massachusetts General Hospital, Boston, Massachusetts

JEFFREY N. MYERS, MD, PhD
Professor, Department of Head and Neck Surgery, The University of Texas MD Anderson Cancer Center, Houston, Texas

MICHELE NESKEY, PA
Department of Thoracic/Head and Neck Medical Oncology, The University of Texas MD Anderson Cancer Center, Houston, Texas

JAMES W. ROCCO, MD, PhD
Daniel Miller Associate Professor of Otology and Laryngology at Harvard Medical School; Director of Head and Neck Research, Department of Otolaryngology, Massachusetts Eye and Ear Infirmary; Department of Surgery, Massachusetts General Hospital Principal Investigator, Massachusetts General Hospital Cancer Center, Boston, Massachusetts

PIERRE SAINTIGNY, MD, PhD
Assistant Professor, Department of Thoracic/Head and Neck Medical Oncology, The University of Texas MD Anderson Cancer Center, Houston, Texas

ERICH M. STURGIS, MD, MPH
Professor, Department of Head and Neck Surgery, The University of Texas MD Anderson Cancer Center, Houston, Texas

MARIETTA TAN, MD
Resident Physician, Department of Otolaryngology-Head and Neck Surgery, Johns Hopkins University School of Medicine, Baltimore, Maryland

RANDAL S. WEBER, MD
Professor and Chairman, Department of Head and Neck Surgery, The University of Texas MD Anderson Cancer Center, Houston, Texas

WILLIAM N. WILLIAM Jr, MD
Assistant Professor, Department of Thoracic/Head and Neck Medical Oncology, The University of Texas MD Anderson Cancer Center, Houston, Texas

MARK E. ZAFEREO, MD
Assistant Professor, Department of Head and Neck Surgery, The University of Texas MD Anderson Cancer Center, Houston, Texas

Contents

Preface: A Tale of Two Cancers: Carcinomas of the Oral Cavity and Oropharynx **xiii**

Jeffrey N. Myers and Erich M. Sturgis

Etiology and Biology

Epidemiology of Oral-Cavity and Oropharyngeal Carcinomas: Controlling a Tobacco Epidemic While a Human Papillomavirus Epidemic Emerges **507**

Mia Hashibe and Erich M. Sturgis

Although tobacco prevalence is declining in most developed countries, less developed countries are still experiencing an increase in tobacco use. Thus the future burden of oral-cavity and oropharyngeal cancers in less developed countries is expected to be heavy. The incidence of human papillomavirus (HPV)-associated oropharyngeal cancer is dramatically increasing in the United States and other developed countries, although trends in less developed countries are not clear at present. HPV vaccine compliance in the United States is low, although it continues to increase each year. Increasing the HPV vaccination rate to control future HPV-associated cancer incidence remains a priority.

Impact of Human Papillomavirus on Oropharyngeal Cancer Biology and Response to Therapy: Implications for Treatment **521**

Juliana Bonilla-Velez, Edmund A. Mroz, Rebecca J. Hammon, and James W. Rocco

Oropharyngeal squamous cell carcinoma (OPSCC) originating from human papillomavirus infection has emerged as a new entity in head and neck cancer, defining a subset of patients with distinct carcinogenesis, risk factor profiles, and clinical presentation that show markedly improved survival than patients with classic OPSCC. De-escalation of therapy and identification of relevant biomarkers to aid in patient selection are actively being investigated. This review addresses the implications of these findings in clinical care.

Oral Cavity and Oropharyngeal Squamous Cell Carcinoma Genomics **545**

Marietta Tan, Jeffrey N. Myers, and Nishant Agrawal

Recent technological advances now permit the study of the entire cancer genome, which can elucidate complex pathway interactions that are not apparent at the level of single genes. In this review, the authors describe innovations that have allowed for whole-exome/genome analysis of genetic and epigenetic alterations and of changes in gene expression. Studies using next-generation sequencing, array comparative genomic hybridization, methylation arrays, and gene expression profiling are reviewed, with a particular focus on findings from recent whole-exome sequencing projects. A discussion of the implications of these data on treatment and future goals for cancer genomics is included.

Why Otolaryngologists Need to be Aware of Fanconi Anemia 567

Jiahui Lin and David I. Kutler

Fanconi anemia (FA) is a rare disorder inherited in an autosomal recessive fashion, with an estimated incidence of 1:360,000 births. Although hematologic complications are the most common manifestation of this disease, cancers, especially of the head and neck, are also prominent. The chromosomal fragility of patients with FA necessitates careful planning of therapy and monitoring, and awareness of this rare disorder is crucial to recognizing it in the clinic.

Evaluation and Therapy

Oral Premalignancy: The Roles of Early Detection and Chemoprevention 579

Jean-Philippe Foy, Chloé Bertolus, William N. William Jr, and Pierre Saintigny

Premalignancy and chemoprevention studies in head and neck cancer typically focus on the oral cavity. Avoiding or cessation of alcohol and smoking, early detection of potentially malignant disorders or cancer, and early detection of recurrent and/or second primary tumor form the basis of prevention of oral cancer. Analysis of tissue prospectively collected in evaluation of retinoids for chemoprevention trials allowed identification of molecular biomarkers of risk to develop oral cancer, loss of heterozygosity being the most validated one. Improving risk assessment and identification of new targets for chemoprevention represent the main challenges in this field.

Evaluation and Staging of Squamous Cell Carcinoma of the Oral Cavity and Oropharynx: Limitations Despite Technological Breakthroughs 599

Mark E. Zafereo

Squamous cell carcinoma of the oral cavity (SCCOC) and squamous cell carcinoma of the oropharynx (SCCOP) represent two distinct disease entities. SCCOC continues to be related to tobacco risk factors, and the current anatomic staging system provides useful prognostic value. Most patients with SCCOP in Western countries now have HPV-associated tumors, and tumor HPV status is considered the most important prognostic factor. Smoking status is emerging as an important prognostic factor for HPV-driven SCCOP, independent of tumor HPV status. Sentinel lymph node biopsy and FDG-PET/CT imaging are diagnostic staging tools useful in select patients with SCCOC and SCCOP.

Surgical Innovations 615

Daniel R. Clayburgh and Neil Gross

This article reviews the evidence behind surgical innovations and effect on treatment-related morbidity to examine how they may be integrated into modern management strategies for oral cavity and oropharyngeal squamous cell carcinoma (SCC). Technologic advances, including transoral laser microsurgery and transoral robotic surgery, along with the application of sentinel lymph node biopsy for oral cavity and oropharyngeal SCC are discussed.

Advances in Radiation Oncology for the Management of Oropharyngeal Tumors 629

G. Brandon Gunn and Steven J. Frank

The major benefits of modern radiation therapy (eg, intensity-modulated [x-ray] radiation therapy [IMRT]) for oropharyngeal cancer are reduced xerostomia and better quality of life. Intensity-modulated proton therapy may provide additional advantages over IMRT by reducing radiation beam–path toxicities. Several acute and late treatment-related toxicities and symptom constellations must be kept in mind when designing and comparing future treatment strategies, particularly because currently most patients with oropharyngeal carcinoma present with human papillomavirus–positive disease and are expected to have a high probability of long-term survival after treatment.

The Role of Systemic Treatment Before, During, and After Definitive Treatment 645

Kathryn A. Gold, Michele Neskey, and William N. William Jr

In locoregionally advanced head and neck squamous cell carcinomas, outcomes using single-modality therapy are usually poor. Although chemotherapy alone is not considered a curative therapy, the addition of chemotherapy to other modalities can lead to improved outcomes. Discussed here is the use of chemotherapy for oropharyngeal and/or oral cavity squamous cell carcinomas in 3 settings: in combination with radiation as definitive therapy, as induction treatment before definitive therapy, and in combination with radiation therapy as adjuvant treatment following surgical resection. The role of the targeted agent cetuximab in combination with radiation therapy for locally advanced disease is also discussed.

Quality of Life and Quality of Care

Functional Assessment and Rehabilitation: How to Maximize Outcomes 657

Katherine A. Hutcheson and Jan S. Lewin

The number of oral cavity and oropharyngeal cancer survivors is rising. By 2030, oropharyngeal cancers are projected to account for almost half of all head and neck cancers. Normal speech, swallowing, and respiration can be disrupted by adverse effects of tumor and cancer therapy. This review summarizes clinically distinct functional outcomes of patients with oral cavity and oropharyngeal cancers, methods of pretreatment functional assessments, strategies to reduce or prevent functional complications, and posttreatment rehabilitation considerations.

Standardizing Treatment: A Crisis in Cancer Care 671

Carol M. Lewis and Randal S. Weber

The Institute of Medicine has emphasized the roles of multidisciplinary treatment planning, evidence-based clinical practice guidelines, and regionalization of healthcare in optimizing the quality of cancer care. We discuss these critical elements as they pertain to head and neck cancer care.

Survivorship—Competing Mortalities, Morbidities, and Second Malignancies 681

Pablo H. Montero-Miranda and Ian Ganly

Mortality of head and neck cancer has declined in the United States over the past 20 years. This improvement has been linked to use of multimodality treatment of advanced disease. Despite this improvement, disease-specific survival remains low. Patients who survive head and neck cancer are exposed to morbidity and mortality secondary to the same factors as the general population. Factors related to cancer and cancer treatment predispose them to increased risk of mortality. Improvements in head and neck cancer treatment have led to a scenario where an increasing proportion of patients die from causes other than the primary cancer, called competing mortalities.

Erratum 711

Index 713

OTOLARYNGOLOGIC CLINICS OF NORTH AMERICA

OTOLARYNGOLOGIC CLINICS OF NORTH AMERICA

FORTHCOMING ISSUES

Surgical Management of Facial Trauma
Kofi Boahene, MD, and
Anthony Brissett, MD, *Editors*

Asthma
Karen Calhoun, MD, *Editor*

Headache
Howard Levine, MD, and
Michael Setzen, MD, *Editors*

TransOral Robotic Surgery (TORS)
Neil Gross, MD, and
F. Christopher Holsinger, MD, *Editors*

RECENT ISSUES

Complementary and Integrative Therapies for ENT Disorders
John Maddalozzo, MD,
Edmund A. Pribitkin, MD, and
Michael D. Seidman, MD, FACS, *Editors*
June 2013

Endoscopic Ear Surgery
Muaaz Tarabichi, João Flávio Nogueira, Daniele Marchioni, Livio Presutti, and David D. Pothier, *Editors*
April 2013

Office Procedures in Laryngology
Milan R. Amin, *Editor*
February 2013

Imaging of Head and Neck Spaces for Diagnosis and Treatment
Sangam G. Kanekar, MD, and
Kyle Mannion, MD, *Editors*
December 2012

NOW AVAILABLE FOR YOUR iPhone and iPad

Preface

A Tale of Two Cancers: Carcinomas of the Oral Cavity and Oropharynx

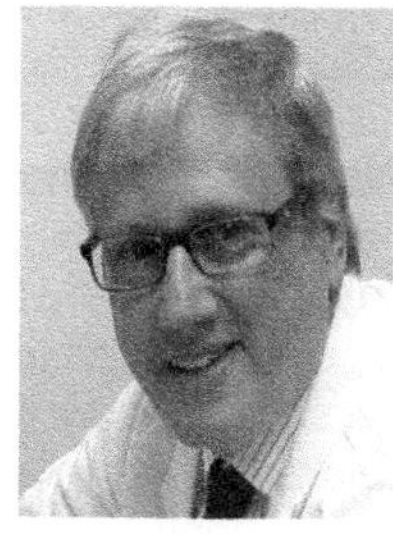

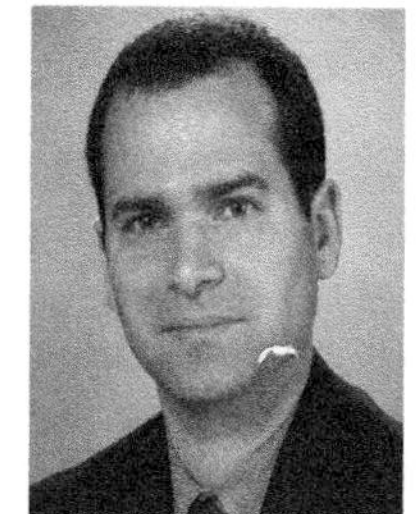

Jeffrey N. Myers, MD, PhD   Erich M. Sturgis, MD, MPH
Editors

KEY POINTS

- Oral cavity cancer and oropharyngeal cancer are now considered 2 distinct diseases with differences in demographics, risk factors, presentation, and clinical behavior and consequently must be studied, evaluated, and treated as different diseases to achieve the best oncologic and functional outcomes.
- The epidemiology, etiology, and biology of these cancers are reviewed. Up-to-date evaluation and treatments are presented. Quality of life/function, treatment standardization, and survivorship are reviewed.

INTRODUCTION

The developed world is experiencing a major shift in the epidemiology of head and neck cancer. Cancers of the oral cavity and oropharynx were once overwhelming found in smokers and drinkers, but recently there has been a rise in the incidence of human papillomavirus (HPV)-associated oropharyngeal cancers, whereas the reduction in cigarette smoking has been reflected in a decline in the incidence of oral cavity cancers and HPV-negative oropharyngeal cancers. These trends have implications for prevention, diagnosis, workup, treatment, and follow-up. This issue of *Otolaryngologic Clinics of North America* is focused on oral cavity and oropharyngeal cancer and the impact of the HPV epidemic on how clinicians view all aspects of these 2 different diseases.

Otolaryngol Clin N Am 46 (2013) xiii–xvi
http://dx.doi.org/10.1016/j.otc.2013.04.012
0030-6665/13/$ – see front matter

OVERVIEW OF ORAL CAVITY AND OROPHARYNGEAL CANCER

Etiology and Biology

Dr Mia Hashibe of Huntsman Cancer Institute and the University of Utah School of Medicine opens our discussion with a review of the changing epidemiology of these 2 diseases. She reviews the evolution of the tobacco epidemic and advances in tobacco control in the United States since the Surgeon General's Warning of 1964. Although this public health success has resulted in a drop in the incidence rates for most types of head and neck cancer, oropharyngeal cancer incidence rates have been on the rise because of an epidemic of HPV-associated oropharyngeal cancer. These HPV-associated malignancies have unique demographic and clinical behaviors distinct from those of classical tobacco-associated and alcohol-associated head and neck cancers. Dr Jim Rocco and colleagues of the Massachusetts Eye and Ear Infirmary and Harvard Medical School provide an in-depth discussion of HPV biology and the HPV-related carcinogenesis. The classic presentation of HPV-associated oropharyngeal cancer appears to be a small base of tongue or tonsil cancer, typically with multiple metastatic lymph nodes, in a middle-aged white man with significant sexual exposures. As reviewed by Dr Rocco and colleagues, these HPV-associated cancers have better response rates to traditional treatment and are associated with much improved survival compared to HPV-negative cancers. However, both controversies and opportunities have arisen. Accurate determination of HPV status and accurate prognostic stratification are areas of intense discussion and investigation, and clinical trials of de-escalated treatment for improved functional outcomes and of novel therapies are under way.

Dr Nishant Agrawal of Johns Hopkins University, together with Dr Myers, presents a review of the genomics of head and neck malignancies and how the current understanding of the somatic genetic changes in these cancers reflect the emerging epidemiologic and clinical picture of 2 diseases, one driven by tobacco carcinogens and the other by the oncogenic effects of HPV. The number and spectrum of somatic mutations differ significantly between HPV-associated and non-HPV-associated tumors, reflecting the differences in pathogenesis and partially explaining the distinct response rates to chemotherapy and radiotherapy. To complete our discussion of the etiology and biology of oral cavity and oropharyngeal cancer, Dr David Kutler of the Weill Cornell Medical Center introduces us to Fanconi anemia, an inherited syndrome that puts individuals at extreme risk for the development of oral cavity cancers. Clinicians should at least consider this diagnosis and referral to a clinical geneticist for patients presenting with squamous carcinoma (particularly of the oral cavity) at oddly young ages and should be aware of the other clinical signs of Fanconi anemia, as patients with this syndrome are at very high risk for severe toxic effects from radiotherapy or chemotherapy.

Evaluation and Therapy

An identifiable lesion that is premalignant but with a high potential for becoming an invasive cancer provides an opportunity for screening, early diagnosis, and less invasive treatments to prevent cancers and reduce cancer mortality. These principles are the basis of public health efforts that led to routine Pap testing in the United States, which has resulted in a dramatic reduction in the incidence of and mortality associated with another HPV-associated tumor type, cervical cancer. Unfortunately, an analogous premalignant lesion for HPV-associated oropharyngeal cancer has yet to be identified, and thus hope for a screening program for oropharyngeal cancer remains elusive. However, oral cavity premalignant lesions are easily identifiable and are treatable by one of several methods. Dr Pierre Saintigny of The University of Texas MD Anderson Cancer Center reviews recent progress in screening, risk assessment, chemoprevention, and treatment of oral premalignancy.

The emergence and recognition of HPV as the causative agent in most cases of squamous cell carcinoma of the oropharynx over the past 2 decades necessitates separate discussions of evaluation/staging of squamous cell carcinoma of the oral cavity and evaluation/staging of squamous cell carcinoma of the oropharynx. Dr Mark Zafereo of MD Anderson Cancer Center addresses both topics and also discusses novel diagnostic and staging approaches, including sentinel lymph node biopsy and FDG-PET/CT imaging. Because HPV status has such a profound influence on oropharyngeal cancer outcomes, the current staging system for oropharyngeal cancer, which does not include this critical biological determinate, appears inadequate.

Drs Daniel Clayburgh and Neil Gross of the Knight Cancer Institute at the Oregon Health and Science University provide an overview of both the traditional and the cutting-edge surgical approaches for oral cavity and oropharyngeal cancers. Sentinel lymph node biopsy has emerged as an alternative to staging neck dissection for a selection of patients with small oral cavity cancers for more aggressive treatment (neck dissection and/or radiotherapy). Transoral surgery with robotic and laser assistance is being touted as a less morbid alternative to radiotherapy for early-stage oropharyngeal cancer or as a means of allowing de-intensified radiotherapy for intermediate-stage oropharyngeal cancer; clinical trials are being initiated to substantiate these claims. The past decade has also seen exciting advances in the field of radiotherapy for oral cavity and oropharyngeal cancer, including new delivery strategies, such as intensity modulated radiotherapy; new types of particles, including protons; and newer fractionation schemes and sensitizing strategies. Drs Brandon Gunn and Steven Frank of MD Anderson Cancer Center review these advances and the opportunities for better treatment of these 2 diseases. Dr William William of MD Anderson Cancer Center discusses systemic therapy for oral cavity and oropharyngeal cancer and the impact of conventional chemotherapy or molecularly targeted agents delivered as induction treatment or concurrently with radiotherapy on the outcomes of patients with these types of tumors.

Quality of Life and Quality of Care

A comprehensive discussion of functional assessment and rehabilitation of patients with oral cavity and oropharyngeal cancer is provided by Drs Kate Hutcheson and Jan Lewin of MD Anderson Cancer Center. Understanding how current and emerging treatments influence speech and swallowing outcomes is critical to treatment selection for individual patients as well as for assessing results of clinical trials. Supportive and rehabilitative care during and after treatment yield measurable long-term functional benefits, and patients should be evaluated before initiation of cancer treatment to ensure maximum rehabilitation and function. Efforts to improve functional and oncologic outcomes will have to fit within health care system reforms that aim to control costs, reduce waste, improve quality, and increase access. Both treatment standardization based on evidence and regionalization of complex care at specialized institutions are central to improved efficiency; Drs Carol Lewis and Randal Weber of MD Anderson Cancer Center review these important issues. Although overall and disease-free survival have improved for patients successfully treated for oral cavity and oropharyngeal cancers, these cancers and their treatment predispose patients to an increased risk of mortality. In addition, cancer survivors are exposed to the same risk factors for other causes of morbidity and mortality as the general population.

Dr Ian Ganly of Memorial Sloan-Kettering Cancer Center addresses these and other survivorship issues for patients with oral cavity and oropharyngeal cancers.

SUMMARY

With the emergence of an epidemic of HPV-associated oropharyngeal cancers and a decline in smoking-related cancers, the field of head and neck oncology has changed dramatically in the past 2 decades. We can no longer think of squamous cell carcinoma of the head and neck as a single disease; rather, we must recognize that cancer of the oropharynx, which is commonly associated with HPV, is a different disease altogether from oral cavity cancer. The epidemiology, molecular biology, genomics, and clinical presentation all contribute to these differences. Perhaps more importantly, patients with oral cavity cancer and those with oropharyngeal cancer have different oncologic and functional outcomes and rates of second primary tumors. It is imperative that treating clinicians understand these differences, so that they can provide the most appropriate care and offer the best oncologic and functional outcomes for their individual patients.

Jeffrey N. Myers, MD, PhD
Department of Head and Neck Surgery
The University of Texas MD Anderson Cancer Center
1515 Holcombe Boulevard, Unit 1445
Houston, TX 77030, USA

Erich M. Sturgis, MD, MPH
Department of Head and Neck Surgery
and Department of Epidemiology
The University of Texas MD Anderson Cancer Center
1515 Holcombe Boulevard, Unit 1445
Houston, TX 77030, USA

E-mail addresses:
jmyers@mdanderson.org (J.N. Myers)
esturgis@mdanderson.org (E.M. Sturgis)

Etiology and Biology

Epidemiology of Oral-Cavity and Oropharyngeal Carcinomas

Controlling a Tobacco Epidemic While a Human Papillomavirus Epidemic Emerges

Mia Hashibe, PhD[a,*], Erich M. Sturgis, MD, MPH[b]

KEYWORDS

• Human papillomavirus • Oropharyngeal cancer • HPV vaccine • Tobacco

KEY POINTS

- Although tobacco prevalence is declining in most developed countries, less developed countries are still experiencing an increase in tobacco use. Thus the future burden of oral-cavity and oropharyngeal cancers in less developed countries is expected to be heavy.
- The incidence of human papillomavirus (HPV)-associated oropharyngeal cancer is dramatically increasing in the United States and other developed countries, although trends in less developed countries appear unclear at present.
- HPV vaccine compliance in the United States is low, although it continues to increase each year.

EVOLUTION OF THE TOBACCO EPIDEMIC

Each year in the world, approximately 264,000 cases of oral-cavity cancer and 136,000 cases of pharyngeal (including nasopharynx, oropharynx, and hypopharynx) cancer are diagnosed.[1] In the United States, 41,380 cases of oral-cavity and pharyngeal cancer are expected to be diagnosed in 2013, and almost 8000 deaths will be attributed to these diseases in 2013.[2] Unfortunately, a shortcoming common to many national and international databases is that an accurate separation of head and neck cancer statistics into specific subsites (oral cavity vs oropharynx vs hypopharynx vs nasopharynx) is difficult or impossible because many cases are categorized under generic terms such as "tongue" or "palate," which include both oral cavity (oral

[a] Division of Public Health, Department of Family & Preventive Medicine, Huntsman Cancer Institute, University of Utah School of Medicine, 375 Chipeta Way, Suite A, Salt Lake City, UT 84108, USA; [b] Department of Head & Neck Surgery, The University of Texas M.D. Anderson Cancer Center, 1515 Holcombe Boulevard, Unit #1445, Houston, TX 77030, USA
* Corresponding author.
E-mail address: mia.hashibe@utah.edu

Otolaryngol Clin N Am 46 (2013) 507–520
http://dx.doi.org/10.1016/j.otc.2013.05.001

tongue and hard palate) and oropharynx (base of tongue and soft palate). In addition, the generic term "pharynx" as commonly used mixes naso-, oro-, and hypopharynx anatomic sites; however, at least 80% of pharyngeal cancers are located within the oropharynx in most countries, with some notable exceptions such as China and Southeast Asia. Tobacco use, including both smoking and chewing of tobacco products, is a well-established risk factor for both oral-cavity and oropharyngeal cancers.[3] Cigarette smoking is generally the most common form of tobacco use, but in certain regions local tobacco products are smoked or chewed. Some examples include smoking bidi or chutta in India, smoking water pipes in North Africa, and smoking kreteks (clove-flavored cigarettes) in Indonesia.[4] Cigarette smoking confers a 4- to 5-fold increase of both oral-cavity and oropharyngeal cancers.[5]

Tobacco as a Risk Factor for Oral Cavity and Pharyngeal Cancers

Approximately 65% of oral-cavity cancers and 66% of pharyngeal cancers (perhaps lower for oropharyngeal cancers and higher for hypopharyngeal cancers) are attributed to tobacco smoking.[6] Thus tobacco use can be considered the most important risk factor for oral-cavity and pharyngeal cancers, because the majority of these cancers can be attributed to tobacco use; however, as discussed in this article, human papillomavirus (HPV) may become the principal risk factor for oropharyngeal cancer. The attributable fraction for chewing tobacco varies considerably by region and sex. Among men cases of oral-cavity cancer that are attributed to chewing tobacco are estimated to be 1.6% in Canada, 6.6% in the United States, 52.5% in India, and 68.2% in Sudan.[7] Among women, approximately 13.6% of cases of oral-cavity cancer in Sudan and 51.6% of cases in India were attributed to chewing tobacco.[7]

Tobacco as a Risk Factor Independent of Alcohol

Tobacco use is a risk factor independent of alcohol drinking, as demonstrated by studies focusing on individuals who had never drank alcohol.[3] When estimating the effect of tobacco use on the risk of oral-cavity and pharyngeal cancer, the effect of alcohol drinking is a concern because it could bias the estimation. Thus alcohol drinking may act as a confounder, because it is a risk factor of the disease and is associated with the exposure of tobacco use. Even when alcohol drinking is adjusted for in statistical models, residual confounding is a concern because it is difficult to assess alcohol exposures over a lifetime. One solution to this issue would be to estimate the effect of tobacco use among those who never drink alcohol, but gathering sufficient patients with oral-cavity and pharyngeal cancer who are not alcohol drinkers has been very difficult. The consortium approach, with collaborations of researchers across studies to pool data has been useful in addressing this issue. The International Head and Neck Cancer Epidemiology (INHANCE) consortium pooled data across 14 case-control studies including 717 patients with oral-cavity cancer and 380 with pharyngeal cancer (both oropharynx and hypopharynx) who were never drinkers. Never drinkers who had smoked for more than 40 years had a 3-fold increase in risk for oral-cavity cancer and an almost 5-fold increase in risk for pharyngeal cancer.[3]

Tobacco and Alcohol Interaction

An interaction between tobacco and alcohol is well established for oral-cavity and pharyngeal cancers.[6] An INHANCE consortium analysis of 2992 cases of oral-cavity cancer and 16,152 controls demonstrated an interaction between tobacco and alcohol on the multiplicative scale.[6] The multiplicative interaction parameter for oral-cavity cancer was 3.1 (95% confidence interval [CI] 1.8–5.2), suggesting that the interaction observed was almost 3-fold greater than the product of the individual effects of tobacco and alcohol. Similarly, for pharyngeal cancer, an analysis of 4038 cases (including both oropharyngeal and hypopharyngeal cancer) and 16,152 controls showed that there was an interaction on the multiplicative scale between tobacco and alcohol, with a multiplicative interaction parameter of 1.9 (95% CI 1.4–2.6).[6] The assessment of attributable fraction for tobacco and alcohol combined showed that most cases would be attributed to tobacco alone or a combination of tobacco and alcohol,[6] whereas very few cases would be attributed to alcohol alone.

Tobacco Epidemic and Variation by Country

In high-income countries, tobacco prevalence has been decreasing over the last several decades, owing to the antismoking campaigns. The tobacco epidemic has been described in 4 stages[8]:

- Stage 1 reflects the beginning of the epidemic with cigarette smoking prevalence less than 20%
- Stage 2 shows an increase in the prevalence to around 40% to 80%
- Stage 3 is characterized by a plateau and beginning decline in prevalence
- Stage 4 shows a final decline in the prevalence

Thus, high-income countries are in stage IV, or the last stage, for both men and women, with an overall tobacco prevalence of 30% among men and 19% among women.[8] In the United States, the male tobacco prevalence decreased from 52% in 1960 to 22% in 2010. Among American women, the tobacco prevalence decreased from 34% in 1960% to 17% in 2010.[8] The major concern is that the low-income and middle-income countries are in stages I and II of the tobacco epidemic, respectively, with prevalence expected to continue to increase. In middle-income countries, the overall male prevalence of tobacco smoking is 34% and the overall female prevalence is 5%.[8] In low-income countries, the male prevalence of tobacco smoking is approximately 21% and the female prevalence is 3%.[8]

Variation in Oral-Cavity and Oropharyngeal Cancer Burden by Country

Cancer is already a major burden in low-income and middle-income countries, and the burden is expected to increase in the next decades because of the growing population, adoption of health behaviors of high-income countries, and a decrease in competing risk of infectious diseases.[9] The future burden of oral-cavity and pharyngeal cancers on lower-income countries is expected to increase greatly based just on demographic effects, with an 80% increase in cases of oral-cavity cancer and an 84% increase in cases of pharyngeal cancer. The projected number of cases of oral-cavity cancer in less developed countries for the year 2030 (307,735) is much greater than the projected number of cases of pharyngeal cancer (161,929). If the tobacco epidemic in the less developed countries is further accounted for in the projections, the case numbers are expected to be a heavy burden.[10] Focusing on the countries with the highest male tobacco-smoking prevalences in the world (**Table 1**), also representing chiefly low-income and middle-income countries, the projected number based on demographic effects again show large increases, although they do not yet have the highest incidence rates in the world. Dramatic increases in cases of oral-cavity and pharyngeal cancer are expected for Papua New Guinea (122%), Tunisia (82%), China (71%), and Albania (63%).

Table 1
Incidence rates and case numbers of oral-cavity and pharyngeal cancer for countries with the top 10 highest tobacco-smoking male prevalences in the world[a]

	Currently Smoking Any Tobacco Product		Oral-Cavity and Pharyngeal Cancer Incidence Rates (per 100,000) in 2008[b]	Oral-Cavity and Pharyngeal Cancer Incident Cases		
Country	Male	Female		2008	2030 Projection	% Change from 2008 to 2030
Greece	63	41.4	2.0	496	651	31.3
Albania	60.1	19.4	8.4	334	545	63.2
Russian Federation	59.4	23.9	6.7	14190	16278	14.7
Papua New Guinea	57.7	30.8	27.2	883	1957	121.6
Indonesia	61.3	3.7	3.4	6939	12907	86.0
Georgia	56.6	5.7	1.9	122	133	9.0
Tunisia	52.7	3.6	2.8	271	493	81.9
Armenia	50.9	2.1	2.4	97	127	30.9
China	50.4	2.1	1.4	22134	37838	70.9
Latvia	50.1	22.3	5.4	208	236	14.4

[a] WHO Tobacco Atlas, 2012.
[b] Age-standardized to the world population, GLOBOCAN 2008.

From the perspective of incidence rates, the highest incidence rates of oral-cavity and pharyngeal cancer are observed in:

- Papua New Guinea (27 per 100,000)
- Chinese Taipei (21 per 100,000)
- Maldives (21 per 100,000)
- Hungary (18 per 100,000)
- Bangladesh (14 per 100,000)

Thus the countries with high smoking prevalence observed in **Table 1** are not consistently those with the highest incidence rates of oral-cavity and pharyngeal cancer; however, there is likely a time lag for the effect of the tobacco epidemic to be observed in cancer incidence rates. This observation also highlights that the etiology of oral-cavity and pharyngeal cancer is complex and multifactorial, including other important risk factors such as alcohol drinking, HPV infection, and chewing other products such as betel quid and areca nut (with or without tobacco). The high incidence rates observed in Central Europe are thought to be due to the combined high prevalence of smoking and alcohol drinking among men, whereas in Taiwan, betel quid and areca nut chewed without tobacco may be the main cause of the high incidence rates of oral-cavity and pharyngeal cancer.

EMERGENCE OF THE HPV-ASSOCIATED CANCER EPIDEMIC

In the United States, per capita tobacco consumption and cigarette current smoking prevalence rates have declined relatively steadily since the mid-1960s, and subsequently the incidences of laryngeal, oral-cavity, and hypopharyngeal cancer have declined since the late 1980s.[11–13] However, during this same period the incidence of oropharyngeal cancer initially plateaued but subsequently rose dramtically.[11–17] These complex trends in the incidence of oropharyngeal cancer are consistent with the control of one etiologic exposure (smoking) but with the emergence of a second, unrelated etiologic exposure during the same period.

Evidence for HPV as Cause of Oropharyngeal Cancer

HPV type 16 is a recognized cause of oropharyngeal cancer. The evidence comes from the well-established cervical carcinogenic model by which HPV is the cause of virtually all cervical cancers and similar molecular events occurring in oropharyngeal cancers associated with HPV, as well as case series and molecular epidemiologic studies that have demonstrated strong and consistent associations between oropharyngeal cancer and various HPV markers (reviewed by Sturgis and Ang[15]). The HPV markers studied were[18]:

1. Antibodies to HPV-16 capsids analyzed by enzyme-linked immunosorbent assay (ELISA) using HPV-16 major capsid protein L1–derived virus-like particles as antigens
2. Antibodies to HPV-16 E6 and E7 analyzed by ELISA; such HPV capsid antibodies are a cumulative marker of past and present HPV infection
3. HPV DNA in cancer specimens or oral cell scrapings analyzed by Southern blotting or highly sensitive polymerase chain reaction (PCR) methods

Limitations in the Study/Literature on HPV and Head and Neck Cancers

Despite the evidence, although approximately three-quarters of individuals develop an HPV infection (and certainly a higher proportion are exposed), only a fraction will seroconvert and, of these, many will lose seropositivity. Consequently, HPV seropositivity may not accurately reflect the HPV status of the cancer of an individual patient. An additional shortcoming of much of the literature regarding the role of HPV in head and neck cancers is that establishing whether an individual's cancer is actually attributable to HPV is not straightforward and has evolved over time, making much earlier literature unclear in retrospect. Although modern PCR methods are indeed highly sensitive for detecting the presence of HPV DNA in tumor specimens, most now believe that evidence of somatic molecular markers (such as p16 overexpression) of HPV oncogenic activity by such HPV DNA is necessary to consider causality. In other words, the mere presence of HPV DNA does not necessarily equate to an HPV-driven or HPV-caused tumor. Finally, much of the epidemiologic literature in this field has either suffered from significant site misclassification or has lacked adequate site separation to allow accurate conclusions regarding HPV's role in oropharyngeal carcinogenesis in comparison with oral-cavity carcinogenesis. Recent literature has mostly clarified this problem, but these issues should be considered when reviewing and interpreting this literature. It is now understood that HPV is a major risk factor for oropharyngeal cancer in the United States and other developed countries, but the role of HPV in oral-cavity cancer appears to be very limited.

Epidemiologic Studies Linking HPV and Oropharyngeal Cancer

The first large study on the association of HPV and head and neck cancer, involving 1670 patients with cancer (1415 with cancer of the oral cavity and 255 with cancer of the oropharynx) and 1732 control subjects, reported a prevalence of HPV DNA in 4% of specimens from the oral cavity and 18% of specimens from the oropharynx.[19] However, the investigators grouped cancers of the base of tongue and soft palate (both oropharyngeal sites) with cancers of the oral cavity, thus making the ratio of oral-cavity cancers to oropharyngeal cancers (>5:1) in this study unusual. Consequently, the tumor positivity rate of oral-cavity cancers is likely overstated while that of oropharyngeal cancers is underestimated, although the degree of impact of this misclassification is unknown because the actual numbers of cancers of the base of tongue and soft palate in the study are not provided. When cases were compared with controls, a strongly increased risk was observed for antibodies against HPV-16 E6 and E7 proteins, for cancer of the oropharynx (odds ratio [OR] = 9.2, 95% CI 4.8–17.7). The investigators suggest a significant increased risk for oral-cavity cancer was associated with seropositivity to HPV-16 E6 and E7, but this is in question given the site misclassification already noted, and indeed the patients whose site was misclassified as oral cavity who actually had cancer at an oropharyngeal site had the highest seroprevalence rate among "oral cavity" patients.

In a study from the United States comprising 204 cases of head and neck cancer and 326 controls, a 5-fold increased risk for HPV-16 E6/E7 antibodies was observed for oral-cavity cancer, although nonsquamous cancers and nonspecified "tongue" cancers were included in this group, and a 70-fold increased risk was observed for cancer of the oropharynx.[20]

In another study from the United States including 137 patients with oral-cavity cancer, 188 patients with oropharyngeal cancer, and 335 cancer-free controls, HPV-16 L1 seropositivity for patients with oral-cavity cancer (10%) was very similar to that of the cancer-free controls (13%); and, after multivariate adjustment, HPV-16 seropositivity showed no suggestion that HPV is a risk for oral-cavity cancer but HPV-16 seropositivity was strongly associated with a significant more than 5-fold risk for oropharyngeal cancer.[21]

In a landmark nested case-control serologic analyses within a Nordic cohort of almost 900,000 individuals, there was an increased frequency of HPV-16 infection among subjects who later (on average 10 years after collection of the blood sample) developed oropharyngeal cancer or "tongue" cancer (a mixed grouping of base of tongue and oral tongue), but no evidence of an association with oral-cavity cancer.[22] Because of the sequential nature of these data (exposure years before cancer development), this study provided strong evidence on the causal nature of the association of HPV with oropharyngeal cancer.[22]

In another landmark study including 100 oropharyngeal cases and 200 controls, risk of oropharyngeal cancer was increased with HPV-16 oral infection (OR = 14.6, 95% CI 6.3–36.6) and with oral infection with any of 27 types of HPV (OR = 12.3, 95% CI 5.4–26.4).[23]

An early meta-analysis including 5 studies reported a borderline summary OR of 1.5 (95% CI 1.0–2.1) for the association between HPV-16 seropositivity and "oral" cancer, and a summary OR of 3.8 (95% CI 1.9–7.9) for oropharyngeal cancer.[24] There may have been a greater potential for site misclassification with some oropharyngeal cancers included in the oral-cavity group in these earlier studies; all 5 studies included in this meta-analysis were published in 2003 or earlier.

Prevalence of HPV DNA in Tumor Tissue

In an early systematic review of HPV DNA prevalence in 5046 head and neck cancer specimens from 60 studies, all published before February 2004, HPV-16 accounted for virtually all of the HPV DNA detected in 969 oropharyngeal cancers (prevalence 31%; 42% for North American studies and 24% for European studies).[25] HPV-16 DNA was detected in 35% of oropharyngeal cancers from Asia, although only 54 oropharyngeal cancers from Asia were included. HPV-16 DNA was detected in 16% of oral-cavity cancers (only 10% for European and North American studies), whereas the prevalence of HPV-18 overall in oral-cavity cancer was 8.0%. HPV-16 DNA prevalence in oral-cavity cancers was much higher (22%) in the Asian studies than in those of Europe or North America; however, given the unusual site distribution of the Asian studies (only 4% of included cancers from Asia were of the oropharynx), the possibility of site misclassification exists.

The most recent meta-analysis on HPV and head and neck cancer included 19,638 patients (5396 with oropharyngeal cancer and 13,972 with non-oropharyngeal head and neck cancer) from 269 studies (206 using PCR, 48 using in situ hybridization, and 11 using both for HPV detection).[26] The overall HPV DNA prevalence in oropharyngeal cancers was highest in North America (60%) in comparison with Europe (40%) and other regions (33%). The investigators also assessed the HPV prevalence over time, and concluded that HPV prevalence was increasing over time in all regions for oropharyngeal cancers but was decreasing over time for head and neck cancers at non-oropharyngeal sites (**Fig. 1**). Across all regions combined, the HPV prevalence in oropharyngeal cancers prior to 2000 was approximately 41%, which then increased to 64% in 2000 to 2004 and 72% in 2005 and later. By contrast, the HPV prevalence among non-oropharyngeal cancer sites of the head and neck decreased over the corresponding time periods from 22% to 17% and to 6% respectively. The investigators suggested that site misclassification of oropharyngeal cancers as oral-cavity cancers in the earlier time periods may have contributed to the decline in HPV prevalence in non-oropharyngeal cancers. This study also assessed HPV detection methods (in situ hybridization based vs PCR based) as a source of heterogeneity in HPV prevalence, but did not detect any significant differences once the results were adjusted for the time period during which the test was performed.

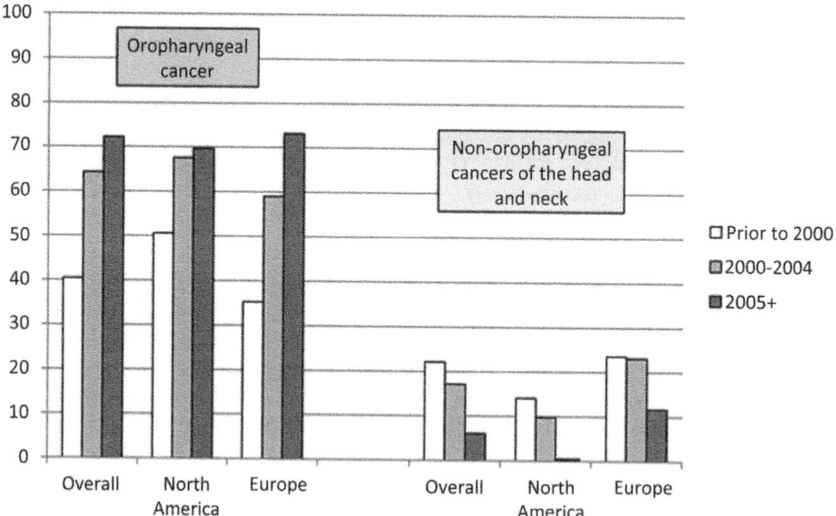

Fig. 1. HPV prevalence among patients with oropharyngeal cancer and non–oropharyngeal cancer by region and time period. (*Data from* Ferlay J, Shin HR, Bray F, et al. GLOBOCAN 2008 v2.0, cancer incidence and mortality worldwide: IARC cancerbase No. 10 [Internet]. Lyon (France): International Agency for Research on Cancer; 2010. Available at: http://globocan.iarc.fr. Accessed August 30, 2012; and Mehanna H, Beech T, Nicholson T, et al. Prevalence of human papillomavirus in oropharyngeal and nonoropharyngeal head and neck cancer—systematic review and meta-analysis of trends by time and region. Head Neck 2013;35(5):747–55.)

The Epidemic of HPV-associated Oropharyngeal Cancer

In an analysis of Surveillance, Epidemiology and End Results (SEER) data (A United States national registry), Chaturvedi and colleagues[14] found that the age-adjusted incidence of head and neck cancer at HPV-related sites (oropharynx) increased significantly between 1973 and 2004, particularly in the most recent time period studied (increase of 5% per year from 2000 to 2004; $P<.016$). By contrast, the age-adjusted incidence of head and neck cancer at HPV-unrelated sites, which in this study was restricted to the oral cavity, decreased during this same time period. Using oropharyngeal cancer specimens from participants from Hawaii, Los Angeles, and Iowa in the SEER Residual Tissue Repositories Program, Chaturvedi and colleagues[16] more recently reported that HPV prevalence in oropharyngeal cancers increased from 16% in the 1980s to 73% in the 2000s. This trend resulted in a 225% population-level increase in incidence of HPV-positive oropharyngeal cancer (from 0.8 cases per 100,000 individuals in 1988 to 2.6 per 100,000 in 2004) and a concomitant 50% decrease in HPV-negative oropharyngeal cancer (from 2.0 cases per 100,000 individuals in 1988 to 1.0 per 100,000 in 2004) (**Fig. 2**).[16] If current trends continue, it is estimated that by 2030 almost half of all head and neck cancers will be HPV-positive oropharyngeal cancer, and that by 2020 the number of cases of HPV-positive oropharyngeal cancer will surpass the number of cases of cervical cancer.

Differing Exposures and Biology Associated with HPV-Positive and HPV-Negative Cancers

As might be expected, the past exposures of patients with HPV-positive oropharyngeal cancers and HPV-negative tumors appear to differ. Since the advent of the epidemic of HPV-related oropharyngeal cancer, patients with oropharyngeal cancer are much more likely to be never/former/light smokers than patients with oropharyngeal cancer diagnosed in earlier decades.[27] Patients with oropharyngeal cancer report more lifetime sexual partners and oral-sex partners than patients with oral-cavity or larynx/hypopharynx cancer.[28] In an important study linking past patient exposures/behaviors to the HPV status of subsequent head and neck cancers, Gillison and colleagues[29] found a significant association between the number of lifetime sexual partners and oral-sex partners and HPV-positive tumors but no association between smoking or alcohol and HPV-positive tumors, whereas HPV-negative tumors were associated with smoking and alcohol but not sexual behaviors.

HPV-associated oropharyngeal cancers also appear to have a different biology and better oncologic outcomes. TP53 mutations are commonly found in HPV-negative oropharyngeal cancers, similar to classic tobacco-related squamous cell carcinomas of the head and neck but in distinction from a low rate of TP53 mutations in HPV-driven oropharyngeal cancers.[30] Furthermore, individuals with HPV-driven oropharyngeal cancer appear to have an increased survival, but the reasons for this have not been fully elucidated.[31]

Better Survival for HPV-driven Oropharyngeal Cancer

A meta-analysis including 13 studies up to January 2007 reported a reduced risk of death from all causes (hazard ratio [HR] = 0.7, 95% CI 0.5–1.0) among patients with oropharyngeal cancer who were positive for HPV-16, and a reduced risk for recurrence of oropharyngeal cancer (HR = 0.5, 95% CI 0.4–0.7).[32] Patients with non-oropharyngeal cancer (oral cavity, hypopharynx, larynx; n = 201) whose tumors were positive for HPV-16 DNA had no apparent survival advantage (HR = 0.8, 95% CI 0.5–1.3). Another meta-analysis of 5 studies on patients with oropharyngeal cancer

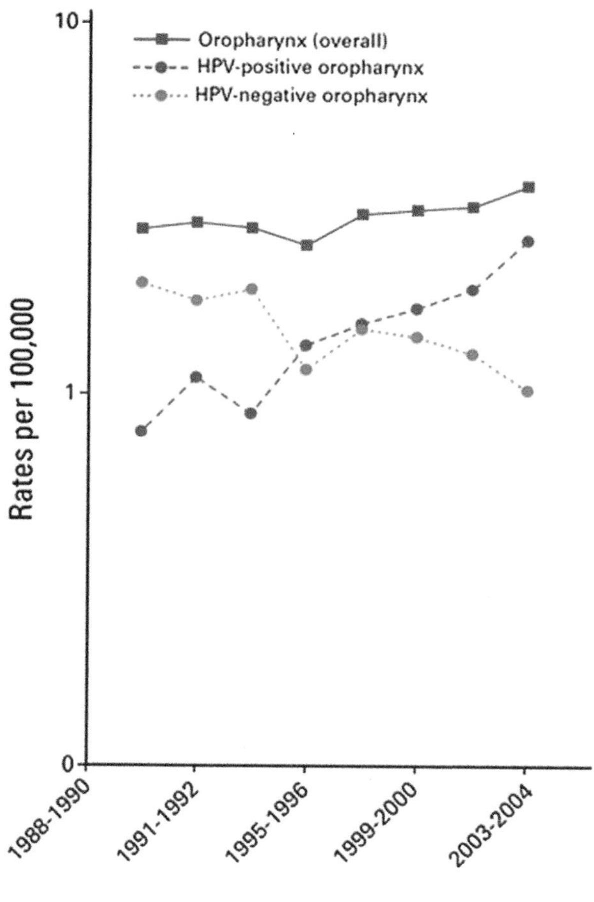

Fig. 2. Incidence rates for oropharyngeal cancer (overall), HPV-positive oropharyngeal cancer, and HPV-negative oropharyngeal cancer. (*Data from* Mehanna H, Beech T, Nicholson T, et al. Prevalence of human papillomavirus in oropharyngeal and nonoropharyngeal head and neck cancer—systematic review and meta-analysis of trends by time and region. Head Neck 2013;35(5):747–55; and Chaturvedi AK, Engels EA, Pfeiffer RM, et al. Human papillomavirus and rising oropharyngeal cancer incidence in the United States. J Clin Oncol 2011;29:4294–301.)

between 2001 and 2008 (only one study in common with the aforementioned meta-analysis) also reported better survival for patients with HPV-positive oropharyngeal cancer (HR = 0.4, 95% CI 0.2–0.6).[33] In addition, this review summarized the demographic, clinical, and exposure characteristics of HPV-related cancers. Compared with patients with HPV-negative cancers, those with HPV-positive cancers were more likely to be middle aged, never smokers, and never drinkers, with higher TNM stage and lymph node metastases. The most recent meta-analysis, including studies published up to 2011, reported significantly better overall, disease-specific, and disease-free survival for patients with HPV-positive oropharyngeal cancer when compared with patients with HPV-negative oropharyngeal cancer in a pooled analysis.[34] Of note, there was no significant difference in disease-free survival among patients with oral-cavity cancer based on HPV status. In addition to these meta-analyses of mostly single-institution retrospective series, many with neither good cancer-site control nor standardized treatment regimens, there are now at least 5 prospective multi-institutional clinical trials now confirming better overall, disease-specific, and/or disease-free survival in patients with HPV-positive oropharyngeal cancer compared with those with HPV-negative oropharyngeal cancers.[31,35–38] In the past at a national level, patients with oropharyngeal cancer had the poorest survival of all patients with head and neck cancer in the United States; however, SEER data show that 5-year survival for patients with oropharyngeal cancer has consistently improved since 1975, and these patients now have better survival than patients with cancers at other head and neck sites.[17]

HPV VACCINATION

The Advisory Committee on Immunization Practices first recommended in 2007 that girls 11 to 12 years of age be vaccinated with the quadrivalent HPV vaccine. The recommendation was updated in 2011 that boys aged 11 or 12 years should also be vaccinated.[39] Females 13 to 26 years of age and males 13 to 21 years of age who were not previously vaccinated are recommended to be vaccinated. For males 22 to 26 years of age, the vaccine is recommended if the individual is immunocompromised, is tested positive for human immunodeficiency virus infection, or has sex with men. The Gardasil vaccine, produced by Merck, targets HPV-6, -11, -16, and -18 (quadrivalent), whereas the Cervarix vaccine, produced by GlaxoSmithKline, targets HPV-16 and -18 and both vaccines are administrated as 3 separate shots.

Vaccine Adherence Rates

According to the National Immunization Survey—Teen 2011 including 23,564 individuals, approximately 35% of females aged 13 to 17 years and 1% of males aged 13 to 17 years completed the 3-dose HPV vaccination.[40] By contrast, 91% completed the 2-dose measles/mumps/rubella vaccine and 92% completed the 3-dose hepatitis B vaccine. The compliance to the HPV vaccination has been improving over the years for girls since it was recommended in 2007, as shown in **Fig. 3.**[41,42] Approximately 53% of the adolescent girls started the HPV vaccination with 1 dose, and of these girls 71% completed the 3-dose series. Among boys, 8% started the HPV vaccination

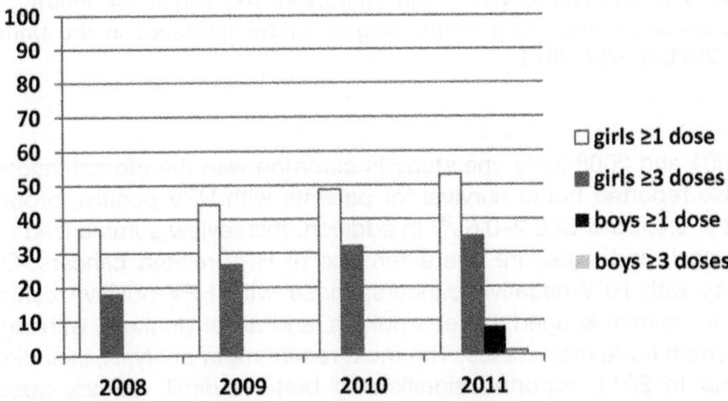

Fig. 3. HPV vaccine adherence proportions among girls and boys aged 13 to 17 years (based on the National Immunization Survey—Teen). (*Data from* Refs.[36–38,40–42])

series with at least 1 dose, 28% of whom completed the 3-dose series. The vaccination completion among adolescent girls by race/ethnicity was 33% in whites, 32% in blacks, 42% in Hispanics, 38% among American Indian/Alaska Natives, and 35% among Asians. Adolescent girls below the poverty level had a higher percentage of HPV-vaccination dose completion (39%) than adolescent girls at or above the poverty level (33%). The states with the lowest compliance for the HPV vaccine completion for girls were Arkansas (16%), Mississippi (20%), Utah (20%), and Kansas (22%), whereas the states with the highest compliance were Rhode Island (57%), Hawaii (51%), South Dakota (50%), and Vermont (50%).

Although the compliance levels for the HPV vaccination are improving each year, the low levels are still a concern. Reasons for not getting vaccinated included concerns about vaccine safety, the provider not making the recommendation, lack of knowledge about the vaccine, and the parental belief that their daughter was not sexually active.[43,44]

FUTURE BURDENS OF ORAL-CAVITY AND OROPHARYNGEAL CANCER

Although high-income countries have experienced a decrease in tobacco prevalence in recent decades, low-income and middle-income countries are still in the early stages of the tobacco epidemic. The future burden of expected cases of oral-cavity and oropharyngeal cancer was already expected to be large because of demographic effects, but with the tobacco epidemic the burden will be very heavy in low-income and middle-income countries. Tobacco use will clearly remain an important risk factor that must be targeted with public health efforts, including preventing youth from starting tobacco use and helping current smokers to quit smoking.

Slowing the increasing incidence of HPV-associated oropharyngeal cancer will be a challenge. Various research efforts are currently focusing on HPV and oropharyngeal cancer in high-income countries. The impact of HPV and incidence of oropharyngeal cancer in low-income and middle-income countries will need to be investigated.

The HPV vaccine may play a role in slowing HPV prevalence and incidence rates of HPV-related cancer, but the current compliance levels are low. Research efforts have been focusing on the barriers to vaccination, and also on research questions such as whether administering the vaccine in 2 doses would be as effective as a 3-dose vaccine, and the possibility of clinical trials with new vaccines covering 9 HPV types.[45]

While HPV remains an important area of focus for cancer research, the overwhelming majority of cases of oral-cavity cancer will be caused by tobacco. HPV is accounting for a rising proportion of oropharyngeal cancers in developed countries, and by the end of the decade will account for more oropharyngeal cancers than cervical cancers in the United States. The proportion of oropharyngeal cancers in developing countries attributable to HPV is currently under investigation. Efforts at tobacco control will continue to be important for preventing oral-cavity and oropharyngeal cancer. Controlling an HPV-associated epidemic of oropharyngeal cancer will be a challenge, and increasing the HPV vaccination rate to control future HPV-associated cancer incidence remains a priority.

REFERENCES

1. Ferlay J, Shin HR, Bray F, et al. GLOBOCAN 2008 v2.0, cancer incidence and mortality worldwide: IARC cancerbase No. 10 [Internet]. Lyon (France): International Agency for Research on Cancer; 2010. Available at: http://globocan.iarc.fr. Accessed August 30, 2012.

2. Siegel R, Naishadham D, Jemal A. Cancer statistics, 2013. CA Cancer J Clin 2013;63:11–30.
3. Hashibe M, Brennan P, Benhamou S, et al. Alcohol drinking in never users of tobacco, cigarette smoking in never drinkers, and the risk of head and neck cancer: pooled analysis in the International Head and Neck Cancer Epidemiology Consortium. J Natl Cancer Inst 2007;99(10):777–89.
4. IARC Monographs on the Evaluation of Carcinogenic Risks to Humans, vol. 83. Lyon (France): IARC Press; 2004. Tobacco smoke and involuntary smoking.
5. Vineis P, Alavanja M, Buffler P, et al. Tobacco and cancer: recent epidemiological evidence. J Natl Cancer Inst 2004;96(2):99–106.
6. Hashibe M, Brennan P, Chuang SC, et al. Interaction between tobacco and alcohol use and the risk of head and neck cancer: pooled analysis in the International Head and Neck Cancer Epidemiology Consortium. Cancer Epidemiol Biomarkers Prev 2009;18(2):541–50.
7. Boffetta P, Hecht S, Gray N, et al. Smokeless tobacco and cancer. Lancet Oncol 2008;9(7):667–75.
8. Thun M, Peto R, Boreham J, et al. Stages of the cigarette epidemic on entering its second century. Tob Control 2012;21(2):96–101.
9. Sloan FA, Gelband H. Cancer control opportunities in low- and middle-income countries. Washington, DC: The National Academies Press; 2007.
10. McCormack VA, Boffetta P. Today's lifestyles, tomorrow's cancers: trends in lifestyle risk factors for cancer in low- and middle-income countries. Ann Oncol 2011;22(11):2349–57.
11. Giovino GA. The tobacco epidemic in the United States. Am J Prev Med 2007; 33(Suppl 6):S318–26.
12. Carvalho AL, Nishimoto IN, Califano JA, et al. Trends in incidence and prognosis for head and neck cancer in the United States: a site-specific analysis of the SEER database. Int J Cancer 2005;114(5):806–16.
13. Sturgis EM, Cinciripini PM. Trends in head and neck cancer incidence in relation to smoking prevalence: an emerging epidemic of human papillomavirus-associated cancers? Cancer 2007;110(7):1429–35.
14. Chaturvedi AK, Engels EA, Anderson WF, et al. Incidence trends for human papillomavirus-related and -unrelated oral squamous cell carcinomas in the United States. J Clin Oncol 2008;26(4):612–9.
15. Sturgis EM, Ang KK. The epidemic of HPV-associated oropharyngeal cancer is here- is it time to change our treatment paradigms? J Natl Compr Canc Netw 2011;9:665–73.
16. Chaturvedi AK, Engels EA, Pfeiffer RM, et al. Human papillomavirus and rising oropharyngeal cancer incidence in the united states. J Clin Oncol 2011;29: 4294–301.
17. Surveillance, Epidemiology and End Results. Fast Stats: an interactive tool for access to SEER cancer statistics. Surveillance Research Program, National Cancer Institute. Available at: http://seer.cancer.gov/faststats. Accessed June 25, 2012.
18. Dillner J. The serological response to papillomaviruses. Semin Cancer Biol 1999; 9(6):423–30.
19. Herrero R, Castellsague X, Pawlita M, et al. Human papillomavirus and oral cancer: the International Agency for Research on Cancer multicenter study. J Natl Cancer Inst 2003;95(23):1772–83.
20. Smith EM, Ritchie JM, Pawlita M, et al. Human papillomavirus seropositivity and risks of head and neck cancer. Int J Cancer 2007;120(4):825–32.

21. Chen X, Sturgis EM, Lei D, et al. HPV seropositivity synergizes with MDM2 variants to increase risk of oral squamous cell carcinoma. Cancer Res 2010; 70(18):7199–208.
22. Mork J, Lie AK, Glattre E, et al. Human papillomavirus infection as a risk factor for squamous-cell carcinoma of the head and neck. N Engl J Med 2001;344(15): 1125–31.
23. D'Souza G, Kreimer AR, Viscidi R, et al. Case-control study of human papillomavirus and oropharyngeal cancer. N Engl J Med 2007;356(19):1944–56.
24. Hobbs CG, Sterne JA, Bailey M, et al. Human papillomavirus and head and neck cancer: a systematic review and meta-analysis. Clin Otolaryngol 2006;31(4):259–66.
25. Kreimer AR, Clifford GM, Boyle P, et al. Human papillomavirus types in head and neck squamous cell carcinomas worldwide: a systematic review. Cancer Epidemiol Biomarkers Prev 2005;14(2):467–75.
26. Mehanna H, Beech T, Nicholson T, et al. Prevalence of human papillomavirus in oropharyngeal and nonoropharyngeal head and neck cancer—systematic review and meta-analysis of trends by time and region. Head Neck 2013;35(5):747–55.
27. Dahlstrom KR, Calzada G, Hanby JD, et al. An evolution in demographics, treatment, and outcomes of oropharyngeal cancer at a major cancer center: a staging system in need of repair. Cancer 2013;119(1):81–9.
28. Dahlstrom KR, Li G, Tortolero-Luna G, et al. Differences in history of sexual behavior between patients with oropharyngeal squamous cell carcinoma and patients with squamous cell carcinoma at other head and neck sites. Head Neck 2011;33(6):847–55.
29. Gillison ML, D'Souza G, Westra W, et al. Distinct risk factor profiles for human papillomavirus type 16-positive and human papillomavirus type 16-negative head and neck cancers. J Natl Cancer Inst 2008;100(6):407–20.
30. Dai M, Clifford GM, le CF, et al. Human papillomavirus type 16 and TP53 mutation in oral cancer: matched analysis of the IARC multicenter study. Cancer Res 2004; 64(2):468–71.
31. Fakhry C, Westra WH, Li S, et al. Improved survival of patients with human papillomavirus-positive head and neck squamous cell carcinoma in a prospective clinical trial. J Natl Cancer Inst 2008;100(4):261–9.
32. Ragin CC, Taioli E. Survival of squamous cell carcinoma of the head and neck in relation to human papillomavirus infection: review and meta-analysis. Int J Cancer 2007;121(8):1813–20.
33. Dayyani F, Etzel CJ, Liu M, et al. Meta-analysis of the impact of human papillomavirus (HPV) on cancer risk and overall survival in head and neck squamous cell carcinomas (HNSCC). Head Neck Oncol 2010;2:15.
34. O'Rorke MA, Ellison MV, Murray LJ, et al. Human papillomavirus related head and neck cancer survival: a systematic review and meta-analysis. Oral Oncol 2012; 48:1191–201.
35. Ang KK, Harris J, Wheeler R, et al. Human papillomavirus and survival of patients with oropharyngeal cancer. N Engl J Med 2010;363:24–35.
36. Rischin D, Young RJ, Fisher R, et al. Prognostic significance of p16INK4A and human papillomavirus in patients with oropharyngeal cancer treated on TROG 02.02 phase III trial. J Clin Oncol 2010;28(27):4142–8.
37. Posner MR, Lorch JH, Goloubeva O, et al. Survival and human papillomavirus in oropharynx cancer in TAX 324: a subset analysis from an international phase III trial. Ann Oncol 2011;22(5):1071–7.
38. Lassen P, Eriksen JG, Krogdahl A, et al, Danish Head and Neck Cancer Group (DAHANCA). The influence of HPV-associated p16-expression on accelerated

fractionated radiotherapy in head and neck cancer: evaluation of the randomised DAHANCA 6&7 trial. Radiother Oncol 2011;100(1):49–55.
39. Available at: http://www.cdc.gov/hpv/vaccine.html. (2012).
40. Centers for Disease Control and Prevention (CDC). National and state vaccination coverage among adolescents aged 13-17 years—United States, 2011. MMWR Morb Mortal Wkly Rep 2012;61:671–7.
41. Centers for Disease Control and Prevention (CDC). National, state, and local area vaccination coverage among adolescents aged 13-17 years—United States, 2009. MMWR Morb Mortal Wkly Rep 2010;59(32):1018–23.
42. Centers for Disease Control and Prevention (CDC). National, state, and local area vaccination coverage among adolescents aged 13-17 years—United States, 2008. MMWR Morb Mortal Wkly Rep 2009;58(36):997–1001.
43. Stokley S, Cohn A, Dorell C, et al. Adolescent vaccination-coverage levels in the United States: 2006-2009. Pediatrics 2011;128(6):1078–86.
44. Kester LM, Zimet GD, Fortenberry JD, et al. A national study of HPV vaccination of adolescent girls: rates, predictors, and reasons for non-vaccination. Matern Child Health J 2012. [Epub ahead of print].
45. Kreimer AR, Rodriguez AC, Hildesheim A, et al. Proof-of-principle evaluation of the efficacy of fewer than three doses of a bivalent HPV16/18 vaccine. J Natl Cancer Inst 2011;103(19):1444–51.

Impact of Human Papillomavirus on Oropharyngeal Cancer Biology and Response to Therapy

Implications for Treatment

Juliana Bonilla-Velez, MD[a], Edmund A. Mroz, PhD[b],
Rebecca J. Hammon, MD[a], James W. Rocco, MD, PhD[a,b,*]

KEYWORDS

• HPV-positive oropharyngeal cancer • Clinical implications • Treatment implications

KEY POINTS

- Human papillomavirus (HPV)-positivity defines a subset of patients with oropharyngeal squamous cell carcinoma (OPSCC) with distinct carcinogenesis, risk factors, clinical presentation and prognosis, representing a different disease from other head and neck squamous cell carcinomas (HNSCC).
- Cancer in these patients is mainly driven by the viral E6 and E7 oncoproteins, which interfere with p53 and pRb tumor-suppressor pathways.
- Patients are typically younger, nondrinkers, and nonsmokers, with risk factors associated with sexual exposure to HPV.
- Patients with HPV-positive OPSCC show better response to treatment, overall survival, and progression-free survival than those with HPV-negative tumors.
- Reasons for improved survival are unknown. Current hypotheses include decreased field cancerization, decreased genetic instability and tumor heterogeneity, reactivation of p53 by chemotherapy and radiotherapy, and improved immune response in HPV-positive cancers.
- The improved outcomes found in HPV-positive OPSCC have confounded clinical trial results in the recent past. Ongoing trials need to include assessment of HPV status in their design.

Continued

Funding Sources and Support: Flight Attendant Medical Research Institute; NIH NIDCR R01 DE022087; NCI R21 CA119591; NIDCD T32 DC000020; 2012 AAO-HNSF Resident Research Award; Principles and Practice of Clinical Research and Latin American Initiative program, Harvard Medical School.
Conflict of Interest: None.
[a] Department of Otolaryngology, Massachusetts Eye and Ear Infirmary, Harvard Medical School, 243 Charles Street, Boston, MA 02114, USA; [b] Center for Cancer Research and Department of Surgery, Massachusetts General Hospital, 55 Fruit Street, Boston, MA 02114, USA
* Corresponding author. Jackson 904G, Massachusetts General Hospital, 55 Fruit Street, Boston, MA 02114.
E-mail address: jrocco@partners.org

Otolaryngol Clin N Am 46 (2013) 521–543
http://dx.doi.org/10.1016/j.otc.2013.04.009 **oto.theclinics.com**
0030-6665/13/$ – see front matter

Continued

- Clinical trials are under way to determine whether de-escalation of therapy is possible in HPV-positive patients with OPSCC to achieve similar survival with reduced short-term and long-term morbidity.
- Biomarkers that may direct different therapeutic approaches are actively being investigated.
- Prevention should be focused on modification of risk factors, with a special emphasis on HPV vaccination.

Abbreviations: Impact of HPV on Oropharyngeal Cancer	
CRT	Chemo-radiotherapy
CT	Chemotherapy
HNSCC	Head and neck squamous cell carcinoma
HPV	Human papillomavirus
IC	Induction chemotherapy
ISH	In situ hybridization
OPSCC	Oropharyngeal squamous cell carcinoma
OS	Overall survival
PFS	Progression free survival
RT	Radiotherapy
TLM	Transoral laser microsurgery
TORS	Transoral robotic surgery

INTRODUCTION

Within the recent epidemic of oropharyngeal squamous cell carcinoma (OPSCC),[1] human papillomavirus (HPV) has been found to play a pivotal role in defining a subset of patients with distinct carcinogenesis,[2,3] risk factors,[4] clinical presentation,[5] and prognosis.[6–8] HPV-positive OPSCC patients, OPSCC seems to be a wholly different disease to that classically described for HPV-negative tumors, which are typically driven by the carcinogenic effects of tobacco and alcohol exposure. Although much effort has been put into describing the subset of HPV-positive patients, research has not yet translated into therapies that address the different biology and its associated better outcomes. The identification of biomarkers to aid in prognostic and therapeutic decisions, the potential for de-escalation of therapy, and the incorporation of therapies targeted to relevant HPV-related pathways are areas that are actively being evaluated in clinical trials. In this review, the implications of these findings in clinical care are addressed.

HPV BASICS

The causal role of HPV in carcinogenesis was first described in cervical cancer, but the virus has also been implicated in oropharyngeal, penile, anal, vaginal, and vulvar cancer.[9] It is estimated that 5.2% of all cancers worldwide are attributable to HPV, and the burden of incidence and costs is increasing for noncervical HPV-related cancers, especially in the oropharynx.[9] The incidence of OPSCC increased from 1988 to 2004, mainly driven by an increase in HPV-positive OPSCC of 225%, whereas HPV-negative disease has declined by 50%.[1] HPV now accounts for 45% to 90% of cases of OPSCC in developed countries, and more than 90% of these are caused by the HPV-16 subtype.[10,11] HPV status has important implications in OPSCC tumor biology, clinical presentation, prognosis, and potential treatment options, but its importance in other subsites is unclear. HPV has been detected in laryngeal (6%), hypopharyngeal (3%), oral cavity (4%), and paranasal (14%) cancers,[4,12] but the significantly lower rates of HPV positivity and inconsistent findings among the studies suggest that HPV may not be playing a causative role in these subsites.[13]

HPV and Carcinogenesis

Human papillomaviruses are small, nonenveloped, double-stranded DNA viruses that show tropism for squamous epithelium.[3] They are classified into high risk (HR, HPV-16, HPV-18, HPV-51, HPV-53) and low risk (LR, HPV-6, HPV-11) based on the ability of the virus to promote progression to cancer.[14] The process of HPV carcinogenesis is well characterized in cervical cancer, in which infection is established in the basal cell layer of the epithelium and leads to either a subclinical infection or a benign or malignant lesion.[15] Although most women have a cervical HPV infection over their lifetime, about 10% of these become persistent and only a few may progress to cancer.[15] For OPSCC, it is now known that 1% of the population has an oral HPV-16 infection, and that this confers a 50-fold increased risk for HPV-positive OPSCC,[16] but the intermediate steps in progression have not been described. The cryptic epithelium that covers the tonsil and tongue base serves as a viral reservoir and facilitates infection through increased access to its basal layer,[17,18] with an apparent predilection of this anatomic site to transformation by HPV similar to the cervical transformation zone.[18]

The process of malignant transformation arises from the continued function of the E6 and E7 oncoproteins expressed by HR-HPV.[3] These oncoproteins target several critical cellular pathways, providing multiple simultaneous oncogenic hits and leading to deregulation of proliferation, evasion of apoptosis, and induction of invasive and metastatic properties.[3] As a result, HPV infection reduces the number of subsequent mutations needed to develop invasive carcinoma. The difference in oncogenic potential between HR-HPV and LR-HPV may rely on more efficient disruption of the biological activities of E6 and E7 proteins.[3,19] Specifically, E7 inhibits the retinoblastoma tumor suppressor protein (pRb) and targets it for degradation, whereas E6 inactivates the p53 tumor suppressor.[3,19] Inhibition of pRb function by viral proteins allows cells to continue dividing, despite signals for cell cycle arrest caused by oncogenic stress, such as those mediated by p53 or p16.[20] High-risk HPV-E6 also induces the expression of vascular endothelial growth factor (VEGF) and activates telomerase, an essential step in immortalization.[3,19] The combined effects of E6 and E7 on the p53/pRb pathways create an environment of genomic instability, which is highly conducive to cancer development.[3,19]

Carcinogenesis in HPV-positive OPSCC is a process of cell cycle deregulation mediated by viral oncoproteins, which is specific to the epithelium under transformation.[2] In contrast, HPV-negative OPSCC usually results from exposure to environmental carcinogens such as tobacco and alcohol, leading to disruption of those same cancer-promoting signaling pathways targeted by HPV. This disruption occurs via the process of field cancerization, or the progressive accumulation of mutations over large regions of aerodigestive mucosa, and leads to a higher probability of developing additional primary tumors.[5] The highly localized carcinogenesis in HPV-positive OPSCC represents a profound difference in tumor biology.

CLINICAL IMPLICATIONS OF HPV-POSITIVE OPSCC

The distinct carcinogenesis of HPV-positive OPSCC leads to important differences in the population at risk for this disease, their clinical presentation, and prognosis. From the physician's standpoint, this information is highly relevant in patient education and counseling. In the future, this information may soon translate into differential workup and tailored treatments for this patient population.

Clinical Presentation

Clinical presentation of HPV-positive OPSCC is different from that of HPV-negative patients. Patients tend to be younger and are more likely to be white, married, and college educated and typically present without a history of smoking or drinking.[4,16] Given that HPV is a sexually transmitted disease, factors that increase oral or genital HPV exposure increase the risk of OPSCC, such as increasing age, increasing number of lifetime vaginal or oral sexual partners, ever having participated in casual sex, infrequent use of barriers during vaginal or oral sex, and ever having had a sexually transmitted disease. Oral HPV infection increases the risk for HPV-positive OPSCC,[4] and this risk is higher among individuals who first performed oral sex at 18 years or younger or with increasing number of cigarettes smoked per day.[16] Other risk factors for HPV-positive OPSCC include immunosuppression, seropositivity for HR-HPV, history of an HPV-associated malignancy, and being the partner of a woman with cervical cancer.[4,5,16] Patients tend to present with low T and high N stage tumors on the American Joint Committee on Cancer TNM staging system,[11,21,22] and histologically, these are usually nonkeratinizing, poorly differentiated, and of basaloid morphology.[6,17,23]

HPV Status Determination

There is no general consensus on which method for diagnosing HPV-positive cancer should be used in HNSCC, because the techniques differ in sensitivity, specificity, and other technical considerations.[24] Real-time polymerase chain reaction (RT-PCR) performed on microdissected tumors can detect small quantities of HPV DNA and describe the subtype, but it gives no information on host cell integration or activity, which are critical for carcinogenesis, and is not available in most clinical laboratories.[24–26] In situ hybridization (ISH) localizes HPV DNA integrated into the host cell genome with high specificity, indicating viral presence and activity, but is less sensitive and more time consuming than RT-PCR and is available only at selected centers.[24,25] Immunohistochemistry (IHC) of p16 has been suggested as a surrogate marker for HPV infection because of the simplicity, low cost, high sensitivity, and good correlation to HPV RT-PCR and ISH.[25–27] However, because p16 has been reported to be constitutively expressed in tonsillar epithelium, can rarely be overexpressed in HPV-negative tumors, and the practice and reporting of IHC varies, its clinical application as a single assay may occasionally be misleading.[2,20,26] With these considerations, an expert panel recommends a cost-efficient algorithm for HPV detection. Initial testing should include p16 IHC with HPV-16 ISH performed concurrently or after a positive IHC for confirmation. In case of discrepancy, a consensus ISH probe that detects an extended panel of HPV types or RT-PCR can be used to determine HPV status and subtype.[28] However, to allow for standardized detection and robust clinical investigations, a true consensus has to be reached on the method of HPV detection in OPSCC.

Prevention

The distinct pathogenesis of HPV-positive OPSCC raises important public health considerations aiming to decrease the increasing incidence of this disease through health promotion and primary prevention strategies. The prevalence of oral HPV-16 infection is 1% in the United States and has been associated with a 50-fold increased risk for HPV-positive OPSCC.[4,16] Infection is more common in smokers, and its increasing incidence has been related to the changing sexual behaviors among the population.[16]

In the primary care setting, efforts toward the modification of risk factors should be directed to reducing high-risk sexual behavior, decreasing oral HPV infection, and smoking cessation.

Because HPV-positive OPSCC is related to only a few HR-HPV subtypes,[10,16] there is potential for the prevention of this disease through vaccination targeting those subtypes. Vaccination is effective only before infection is established, because it induces neutralizing antibodies that prevent virion entry but do not halt the progression of existing lesions.[15,19] The 2 vaccines (HPV bivalent[29] and quadrivalent[30] vaccines) approved by the US Food and Drug Administration prevent persistent cervical HPV-16 infection.[15] The bivalent vaccine is indicated for the prevention of cervical cancer in women, whereas the quadrivalent vaccine has in addition been approved for the prevention of genital warts and genital cancers in both sexes up to age 26 years. Vaccination may have higher impact in OPSCC than in cervical cancer, given that, unlike cervical cancer, there is no screening strategy for OPSCC and incidence is estimated to surpass that of cervical cancer by 2020.[1] Parents of children of both sexes should be informed that vaccination is available and, although not approved for this indication, it may reduce the risk of other HPV-related cancers, including OPSCC.

IMPLICATIONS OF HPV FOR TREATMENT AND OUTCOMES

Survival in HPV-positive OPSCC

Over the last few decades, there has been improved survival in OPSCC and a resultant move toward organ preservation therapy as the primary treatment choice for these patients. Older studies looking at the effect of HPV on survival had mixed results, but the data that have accrued over the intervening years are increasingly convincing that HPV-positive OPSCC has a more favorable prognosis.[31] A recent historical demographic analysis of patients with OPSCC at a single institution by Dahlstrom and colleagues (**Table 1**)[32] showed that, after 1995, patients with OPSCC were more likely to be male, white, never-smokers or former smokers, and have low T and high N stage tumors. These characteristics are now known to be closely associated with HPV-positive tumors. Thus, it seems that the changing demographics are caused by the increase in the proportion of HPV-positive OPSCC, and that survival also improved in their cohort of patients. However, the external validity of these results is limited by the inability to control for confounders, such as treatment regimens, in this historical analysis.

Randomization to treatment regimens

Only recently have clinical trials begun to include HPV status in their patient stratification, but retrospective subgroup analyses have been performed in several phase III, multicenter trials involving the prospective randomization of patients with HNSCC to different treatment regimens. In each, a post hoc analysis has been performed to investigate the effect of HPV status on patient survival. Ang and colleagues[7] investigated the RTOG (Radiation Therapy and Oncology Group) 0219 trial, which randomized patients to concurrent chemoradiation with either standard fractionation or accelerated fractionation radiotherapy (RT). The subgroup of patients with OPSCC had an increase in overall survival (OS) and progression-free survival (PFS) for HPV-positive compared with HPV-negative OPSCC (**Table 1**). Rischin and colleagues[33] had similar results in their analysis of the HeadSTART trial, which compared the effect of the addition of tirapazamine with chemoradiotherapy (CRT) on outcome in OPSCC. These investigators also noted improved survival at 2 years in the HPV-positive subgroup as well as lower rates of locoregional failure compared with the HPV-negative subgroup (see **Table 1**). More recently, Posner and colleagues[22] looked at

Table 1
Selected studies evaluating the effect of HPV status on survival. Studies or presented results limited to previously untreated OPSCC except as noted

Study	Study Design	Results		
			HR (95% CI) or %	*P*
Dahlstrom et al,[32] 2013	Retrospective study comparing patients before and after 1995 in 1 center	Tumor subsite		
	N = 3891	BOT	0.6 (0.5–0.8)	.001
	HR: overall survival analysis with the earlier cohort as reference	Tonsil	0.6 (0.5–0.8)	<.001
		CRT	0.4 (0.3–0.6)	<.001
		N status		
		N1	0.5 (0.4–0.8)	.001
		N2	0.5 (0.4–0.6)	<.001
		TNM stage		
		Stage III	0.5 (0.4–0.8)	<.001
		Stage IV	0.5 (0.4–0.6)	<.001
Ang et al,[7] 2010	Retrospective analysis (RTOG 0129 trial: accelerated vs standard fractionation RT each with concurrent cisplatin)	OS at 3 y		
	N = 323 patients with HPV data	HPV+	82	
		HPV–	57.1	
			0.42 (0.27–0.66)	<.001
		PFS at 3 y		
		HPV+	73.7	
		HPV–	43.4	
			0.49 (0.33–0.74)	<.001
		LR recurrence		
		HPV+	13.6	
		HPV–	35.1	<.001
		Second primary tumors		
		HPV+	5.9	
		HPV–	14.6	.02

Rischin et al,[33] 2010	Retrospective analysis (TROG 02.02 trial. CRT with or without tirapazamine) N = 185 patients with HPV data	OS at 2 y		
		HPV+	91	
		HPV−	74	
			0.36 (0.17–0.74)	.004
		PFS at 2 y		
		HPV+	87	
		HPV−	72	
			0.39 (0.2–0.74)	.003
		LR recurrence		
		HPV+	93	
		HPV−	86	
			0.43 (0.17–1.11)	.091
Posner et al,[22] 2011	Retrospective analysis (TAX 324 trial: IC TPF vs PF, both followed by CRT) N = 111 patients with HPV data	OS at 5 y		
		HPV+	82	
		HPV−	35	<.0001
		PFS at 5 y		
		HPV+	78	
		HPV−	28	<.0001
		LR recurrence		
		HPV+	13	
		HPV−	42	.0006
Fakhry et al,[6] 2008	Prospective analysis (ECOG 2399 trial. Sequential therapy to CRT or surgery) N = 101, includes larynx cancer	Response to IC		
		HPV+	82	
		HPV−	55	.01
		Response to CRT		
		HPV+	84	
		HPV−	57	.007
		OS at 2 y		
		HPV+	95	
		HPV−	62	
			0.36 (0.15–0.85)	.02
		PFS at 2 y		
		HPV+	86	
		HPV−	53	
			0.27 (0.10–0.75)	.01
O'Rorke et al,[31] 2012	Meta-analysis N = 42 studies, 4834 patients	OS	0.47 (0.35–0.62)	.08
		PFS	0.48 (0.33–0.69)	.87

Abbreviations: BOT, base of tongue; CI, confidence interval; CRT, chemoradiation; HPV+, HPV-positive; HPV−, HPV-negative; HR, hazard ratio HPV+ versus HPV− unless as noted; IC, induction chemotherapy; LR, locoregional; PF, cisplatin+fluorouracil; TPF, docetaxel+cisplatin+fluorouracil.

HPV-related outcomes in the TAX 324 trial, which compared the addition of docetaxel to a standard induction chemotherapy (IC) regimen. Their results show increased OS and PFS in HPV-positive compared with HPV-negative OPSCC, along with a decreased risk of death and a significant reduction in locoregional failure rates (see **Table 1**). Overall, these retrospective analyses of prospectively treated patients strongly suggest that there is a survival benefit in HPV-positive OPSCC. However, the generalizability of these results is limited by their retrospective nature and post hoc analysis; in addition, the ability of all 3 studies to determine HPV status was limited by tissue availability.

Oropharyngeal and laryngeal cancer

Published data on the effect of HPV on survival have been provided in a prospective fashion in a single study. In 2008, Fakhry and colleagues[6] reported the results of a substudy in ECOG 2399, a phase II trial on the use of sequential therapy for organ preservation in resectable advanced stage oropharyngeal and laryngeal cancer. HPV status was determined prospectively in both subsites, and none of the laryngeal tumors was HPV positive. These investigators found that HPV-positive patients had higher response rates to IC and CRT, as well as improved OS and PFS (see **Table 1**). However, this effect did not reach statistical significance for the oropharyngeal subsite alone, because it was underpowered for subgroup analysis. At the time of the study design, it was believed that HPV was a cause of laryngeal cancer as well, so those patients were included in the trial. By the time of the data analysis, this hypothesis had largely been disproved, but the number of oropharyngeal patients alone was insufficient for the results of the multivariate analysis to remain statistically significant.

Survival disparity

Awareness of the increase in incidence of HPV-positive OPSCC has also solved one of the survival conundrums in OPSCC. Multiple studies had reported a disparity in survival rates between African American and white patients, despite controlling for tumor site, age, and other risk factors.[34,35] However, using data from the TAX 324 trial, Settle and colleagues[12] concluded that the disparity in survival between African American and white patients with OPSCC was entirely caused by significant differences in rates of HPV infection between the 2 groups. A more recent report confirms that the shorter PFS in African American patients with OPSCC may be caused by HPV status, treatment type, and higher T stage at presentation but is not caused by race.[36]

HPV-positive OPSCC has improved survival, lower rate of disease progression, and lower chance of locoregional recurrence when compared with HPV-negative OPSCC. There have not been significant differences in the rates of distant failure, which may or may not be related to insufficient power to detect a difference.[6,7,22,33] Furthermore, a recent meta-analysis by O'Rorke and colleagues,[31] the most comprehensive to date, reported a 53% better OS and 74% better disease-specific survival for HPV-positive OPSCC, as well as statistically significant improvement in PFS and disease-free survival (DFS). Prospective data are limited; however, there are ongoing clinical trials that include HPV status stratification in their trial design (**Table 2**). Several of the recent trends observed in OPSCC (improved survival, change in patient demographics, and suspected racial outcome disparities) are likely caused by differences in incidence of HPV-positive OPSCC.

Possible Mechanisms Underlying the Survival Benefit in HPV-Positive OPSCC

The unique carcinogenesis of HPV-positive OPSCC provides several possible explanations for the survival benefit seen in these patients. For instance, the lack of field cancerization in HPV-positive patients with OPSCC may explain the improved locoregional control, reduced risk of recurrence, and reduced risk of second primary tumors compared with HPV-negative cancers.[5,7,37,38] Others have proposed an increased sensitivity to RT and chemotherapy in HPV-positive cancers as an explanation for improved survival.[38–40] In vitro data from cervical cancer cell lines showed that cisplatin treatment induced apoptosis by both p53-dependent and p53-independent pathways,[39] suggesting that p53 could be reactivated and enable the cell to respond to DNA damage after chemotherapy-mediated repression of viral E6 and E7. HPV-positive OPSCC has also shown better survival and higher local control rates after treatment with RT (risk ratio for local treatment failure of 0.33), which may result from persistent, functional p53.[38]

Genomic differences

Another mechanism for improved survival may be genomic differences between HPV-positive and HPV-negative tumors. Sequencing of HNSCC reveals fewer mutations in protein-encoding genes in HPV-positive cancers, suggesting that genetic instability is less pronounced.[41,42] There may also be a difference in the degree of intratumor heterogeneity between HPV-positive and HPV-negative OPSCC. Intratumor heterogeneity refers to the number of subpopulations of tumor cells within a single tumor that have different genotypes. Considering that therapy can select for subpopulations of cells that resist that particular treatment,[43] high intratumor heterogeneity is increasingly recognized as a risk for treatment failure or recurrence. A measure of genomic intratumor heterogeneity based on next-generation DNA sequencing indicates that HPV-positive tumors have less intratumor heterogeneity than do HPV-negative tumors, and thus may be more likely to respond to therapy without recurrence.[44]

Immune system

The immune system may also contribute to the increased survival observed in HPV-positive OPSCC. A robust cytotoxic lymphocytic response related to HPV-positive tumors is associated with better response to therapy and increased survival.[40,45,46] Preclinical models suggest that improved treatment response in HPV-positive tumors results from the combination of treatment effect and immune response, rather than to an intrinsic sensitivity of the cells to therapy.[47] In the absence of the immune system, HPV-positive cell lines were more resistant to therapy, although in vivo, an immunocompetent environment was required to achieve complete tumor clearance.[47] However, the investigators did not evaluate the role of the immune system in response to therapy in the HPV-negative setting, so it is unclear if they were measuring a general antitumor response or one specific to HPV. Clinically, several mechanisms have been described to suggest that the improved response of HPV-positive tumors to RT may be related to enhancement of the immune response.[40] The proposed mechanisms underlying the improved survival in HPV-positive OPSCC have not been clinically validated, but it is likely that they all contribute with varying degrees.

Current Treatment Implications for HPV-Positive OPSCC and Unknown Primary

Because HPV delineates a distinct type of OPSCC, HPV status should be routinely tested in all patients presenting with OPSCC or an unknown primary. HPV positivity in OPSCC offers more accurate prognostic information than that given by TNM staging alone,[32,37] because nodal involvement leads to overstaging of disease that does not represent the same risk when compared with other head and neck cancers with the same stage.[37] In the setting of an unknown primary, studies have shown that HPV positivity in a lymph node biopsy may be used to localize the primary with high

Table 2
Summary of selected OPSCC HPV-related trials

Trial	Study Design	Population[a]	HPV Assay	Primary Outcome	Status and Projected End Date[b]	Relevance
NCT01598792	REALISTIC: dose escalation trial of recombinant *Listeria monocytogenes*–based vaccine encoding HPV-16 target antigens (ADXS11-001) Phase I	In remission after standard treatment	p16 IHC	Systemic or local adverse events	10/2014	Novel immune modulation strategy
NCT01064921	Dose escalation study of vorinostat administered with CRT (standard RT+P) Phase I	Advanced, unresectable	HPV tested, method not reported	Maximum tolerated dose and toxicity	01/2013	Novel targeted therapy
NCT01088802	De-escalation CRT (IMRT: 70 Gy, 63 Gy and 58.1 Gy to primary and neck. Chemotherapy: P/CP) Phase I/II	Resectable	HPV tested, method not reported	2-y toxicity and locoregional control	02/2015	Decrease morbidity
NCT01585428	Lymphodepletion followed by autologous tumor-infiltrating lymphocytes and high-dose aldesleukin Phase II	M1 or locally advanced, refractory or recurrent HPVAC	HPV ISH PCR	Objective tumor response and duration	04/2014	Novel immune modulation strategy
NCT01590355	ORATOR: TORS + ND vs RT/CRT ± surgical salvage. Phase II	Early stage	HPV tested, method not reported	Quality of life 1 y after treatment	06/2021	Novel surgical technique, decrease morbidity. Attempt to identify genetic markers of treatment failure and toxicity

specificity to the oropharynx, providing diagnostic information that may change RT planning.[48] For an HPV-positive unknown primary, RT might be limited to the oropharynx and neck as opposed to a wider field, potentially from the nasopharynx down to the larynx, depending on neck disease localization, thus significantly decreasing treatment-related morbidity and complications.[49]

De-escalation of Treatment and New Targets

Knowledge that HPV-positive OPSCC may result in better response to therapy, improved locoregional control, and better survival may open an avenue to specialized treatment regimens that achieve the same oncologic outcomes with decreased morbidity. Currently available treatment modalities (CRT, sequential therapy or surgery)[49] achieve comparable survival, but differ in associated risks and complications. Surgical approaches carry risks common to invasive procedures, although current acute and late complications associated to RT-based modalities negatively affect patient quality of life.[50] In addition, the long-term side effects of cancer treatment seen in survivors of other malignancies will likely increase in this patient population. RT-induced cardiovascular disease has become the leading noncancer cause of mortality among survivors of some cancers, and significant trends in RT-induced malignancies have been reported among survivors of adult-onset cancers for several malignancies.[51] Risk of stroke and occlusive carotid artery disease is particularly increased in patients with HNSCC.[51] The HPV-positive population is younger, higher-functioning, and has fewer comorbidities and less smoking and alcohol exposure, with subsequent decreased cardiovascular risk.[4,16] These individuals are also likely to achieve better survival regardless of treatment modality.[7] We are facing a subgroup of patients who will likely achieve complete response and outlive their cancer by 10 to 30 years and will have to endure the side effects of cancer treatment for their lifetime. Thus, evaluating the possibility of treatment de-escalation to optimize long-term quality of life is of paramount importance.

Several trials are under way evaluating different de-escalation regimens for HPV-positive OPSCC. Strategies include modifying existing treatment modalities, evaluating novel targeted therapies, or inducing immunologic responses to HPV-positive tumors (see **Table 2**). An initial approach is to reduce the radiation dose of CRT regimens. A phase I/II trial is evaluating reduced radiation doses to the primary tumor and neck with concurrent platinum therapy in patients with resectable OPSCC (see **Table 2**). Another phase II trial is evaluating reduced dosing of CRT followed by surgery in previously untreated OPSCC (see **Table 2**). These studies will address whether reduced chemotherapy or RT dosing schemes result in equivalent survival with decreased morbidity in CRT regimens.

IC

The role of IC in treatment of HNSCC remains unclear. IC has not shown a survival advantage in HNSCC, but some evidence suggests that it may contribute to improved survival in OPSCC.[52] Three phase II trials are active to address this question. One study uses IC to select patients to reduced-dose RT or standard CRT; a second trial evaluates IC followed by cetuximab with reduced or standard RT; and a third trial administers IC followed by reduced or standard RT with concurrent platinum and cetuximab. These trials will determine if sequential therapy is effective in OPSCC and may provide insight into the relative efficacy of IC followed by platinum-only, cetuximab-only, or combined platinum-cetuximab regimens concurrent to standard or reduced-dose RT, and their differential effects on morbidity and oncologic outcomes (see **Table 2**).

Surgical alternatives

New surgical alternatives in the treatment of OPSCC include transoral laser microsurgery (TLM) and transoral robotic surgery (TORS), and offer an additional pathway to organ preservation. TLM has become 1 standard of care for early laryngeal cancer, with usefulness in the oropharynx.[53] TLM uses surgical tools available in most hospitals, maximizes conservation of normal mucosa, and achieves adequate outcomes.[53] The line-of-sight limitation posed by the laser while accessing the oropharynx has been partially addressed by the development of fiber-optic delivery systems.[53] However, because tumor is typically removed by piecemeal resection, novel pathologic techniques are often required to adequately assess margin status. Alternatively, TORS provides improved surgical access to the oropharynx and enhanced visual evaluation of margins because of improved infield optics, three-dimensional imagery, tremor filtration, and high-precision movements, although at increased cost.[54,55] TORS shows promising oncologic outcomes shown by the 1-year and 2-year OS rates of 90% and 80% to 90%, respectively, in the initial retrospective studies on highly selected patients.[54] TORS offers the additional benefit of complete pathologic staging information via en bloc resection, with markedly decreased morbidity compared with CRT regimens.[54,56] In addition, successful control of the primary tumor burden opens avenues for de-escalation regimens, which could decrease or avoid adjuvant treatment requirements.[54] This surgical approach is under investigation as a de-escalation modality in OPSCC, in which patients with resectable OPSCC will be randomized to TORS with neck dissection or RT plus or minus chemotherapy with surgical salvage for persistent disease. This study will offer a direct comparison of TORS with RT or CRT and determine if TORS achieves better functional outcomes in early-stage OPSCC (see **Table 2**).

Novel targeted therapies

The increased understanding of molecular signaling pathways in HNSCC has led to studies of novel targeted therapies, which may decrease the morbidity associated with conventional treatment of HNSCC. The first FDA-approved targeted therapy for HNSCC is cetuximab, a monoclonal antibody against epidermal growth factor receptor (EGFR). It showed a 5-year survival benefit when added to RT (RT: 36.4%, RT and cetuximab: 45.6%, hazard ratio: 0.73, $P = .018$) with decreased morbidity and an improvement in quality of life, although at a significantly higher cost.[57,58] The survival benefit was restricted to patients with clinical and tumor characteristics associated with HPV-positive OPSCC (**Fig. 1**).[59] This finding may suggest that the benefit of cetuximab as initial treatment is limited to HPV-positive patients. However, these results may merely portray the known improved survival in HPV-positive patients, their better response to treatment, or a marked imbalance of HPV-positive patients between the intervention groups despite randomization.[60]

In contrast, panitumumab, another EGFR inhibitor, may benefit HPV-negative patients only in the recurrent/metastatic setting, according to an initial report.[61] Differences in clinical setting (primary vs recurrent/metastatic tumors) or treatment regimen (chimeric vs humanized anti-EGFR antibody, radiation vs chemotherapy) may explain these apparently contradictory findings.[62] More studies are needed to determine how HPV status affects response to EGFR inhibitors in HNSCC (see **Table 2**).

The RTOG-1016 trial is performing a direct comparison of RT with cisplatin or cetuximab in patients with OPSCC with prospective HPV testing that will address the efficacy of cetuximab as single agent in CRT regimens, compare the toxicity profiles, and possibly the relative efficacy in HPV-positive and HPV-negative patients (see **Table 2**).

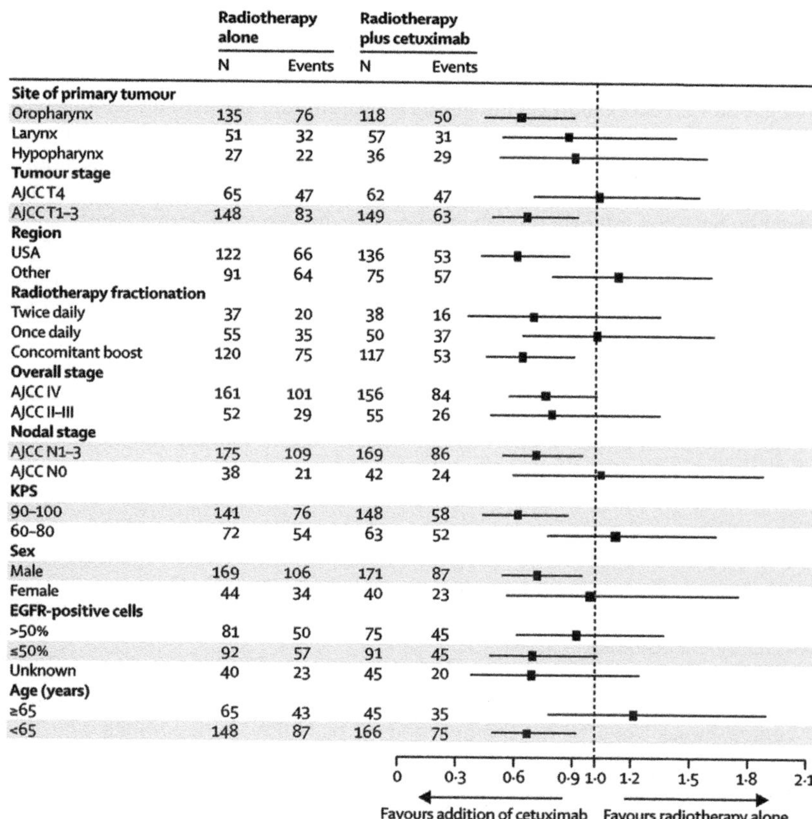

Fig. 1. Hazard ratios for overall survival based on patient pretreatment characteristics. Marked categories represent characteristics associated with HPV-positive OPSCC. (*Adapted from* Bonner JA, Harari PM, Giralt J, et al. Radiotherapy plus cetuximab for locoregionally advanced head and neck cancer: 5-year survival data from a phase 3 randomised trial, and relation between cetuximab-induced rash and survival. Lancet Oncol 2010;11(1):25; with permission.)

Histone deacetylase inhibitors have emerged as another potential drug to reverse aberrant epigenetic changes associated with cancer.[63] One of these drugs, vorinostat, is being evaluated for safety and maximum tolerated dose when administered concurrently with CRT in the treatment of OPSCC (see **Table 2**). Several additional biochemical pathways such as VEGF and intracellular signaling pathways are being targeted for treatment with drugs currently in various stages of development for the treatment of HNSCC.[58] These drugs may lead to new treatment alternatives for OPSCC.

Specific targeting of HPV-positive tumor cells may be achieved as a result of the unique expression of E6 and E7 oncoproteins by HPV-positive OPSCC. For example, suppression of cellular E6 and E7 protein levels by short hairpin RNA is able to restore p53 and pRb function and induce apoptosis in cell line studies.[64] As a consequence, small molecule inhibitors that inhibit the protein-protein interaction of the viral oncoproteins E6 and E7 are actively being investigated, which may sensitize tumor cells to other therapies.[58] Tumor expression of E6 and E7 may also provide the possibility to induce or enhance cell-mediated immunity against tumor cells. This strategy is being investigated in several phase I and II trials in HNSCC (NCT01493154, NCT00019110, and NCT01462838, available at http://www.clinicaltrials.gov). Specifically in OPSCC, 1 study is using a *Listeria monocytogenes*–based vaccine to deliver HPV antigens for recognition by the immune system and elicit an immune response (see **Table 2**).[65] Another approach is harvesting, expanding, and readministering tumor-infiltrating lymphocytes to patients to enhance the cytotoxic antitumoral immune response as a treatment strategy in HPV-related cancers (see **Table 2**). These approaches have the intrinsic benefit of using physiologic antitumoral responses as a treatment modality that theoretically carries decreased risk and morbidity. Further research will allow us to evaluate the safety and efficacy of novel treatment strategies and to gain understanding into the mechanisms involved in the response to treatment of HPV-positive and HPV-negative OPSCC.

Biomarkers and Risk Stratification for Patient Selection

There has also been a recent effort to use biomarkers to identify which patients will benefit from de-escalation of therapy and which patients will require standard treatments. Approaches using IC as a stratification marker to select patients for early surgical intervention, if there is an insufficient response, have been unsatisfying.[17] It is unclear whether IC achieves effective downstaging of the tumor, making RT more effective, or more likely selects potentially curable patients.[52] Furthermore, this selection method is time consuming, carries additional costs and morbidity, and has not shown a survival advantage in HNSCC.[17,52]

A second strategy is to identify biomarkers that can prospectively distinguish between those patients with a high probability to respond to treatment and achieve cure versus those likely to fail therapy and at high risk of recurrence and death. HPV status is one widely used biomarker and the most accepted means of stratification, but alone it is insufficient to direct therapy outside clinical trials. There is also a need to find complementary biomarkers to further stratify HPV-positive patients, because the ever-increasing incidence of HPV-positive cases translates into approximately half of all OPSCC recurrences presenting in HPV-positive patients, despite the improved outcomes.[37,66]

Approaches to stratifying HPV-positive patients

Several approaches have been proposed with this objective. Kumar and colleagues[67] studied how HPV status and expression of EGFR, p16, p53, Bcl-xL, and p53 mutations on pretreatment biopsies affected OS and DFS in patients with advanced OPSCC enrolled in an organ-sparing trial. Treatment consisted of IC followed by CRT and adjuvant paclitaxel or surgery and RT. Patients with favorable expression profiles (low EGFR and high HPV titer/p16, or low p53 with low Bcl-xL), showed significantly better OS and DFS (**Fig. 2**).[67] This study shows how in a group of homogeneously treated patients, the combination of HPV status and EGFR expression could accurately stratify survival. Moreover, p53 and Bcl-xL were found to be predictors of survival independent of HPV status, which points toward a molecular mechanism that may underlie these findings. Inhibition of apoptosis by high Bcl-xL favors DNA repair by the increased p53 level, allowing the cells to continue to grow despite cisplatin-induced DNA damage.[67] Furthermore, the percentage of HPV-positive patients who fail treatment is similar to the percentage of HPV-positive tumors reported to harbor p53 mutations,[23,67,68] suggesting that mutant p53 may be used as a marker to further stratify the HPV-positive population.

Ang and colleagues[7] constructed an algorithm to classify patients into distinct risk categories after CRT. HPV status was the major determinant of OS, followed by

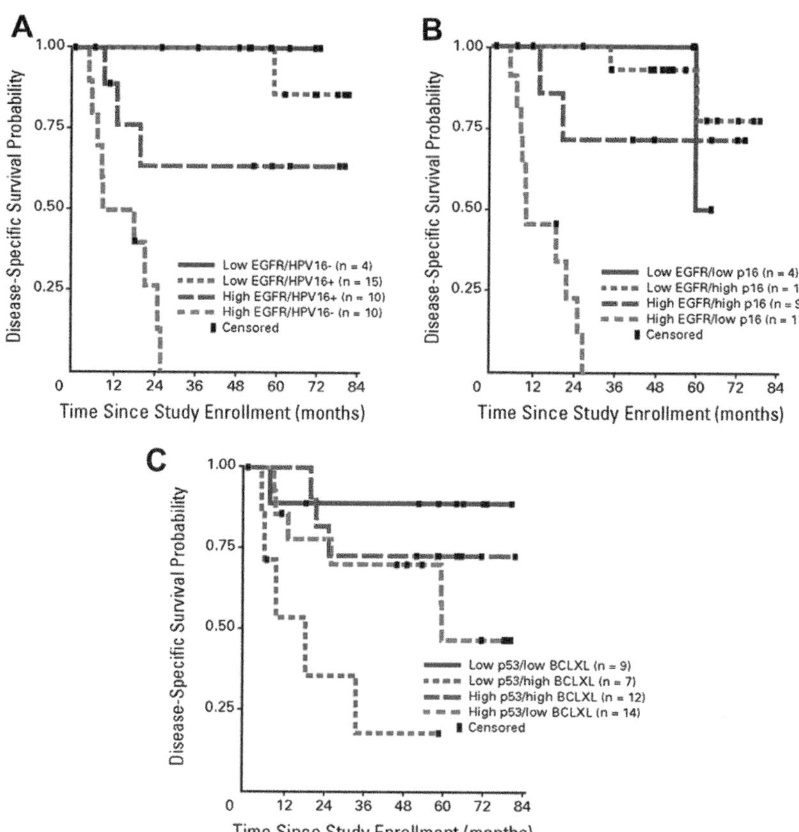

Fig. 2. Kaplan-Meier curves for DFS based on risk stratification by (*A*) EGFR and HPV-16, (*B*) EGFR and p16, (*C*) p53 and Bcl-xL. (*From* Kumar B, Cordell KG, Lee JS, et al. EGFR, p16, HPV Titer, Bcl-xL and p53, sex, and smoking as indicators of response to therapy and survival in oropharyngeal cancer. J Clin Oncol 2008;26(19):3134; with permission.)

pack-years of smoking. These subgroups were further classified according to N stage for HPV-positive tumors and T stage for HPV-negative tumors. Patients were then classified into low, intermediate, or high risk of death categories, which correlate with a 3-year OS of 93%, 70.8%, and 46.2%, respectively (**Fig. 3**).[7] Classification into HR and intermediate-risk groups showed a 7-fold and 4-fold higher risk of death than LR patients.[7] This is a simple method to estimate individual patient risk of death after treatment with CRT, which is easily translatable to the clinic, because HPV status, TNM staging, and smoking history are readily available to clinicians.

Nichols and colleagues[66] evaluated retrospectively whether Bcl-2 and HPV status could be used as markers for therapeutic response in a cohort of newly diagnosed patients with OPSCC for whom pretreatment biopsies were available and had either a minimum 2-year follow-up, death, or recurrence. HPV infection and Bcl-2 were found to be independent predictors of improved DFS and OS. Patients with high Bcl-2 tumors had approximately a 7-fold increased risk of recurrence and death after adjusting for HPV status. The data also suggested that Bcl-2 was specifically associated with increased risk of distant metastasis, with no relation to locoregional recurrence.

NCT01530997	De-escalation CRT (RT:v54–60 Gy, P:30 mg/m^2) followed by surgery (salvage for residual primary, SND for pretreatment nodal disease) Phase II		p16 IHC	CR after de-escalated CRT	01/2014	Decrease morbidity
NCT01525927	IC (T, CP, FU) followed by reduced-dose RT/CRT for responders or standard CRT (EBRT/IMRT $\pm$ P/Carbo) for nonresponders Phase II		p16 IHC HPV ISH	Response 3 mo after therapy (CR+PR)	07/2013	Decrease morbidity. Determine efficacy of sequential therapy in OPSCC
NCT01084083	ECOG-E1308: IC (PT+P+cetuximab) followed by cetuximab+low/standard dose IMRT Phase II	Advanced, resectable	HPV ISH p16 IHC	2-y PFS	Active, not recruiting 03/2015	Decrease morbidity. Determine efficacy of sequential therapy in OPSCC
NCT01221753	IC (T+P+FU) followed by CRT (low vs standard dose IMRT with CP+cetuximab) Phase II	Locally advanced	HPV ISH p16 IHC	Locoregional control at 2 and 5 y	09/2015	Decrease morbidity. Determine efficacy of sequential therapy in OPSCC
NCT01302834	RTOG-1016: IMRT+cetuximab vs IMRT+P Phase III		p16 IHC	5-y OS	01/2015	Decrease morbidity. Direct comparison cetuximab vs cisplatin for CRT

Abbreviations: +, and; /, or; $\pm$, with or without; APC, antigen-presenting cells; CP, carboplatin; CR, complete response; EBRT, external beam radiation therapy; FU, 5-fluorouracil; HPVAC, HPV-associated cancer (cervical, oropharyngeal, vaginal, anal, or penile cancer); IMRT, intensity modulated radiation therapy; ND, neck dissection; PR, partial response; PT, paclitaxel; P, cisplatin; SND, selective neck dissection; T, docetaxel; TORS, transoral robotic surgery.

[a] Primary untreated HPV+ OPSCC except as noted.

[b] Trials are active and recruiting except as noted, with estimated primary completion date as reported on www.clinicaltrials.gov.

Data from U.S. National Institutes of Health. Available at: http://www.clinicaltrials.gov.

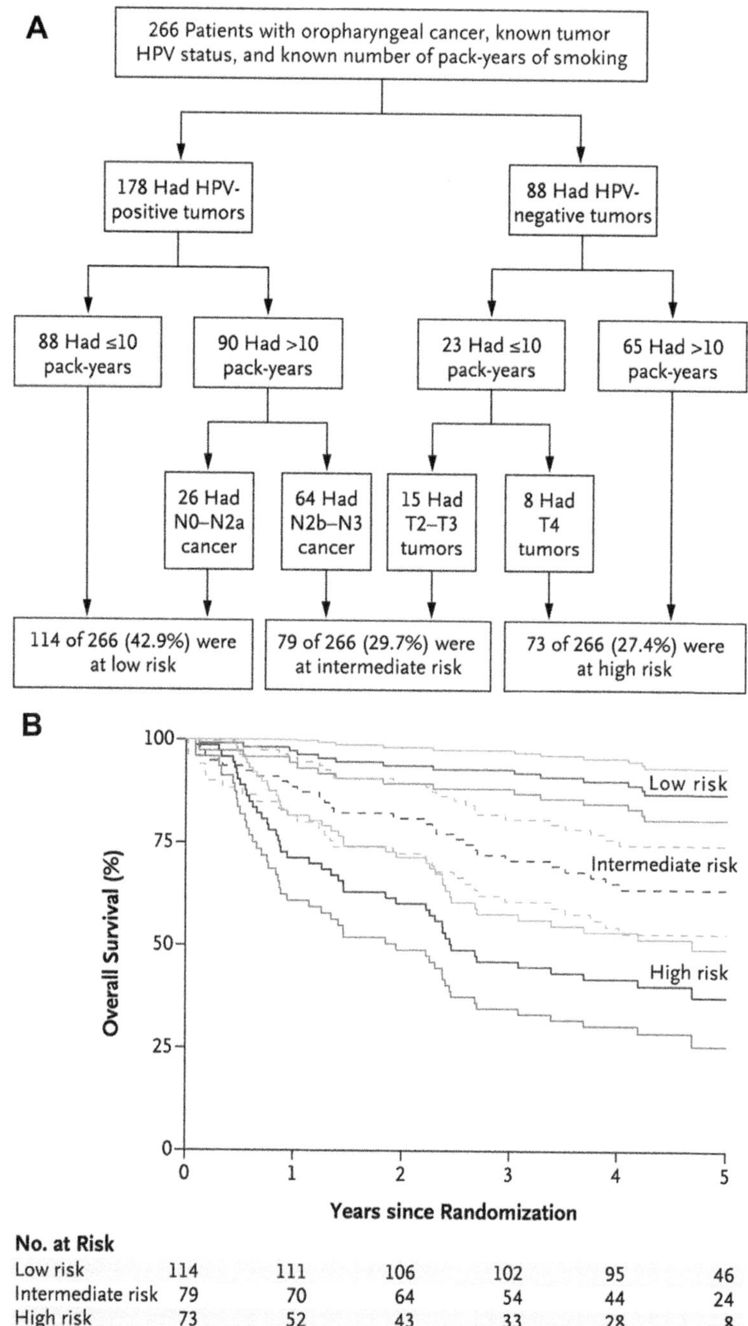

No. at Risk

	0	1	2	3	4	5
Low risk	114	111	106	102	95	46
Intermediate risk	79	70	64	54	44	24
High risk	73	52	43	33	28	8

Fig. 3. Risk classification scheme (*A*) and corresponding Kaplan-Meier curves for OS with their 95% confidence interval (*B*). (*From* Ang KK, Harris J, Wheeler R, et al. Human papillomavirus and survival of patients with oropharyngeal cancer. N Engl J Med 2010;363(1):33; with permission.)

Based on HPV and Bcl-2, patients were segregated into 3 risk groups: those with 2 favorable markers showed excellent survival (HPV-positive and low Bcl-2); patients with 1 favorable and 1 unfavorable marker showed intermediate survival (HPV-positive and high Bcl-2, or HPV-negative and low Bcl-2); and those with both unfavorable markers showed poor survival (HPV-negative and high Bcl-2) (**Fig. 4**).[66] The high percentage of HPV-positive tumors that had high Bcl-2 (40%) suggests that this biomarker will become increasingly useful over time.[66] Small molecule inhibitors of Bcl-2 are under investigation and may play an important role in defining new treatment regimens for patients with OPSCC at high risk of recurrence and death. Because Bcl-2 may also identify patients at higher risk for distant metastasis, it has the potential to be used as a marker for intensification of systemic treatment, such as the addition of IC before CRT rather than CRT alone.

Several other markers have been studied with different degrees of reliability in HNSCC, and although their relation to HPV-positive OPSCC has not been established, they may have future implications for risk stratification in this cancer.[17,69] The studies presented were limited in some instances by their retrospective nature and, overall, by the small sample sizes and limited generalizability, given the different populations and variety of interventions studied. Nonetheless, these promising findings point the way toward future prospective studies in more general clinical scenarios.

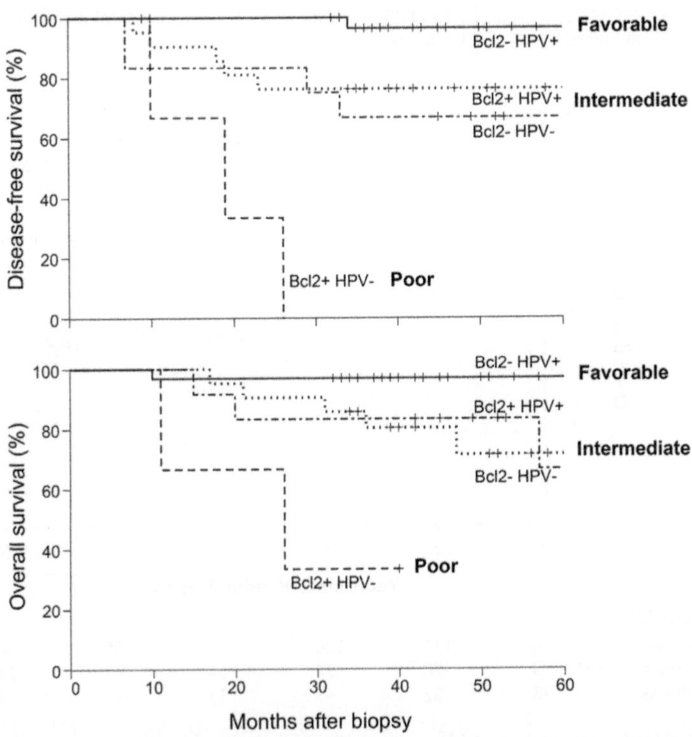

Fig. 4. Kaplan-Meier curves for DFS and OS based on risk classification by HPV status and Bcl-2. (*Adapted from* Nichols AC, Finkelstein DM, Faquin WC, et al. Bcl2 and human papilloma virus 16 as predictors of outcome following concurrent chemoradiation for advanced oropharyngeal cancer. Clin Cancer Res 2010;16(7):2144; with permission.)

SUMMARY

In the past decade, otolaryngologists and related specialists have seen the emergence and characterization of a new entity, HPV-positive oropharyngeal cancer, which has changed the way we understand and manage cancer of the head and neck. HPV-positive OPSCC has a distinct pathogenesis and develops in a localized environment of genomic instability and malignant transformation driven by the expression of the E6 and E7 viral oncoproteins. In contrast to HPV-negative OPSCC, it is a disease of younger patients, with a distinct subset of risk factors related to sexual practices that have evolved over the past several decades. These patients show better oncologic outcomes than their historical cohort, as shown by their favorable response to treatment and improved PFS and OS, although the mechanism underlying this benefit remains unknown.

There are several important treatment implications. Could we identify patients with OPSCC who will show complete response to treatment a priori and decrease the morbidity of treatment safely and with the same oncologic outcomes to achieve better quality of life? Can we also predict which patients will fail treatment, allowing us to test more intensified regimens in the population at risk to increase the probability of initial cure? What should these intensified and deintensified regimens be? Which biomarkers will allow us to make these predictions to be able to offer personalized therapy? Does organ preservation therapy work in the absence of HPV infection?

Different organ preservation regimens, surgical approaches, and novel targeted therapy strategies that address cancer-related pathways and HPV-specific targets are being studied to begin offering some insight into these challenging questions. Some changes to clinical practice have already been recommended, such as determining HPV status for all patients with oropharyngeal cancer or unknown primary. Patients with OPSCC should also be strongly encouraged to participate in clinical trials. The success of trials evaluating different treatment modalities as well as de-escalation of therapy will depend on adequate recruitment; thus we encourage active enrollment of patients to be able to determine new standards of care. There is great potential for the prevention of this disease through modification of risk factors and potentially with vaccination, such that the impact of this cancer epidemic may be stabilized or decreased.

ACKNOWLEDGMENTS

We are grateful to the Principles and Practice of Clinical Research Course and Latin American Initiative Program for training support to JBV.

REFERENCES

1. Chaturvedi AK, Engels EA, Pfeiffer RM, et al. Human papillomavirus and rising oropharyngeal cancer incidence in the United States. J Clin Oncol 2011;29(32): 4294–301.
2. Begum S, Cao D, Gillison M, et al. Tissue distribution of human papillomavirus 16 DNA integration in patients with tonsillar carcinoma. Clin Cancer Res 2005; 11(16):5694–9.
3. McLaughlin-Drubin ME, Munger K. Oncogenic activities of human papillomaviruses. Virus Res 2009;143(2):195–208.
4. Gillison ML, D'Souza G, Westra W, et al. Distinct risk factor profiles for human papillomavirus type 16-positive and human papillomavirus type 16-negative head and neck cancers. J Natl Cancer Inst 2008;100(6):407–20.

5. Fakhry C, Gillison ML. Clinical implications of human papillomavirus in head and neck cancers. J Clin Oncol 2006;24(17):2606–11.
6. Fakhry C, Westra WH, Li S, et al. Improved survival of patients with human papillomavirus-positive head and neck squamous cell carcinoma in a prospective clinical trial. J Natl Cancer Inst 2008;100(4):261–9.
7. Ang KK, Harris J, Wheeler R, et al. Human papillomavirus and survival of patients with oropharyngeal cancer. N Engl J Med 2010;363(1):24–35.
8. Ragin CC, Taioli E. Survival of squamous cell carcinoma of the head and neck in relation to human papillomavirus infection: review and meta-analysis. Int J Cancer 2007;121(8):1813–20.
9. Chaturvedi AK. Beyond cervical cancer: burden of other HPV-related cancers among men and women. J Adolesc Health 2010;46(Suppl 4):S20–6.
10. D'Souza G, Dempsey A. The role of HPV in head and neck cancer and review of the HPV vaccine. Prev Med 2011;53(Suppl 1):S5–11.
11. Marur S, D'Souza G, Westra WH, et al. HPV-associated head and neck cancer: a virus-related cancer epidemic. Lancet Oncol 2010;11(8):781–9.
12. Settle K, Posner MR, Schumaker LM, et al. Racial survival disparity in head and neck cancer results from low prevalence of human papillomavirus infection in black oropharyngeal cancer patients. Cancer Prev Res (Phila) 2009;2(9):776–81.
13. Joseph AW, D'Souza G. Epidemiology of human papillomavirus-related head and neck cancer. Otolaryngol Clin North Am 2012;45(4):739–64.
14. Chow LT, Broker TR, Steinberg BM. The natural history of human papillomavirus infections of the mucosal epithelia. APMIS 2010;118(6–7):422–49.
15. Schiffman M, Castle PE, Jeronimo J, et al. Human papillomavirus and cervical cancer. Lancet 2007;370(9590):890–907.
16. Gillison ML, Broutian T, Pickard RK, et al. Prevalence of oral HPV infection in the United States, 2009-2010. JAMA 2012;307(7):693–703.
17. Grimminger CM, Danenberg PV. Update of prognostic and predictive biomarkers in oropharyngeal squamous cell carcinoma: a review. Eur Arch Otorhinolaryngol 2011;268(1):5–16.
18. Vidal L, Gillison ML. Human papillomavirus in HNSCC: recognition of a distinct disease type. Hematol Oncol Clin North Am 2008;22(6):1125–42, vii.
19. Moody CA, Laimins LA. Human papillomavirus oncoproteins: pathways to transformation. Nat Rev Cancer 2010;10(8):550–60.
20. Mroz EA, Baird AH, Michaud WA, et al. COOH-terminal binding protein regulates expression of the p16INK4A tumor suppressor and senescence in primary human cells. Cancer Res 2008;68(15):6049–53.
21. Mellin H, Friesland S, Lewensohn R, et al. Human papillomavirus (HPV) DNA in tonsillar cancer: clinical correlates, risk of relapse, and survival. Int J Cancer 2000;89(3):300–4.
22. Posner MR, Lorch JH, Goloubeva O, et al. Survival and human papillomavirus in oropharynx cancer in TAX 324: a subset analysis from an international phase III trial. Ann Oncol 2011;22(5):1071–7.
23. Gillison ML, Koch WM, Capone RB, et al. Evidence for a causal association between human papillomavirus and a subset of head and neck cancers. J Natl Cancer Inst 2000;92(9):709–20.
24. Jordan RC, Lingen MW, Perez-Ordonez B, et al. Validation of methods for oropharyngeal cancer HPV status determination in US cooperative group trials. Am J Surg Pathol 2012;36(7):945–54.
25. Palka KT, Slebos RJ, Chung CH. Update on molecular diagnostic tests in head and neck cancer. Semin Oncol 2008;35(3):198–210.

26. El-Naggar AK, Westra WH. p16 expression as a surrogate marker for HPV-related oropharyngeal carcinoma: a guide for interpretative relevance and consistency. Head Neck 2012;34(4):459–61.
27. Singhi AD, Westra WH. Comparison of human papillomavirus in situ hybridization and p16 immunohistochemistry in the detection of human papillomavirus-associated head and neck cancer based on a prospective clinical experience. Cancer 2010;116(9):2166–73.
28. Adelstein DJ, Ridge JA, Gillison ML, et al. Head and neck squamous cell cancer and the human papillomavirus: summary of a National Cancer Institute State of the Science Meeting, November 9-10, 2008, Washington, D.C. Head Neck 2009;31(11):1393–422.
29. US Food and Drug Administration. Approved products. Cervarix. 2012. Available at: http://www.fda.gov/BiologicsBloodVaccines/Vaccines/ApprovedProducts/ucm186957. Accessed July 23, 2012.
30. US Food and Drug Administration. Approved products. Gardasil. 2012. Available at: http://www.fda.gov/BiologicsBloodVaccines/Vaccines/ApprovedProducts/UCM094042. Accessed July 23, 2012.
31. O'Rorke MA, Ellison MV, Murray LJ, et al. Human papillomavirus related head and neck cancer survival: a systematic review and meta-analysis. Oral Oncol 2012;48(12):1191–201.
32. Dahlstrom KR, Calzada G, Hanby JD, et al. An evolution in demographics, treatment, and outcomes of oropharyngeal cancer at a major cancer center: a staging system in need of repair. Cancer 2013;119(1):81–9.
33. Rischin D, Young RJ, Fisher R, et al. Prognostic significance of p16INK4A and human papillomavirus in patients with oropharyngeal cancer treated on TROG 02.02 phase III trial. J Clin Oncol 2010;28(27):4142–8.
34. Goodwin WJ, Thomas GR, Parker DF, et al. Unequal burden of head and neck cancer in the United States. Head Neck 2008;30(3):358–71.
35. Settle K, Taylor R, Wolf J, et al. Race impacts outcome in stage III/IV squamous cell carcinomas of the head and neck after concurrent chemoradiation therapy. Cancer 2009;115(8):1744–52.
36. Chernock RD, Zhang Q, El-Mofty SK, et al. Human papillomavirus-related squamous cell carcinoma of the oropharynx: a comparative study in whites and African Americans. Arch Otolaryngol Head Neck Surg 2011;137(2):163–9.
37. Mroz EA, Forastiere AA, Rocco JW. Implications of the oropharyngeal cancer epidemic. J Clin Oncol 2011;29(32):4222–3.
38. Licitra L, Perrone F, Bossi P, et al. High-risk human papillomavirus affects prognosis in patients with surgically treated oropharyngeal squamous cell carcinoma. J Clin Oncol 2006;24(36):5630–6.
39. Butz K, Geisen C, Ullmann A, et al. Cellular responses of HPV-positive cancer cells to genotoxic anti-cancer agents: repression of E6/E7-oncogene expression and induction of apoptosis. Int J Cancer 1996;68(4):506–13.
40. Vu HL, Sikora AG, Fu S, et al. HPV-induced oropharyngeal cancer, immune response and response to therapy. Cancer Lett 2010;288(2):149–55.
41. Agrawal N, Frederick MJ, Pickering CR, et al. Exome sequencing of head and neck squamous cell carcinoma reveals inactivating mutations in NOTCH1. Science 2011;333(6046):1154–7.
42. Stransky N, Egloff AM, Tward AD, et al. The mutational landscape of head and neck squamous cell carcinoma. Science 2011;333(6046):1157–60.
43. Salk JJ, Fox EJ, Loeb LA. Mutational heterogeneity in human cancers: origin and consequences. Annu Rev Pathol 2010;5:51–75.

44. Mroz EA, Rocco JW. MATH, a novel measure of intratumor genetic heterogeneity, is high in poor-outcome classes of head and neck squamous cell carcinoma. Oral Oncol 2013;49(3):211–5.
45. Wansom D, Light E, Worden F, et al. Correlation of cellular immunity with human papillomavirus 16 status and outcome in patients with advanced oropharyngeal cancer. Arch Otolaryngol Head Neck Surg 2010;136(12):1267–73.
46. Wansom D, Light E, Thomas D, et al. Infiltrating lymphocytes and human papillomavirus-16–associated oropharyngeal cancer. Laryngoscope 2012;122(1):121–7.
47. Spanos WC, Nowicki P, Lee DW, et al. Immune response during therapy with cisplatin or radiation for human papillomavirus-related head and neck cancer. Arch Otolaryngol Head Neck Surg 2009;135(11):1137–46.
48. Begum S, Gillison ML, Ansari-Lari MA, et al. Detection of human papillomavirus in cervical lymph nodes: a highly effective strategy for localizing site of tumor origin. Clin Cancer Res 2003;9(17):6469–75.
49. National Comprehensive Cancer Network. The NCCN clinical practice guidelines in oncology. Head and neck cancers (version 1.2012). Available at http://www.nccn.org/professionals/physician_gls/f_guidelines.asp#site. Accessed June 12, 2012.
50. Wang X, Hu C, Eisbruch A. Organ-sparing radiation therapy for head and neck cancer. Nat Rev Clin Oncol 2011;8(11):639–48.
51. Travis LB, Ng AK, Allan JM, et al. Second malignant neoplasms and cardiovascular disease following radiotherapy. J Natl Cancer Inst 2012;104(5):357–70.
52. Licitra L, Vermorken JB. Is there still a role for neoadjuvant chemotherapy in head and neck cancer? Ann Oncol 2004;15(1):7–11.
53. Holsinger FC, Sweeney AD, Jantharapattana K, et al. The emergence of endoscopic head and neck surgery. Curr Oncol Rep 2010;12(3):216–22.
54. Dowthwaite SA, Franklin JH, Palma DA, et al. The role of transoral robotic surgery in the management of oropharyngeal cancer: a review of the literature. ISRN Oncol 2012;2012:945162.
55. Hartl DM, Ferlito A, Silver CE, et al. Minimally invasive techniques for head and neck malignancies: current indications, outcomes and future directions. Eur Arch Otorhinolaryngol 2011;268(9):1249–57.
56. de Almeida JR, Genden EM. Robotic surgery for oropharynx cancer: promise, challenges, and future directions. Curr Oncol Rep 2012;14(2):148–57.
57. Bonner JA, Harari PM, Giralt J, et al. Radiotherapy plus cetuximab for locoregionally advanced head and neck cancer: 5-year survival data from a phase 3 randomised trial, and relation between cetuximab-induced rash and survival. Lancet Oncol 2010;11(1):21–8.
58. Fung C, Grandis JR. Emerging drugs to treat squamous cell carcinomas of the head and neck. Expert Opin Emerg Drugs 2010;15(3):355–73.
59. Brockstein BE, Vokes EE. Head and neck cancer in 2010: maximizing survival and minimizing toxicity. Nat Rev Clin Oncol 2011;8(2):72–4.
60. Eriksen JG, Lassen P, Overgaard J. Do all patients with head and neck cancer benefit from radiotherapy and concurrent cetuximab? Lancet Oncol 2010;11(4):312–3.
61. Vermorken J, Stöhlmacher K, Oliner K, et al. Safety and efficacy of panitumumab (pmab) in HPV positive (+) and HPV negative (−) recurrent/metastatic (R/M) Squamous cell carcinoma of the head and neck (SCCHN): analysis of the phase 3 SPECTRUM trial. Eur J Cancer 2011;47(Suppl 2):13.
62. Mroz EA, Rocco JW, Forastiere A. Reply to D.C. Gilbert et al. J Clin Oncol 2012;30(8):891–2.

63. Iglesias-Linares A, Yanez-Vico RM, Gonzalez-Moles MA. Potential role of HDAC inhibitors in cancer therapy: insights into oral squamous cell carcinoma. Oral Oncol 2010;46(5):323–9.
64. Rampias T, Sasaki C, Weinberger P, et al. E6 and e7 gene silencing and transformed phenotype of human papillomavirus 16-positive oropharyngeal cancer cells. J Natl Cancer Inst 2009;101(6):412–23.
65. Shahabi V, Maciag PC, Rivera S, et al. Live, attenuated strains of *Listeria* and *Salmonella* as vaccine vectors in cancer treatment. Bioeng Bugs 2010;1(4): 235–43.
66. Nichols AC, Finkelstein DM, Faquin WC, et al. Bcl2 and human papilloma virus 16 as predictors of outcome following concurrent chemoradiation for advanced oropharyngeal cancer. Clin Cancer Res 2010;16(7):2138–46.
67. Kumar B, Cordell KG, Lee JS, et al. EGFR, p16, HPV Titer, Bcl-xL and p53, sex, and smoking as indicators of response to therapy and survival in oropharyngeal cancer. J Clin Oncol 2008;26(19):3128–37.
68. Westra WH, Taube JM, Poeta ML, et al. Inverse relationship between human papillomavirus-16 infection and disruptive p53 gene mutations in squamous cell carcinoma of the head and neck. Clin Cancer Res 2008;14(2):366–9.
69. Langer CJ. Exploring biomarkers in head and neck cancer. Cancer 2012; 118(16):3882–92.

Oral Cavity and Oropharyngeal Squamous Cell Carcinoma Genomics

Marietta Tan, MD[a], Jeffrey N. Myers, MD, PhD[b],
Nishant Agrawal, MD[a,*]

KEYWORDS

• Oral cavity • Genomics • Oropharyngeal squamous cell carcinoma
• Head and neck squamous cell carcinoma

KEY POINTS

- The study of head and neck squamous cell carcinoma (HNSCC) tumor development and progression is complicated by the biologic complexity and heterogeneity of the disease.
- Recent technological advances now permit the study of the entire cancer genome, which can elucidate complex pathway interactions that are not apparent at the level of single genes.
- Next-generation sequencing technology allows for the detection of base substitutions, deletions, insertions, copy number variations, and chromosomal translocations of entire exomes or genomes.
- Two recent whole-exome sequencing studies reported frequent mutations in *TP53*, *NOTCH1*, *CDKN2A*, *PIK3CA*, and *HRAS* in HNSCC tumors.
- Standard or array-based comparative genomic hybridization can detect variations in chromosomal structure with greater resolution than traditional cytogenetic techniques.
- Methylation and gene expression arrays can be used for gene discovery or for the identification of tumor-specific profiles that may serve as biomarkers with diagnostic or prognostic value.

INTRODUCTION

Head and neck squamous cell carcinoma (HNSCC) results from the accumulation of multiple genetic and epigenetic changes in a variety of cellular pathways. The processes of genetic alteration and selection result in the clonal expansion of those cells

---

Disclosures: The authors have no financial disclosures to report.
[a] Department of Otolaryngology, Head and Neck Surgery, Johns Hopkins University School of Medicine, 601 North Caroline Street, Baltimore, MD 21287, USA; [b] Department of Head and Neck Surgery, The University of Texas MD Anderson Cancer Center, 1515 Holcombe Boulevard, Houston, TX 77030, USA
* Corresponding author. 601 North Caroline Street, 6th Floor, Baltimore, MD 21287.
E-mail address: nagrawal@jhmi.edu

Otolaryngol Clin N Am 46 (2013) 545–566
http://dx.doi.org/10.1016/j.otc.2013.04.001 oto.theclinics.com
0030-6665/13/$ – see front matter

Abbreviations	
BAC	Bacterial artificial chromosome
CDK	Cyclin-dependent kinases
CGH	Comparative genomic hybridization
EGF	Epidermal growth factor
EGFR	Epidermal growth factor receptor
FTI	Farnesyltransferase inhibitors
HNSCC	Head and neck squamous cell carcinoma
HPV	Human papillomavirus
MSRE	Methylation-specific restriction enzyme
NGS	Next-generation sequencing
NICD	NOTCH1 intracellular domain
Rb	Retinoblastoma
RLGS	Restriction landmark genomic scanning

with the most favorable genetic aberrations, resulting in tumor development and eventual progression to invasive carcinoma.[1,2]

The development and progression of cancer involves changes within multiple pathways with complex interactions.[3,4] The study of the molecular underpinnings of HNSCC is further complicated by the biologic complexity of the disease. HNSCC is now known to be heterogeneous at both the histopathologic and molecular levels.[5–7] The most prominent distinction is between human papillomavirus (HPV)-positive and HPV-negative tumors, but other subclasses also exist. Even within a single tumor, identification of the genes involved in carcinogenesis is hampered by tumor heterogeneity and by the interaction of tumor cells with the underlying stroma.

Cancer research has traditionally focused on the roles of individual genes in carcinogenesis. However, the study of single genes has several limitations. The process of single-gene investigation can be biased as well as labor and time intensive. Advances in technology, however, now allow for the study of the entire exome or genome. The study of the cancer genome elucidates pathways and other complex interactions that may not be apparent at the level of single genes. Whole exome/genome approaches permit the unbiased assessment of which genes and pathways have been altered. All known human genes may now be evaluated in large numbers of tumors, resulting in a more comprehensive understanding of the complex changes that occur in the formation and progression of cancer.[3]

In this review, the authors briefly describe the recent technological advances that have allowed for whole-exome/genome analysis of genetic and epigenetic alterations as well as changes in gene expression profiles. The authors also describe some of the genes that have been implicated in HNSCC using these techniques. Finally, the authors explore implications for therapy as well as future directions for the field.

GENETIC ALTERATIONS

Genetic alterations in cancer may occur in the form of small intragenic mutations, such as point mutations and insertions/deletions, or large alterations, including genomic deletions, amplifications, and chromosomal rearrangements. Whole cancer exomes/genomes can be evaluated for genetic aberrations using either next-generation sequencing (NGS) or comparative genomic hybridization (CGH) technologies.

NGS

NGS technology allows for massively parallel sequencing, producing data with greater speed and at a lower cost compared with more traditional methods. NGS instruments can process up to several million sequence reads in parallel, compared with the 96 reads produced by capillary-based instruments. In addition, template preparation, sequencing, and imaging steps for NGS platforms are highly automated and streamlined, requiring less time and additional equipment than high-throughput capillary-based sequencing systems.[8,9]

NGS has several other advantages over capillary-based methods, such as Sanger sequencing. Sanger sequencing has generally been limited to the analysis of either single genes or select hot-spot regions within the genome. In contrast, NGS allows the detection of base substitutions, deletions, insertions, copy number variations, and chromosomal translocations. NGS technologies have increased sequencing rates by several orders of magnitude and significantly reduced the cost per base, making it possible to sequence all known genes in multiple tumors of a given cancer type or in matched tumor and normal tissues.[8–10]

Sequencing of either whole exomes or genomes can be performed using NGS platforms. Protein-coding regions constitute only about 1% of the human genome but are thought to account for 85% of mutations resulting in disease.[11] Because it targets that part of the genome enriched for causative genes, whole-exome sequencing is efficient, affordable, and allows many more samples to be sequenced. In addition, because of the exome enrichment and higher base coverage, whole-exome platforms are currently more sensitive than whole-genome technologies for the detection of variants within coding regions.[12] However, whole-exome sequencing cannot identify variants in noncoding regions or genomic structural variations, whereas whole-genome sequencing can identify both. Although greater genomic coverage may be useful, whole-genome sequencing generates vast amounts of data of yet unknown functional and clinical significance.

Recently, 2 studies were published in which whole-exome sequencing was performed in a total of 106 primary HNSCC tumors with matched normal DNA. Mutations were confirmed in several genes, including in *TP53*, *CDKN2A*, *FAT1*, *PTEN*, *HRAS*, *PIK3CA*, and *EGFR*, that had been previously implicated in HNSCC. Both studies also identified mutations in *NOTCH1*, which had never previously been associated with HNSCC (**Fig. 1**).[7,13]

The authors briefly review the most commonly mutated genes in HNSCC, as identified in these two studies (**Table 1**).

Tumor suppressor genes

TP53 The NGS studies confirmed the well-established role of *TP53*, a tumor suppressor gene on chromosome 17p12, in HNSCC. Mutated in approximately half of all HNSCC tumors,[7,13–15] *TP53* is the most commonly mutated gene in HNSCC. Functional loss of p53 has been demonstrated in many human cancers and plays a critical role in malignant transformation.[16,17] In fact, in the carcinogenesis of HNSCC, mutations in *TP53* occur early. *TP53* mutations are present in dysplastic premalignant lesions of the oral cavity, and the prevalence of these mutations increases with histopathologic progression of the tumor from dysplasia to invasive carcinoma.[18,19]

Under normal circumstances, in response to DNA damage, p53 accumulates within the nucleus and causes cell cycle arrest via transcriptional induction of downstream effectors.[20,21] If DNA repair is unsuccessful, p53 triggers apoptosis or senescence.[21] However, cells harboring mutations in *TP53* will not undergo cell cycle arrest, apoptosis, or senescence. The p53-deficient cells can replicate in the presence of damaged DNA and accumulate additional genetic mutations, leading to unchecked cell division and tumor formation and progression.

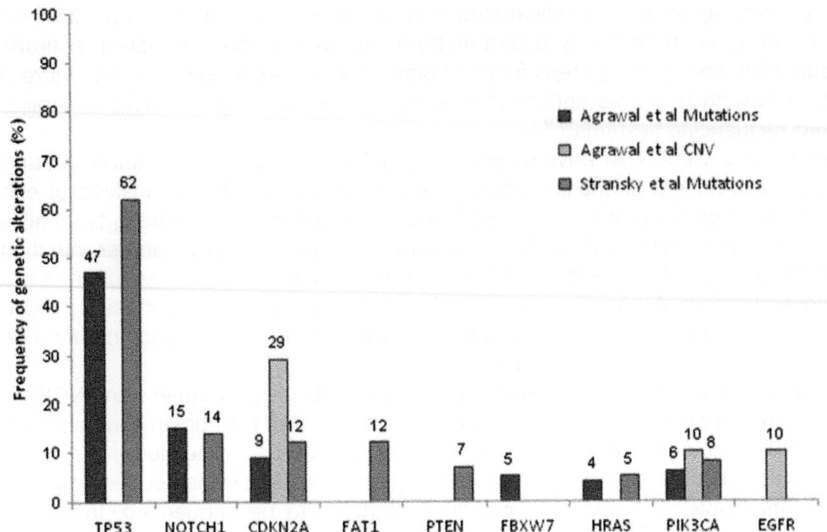

Fig. 1. Frequencies of genetic alterations identified by whole-exome sequencing and copy number analysis studies. CNV, copy number variation. (*Data from* Agrawal N, Frederick MJ, Pickering CR, et al. Exome sequencing of head and neck squamous cell carcinoma reveals inactivating mutations in NOTCH1. Science 2011:333;1154; and Stransky N, Egloff AM, Tward AD, et al. The mutational landscape of head and neck squamous cell carcinoma. Science 2011;333:1157.)

TP53 mutations in HNSCC have been associated with poor clinical outcomes as well as poor response to treatment. A large prospective multicenter trial including 420 patients found that mutations disruptive to the DNA-binding domain of p53 decreased overall survival by 1.7 times compared with patients without disruptive mutations.[14] Poor tumor response to radiation or chemotherapy has also been associated with mutations in *TP53*. Alterations of p53 by mutation, deletion, or other mechanisms of inactivation have been found in 95% of HNSCC tumors refractory to radiation.[22] The risks of locoregional recurrence and death after either primary or postoperative radiation therapy have both been found to be significantly greater for patients with mutations in *TP53*.[23–25] *TP53* mutations have also been associated with poor response to cisplatin and fluorouracil.[26] In a prospective study of 106 patients with HNSCC, *TP53* mutations were more frequent in patients who did not respond to cisplatin and fluorouracil than in patients who did respond. *TP53* mutation status was found to be an independent predictor of response to chemotherapy.[27]

NOTCH1 *NOTCH1* is the second most commonly mutated gene in HNSCC, with a mutation rate of 14% to 15%.[7,13] *NOTCH1* is important in regulating normal cell differentiation, lineage commitment, and embryonic development.[28] It seems to function as a tumor suppressor gene in HNSCC based on the position and characteristics of the mutations and the inactivation of both alleles.[7] *NOTCH1* is thought to act as a tumor suppressor gene in several other human cancers, including cutaneous squamous cell carcinoma (SCC),[29] lung SCC,[30] and chronic myelomonocytic leukemia,[31] although it seems to function as an oncogene in other leukemias.[32]

The NOTCH1 protein is a transmembrane ligand receptor with intracellular and extracellular domains. On ligand binding, the NOTCH1 intracellular domain (NICD) is cleaved and translocates to the nucleus. In the nucleus, the NICD activates transcription by binding to CBF1 in the presence of coactivators from the Mastermindlike family. Downstream target genes of NOTCH1 signaling are crucial for cell differentiation and normal embryonic development.[28]

Activating and loss-of-function mutations preferentially occur in different regions of the *NOTCH1* gene (**Fig. 2**). Most *NOTCH1* mutations observed in HNSCC affect the epidermal growth factor (EGF)-like ligand-binding domain and are thought to lead to loss of function.[7] Inactivating mutations in these regions of the gene have also been reported in skin and lung SCC.[30] In contrast, mutations of the intracellular proline, glutamic acid, serine/threonine-rich motifs regulatory domain or the extracellular heterodimer domain are thought to result in constitutive activation of NOTCH1 signaling.[33]

Mutations in the gene *FBXW7* have also been identified in 5% of HNSCC specimens.[7] FBXW7 is a member of the F-box protein family and is a component of the ubiquitin ligase complex that can mediate NOTCH1 degradation. *FBXW7* mutations could, therefore, also affect the *NOTCH1* pathway, although FBXW7 is also known to target other oncogenic pathways, such as cyclin E and c-myc.[33]

Cyclin-dependent kinase inhibitor 2A (CDKN2A) Alterations of *CDKN2A*/p16^{INK4A}, a tumor suppressor gene located on chromosome 9p21, have long been recognized in HNSCC.[34,35] In the NGS studies, *CDKN2A* mutations were identified in 9% to 12% of all tumors.[7,13] Gene copy number analyses also revealed frequent loss of heterozygosity and deletions of *CDKN2A*.[7] In addition to deletions and point mutations, *CDKN2A* is also inactivated by methylation of the 5′ CpG region.[36]

The protein product of *CDKN2A*, p16, plays a critical role in cell cycle regulation via its interaction with the retinoblastoma (Rb) tumor suppressor. The p16 protein inhibits cyclin-dependent kinases (CDK) 4 and 6, which are in turn necessary for the phosphorylation of Rb. Hypophosphorylated Rb induces G1 arrest of the cell cycle.[37–39]

Alterations of *CDKN2A*, although they are common events in early HNSCC development, alone are likely insufficient to drive tumorigenesis. This point is supported by the fact that *CDKN2A* mutations have been reported in benign epithelial lesions with low potential for malignant transformation.[40]

FAT1 *FAT1* is a tumor suppressor gene in the cadherin family of integral membrane proteins and is involved in cell adhesion, migration, and invasion.[41] It was found to have a 12% incidence of mutation.[13] In previous studies, homozygous deletions in *FAT1* were identified in most oral SCCs.[42]

PTEN *PTEN* is a negative regulator of PI3K, and its loss results in activation of the PI3K/Akt pathway, which is discussed later. Inactivating mutations were found in *PTEN* in 7% of tumors,[13] consistent with previous reports of mutation rates as high as 10%.[43]

Oncogenes

HRAS The true incidence of *Ras* mutations in HNSCC has been unclear. The reported frequency of mutations in the *Ras* family gene *HRAS* in HNSCC has varied from 0% in Western populations to as high as 35% in Indian populations.[44–46] It is thought that these differences in mutation frequencies are related to the use of tobacco chewing and betel quid habits in Indian and other Asian countries, although it may also reflect underlying genetic variations between ethnic groups.[47] Both of the NGS projects confirmed the presence of *HRAS* mutations in HNSCC, with a frequency of 4% to 5%.[7,13]

Ras proteins are GTPases that function as signaling switches by alternating between the guanosine triphosphate–bound active state and the guanosine diphosphate–bound

Table 1
Frequently altered genes in HNSCC

Gene Symbol	Gene Name	Chromosomal Location	Gene Function	Mutation Rate	Copy Number Variation	References
Tumor Suppressor Genes						
TP53	Tumor protein p53	17p13.1	Tumor suppressor that assists in cell cycle arrest, DNA damage repair, apoptosis, and senescence.	40%–62%	N/A	7,13–27
NOTCH1	Notch1	9p34.3	Tumor suppressor or oncogene (tissue dependent) that is important in regulation of cell differentiation, lineage commitment, and embryonic development.	14%–15%	N/A	7,13,28–33
CDKN2A	Cyclin-dependent kinase inhibitor 2A	9p21.3	Tumor suppressor that is important in cell cycle regulation.	9%–12%	29%	7,13,34–40
FAT1	FAT tumor suppressor homolog 1 (*Drosophila*)	4q35.2	Tumor suppressor that is a member of cadherin family and involved in cell adhesion, migration, and invasion.	12%–80%	N/A	13,41,42
PTEN	Phosphatase and tensin homolog	10q23.3	Tumor suppressor that is a negative regulator of PI3K.	7%–10%	N/A	13,43

FBXW7	F-box and WD repeat domain-containing protein 7	4q31.3	Tumor suppressor that is a member of the F-box protein family and component of the ubiquitin ligase complex that can mediate NOTCH1, cyclin E and c-myc degradation.	5%	N/A	[7,33]
Oncogenes						
HRAS	Harvey rat sarcoma viral oncogene homolog	11p15.5	Oncogene; GTPase that is important in promoting cell proliferation, differentiation, and survival through downstream effector pathways.	4%–35%	N/A	[7,13,44–50]
PIK3CA	Phosphoinositide-3-kinase catalytic alpha polypeptide	3q26.32	Oncogene that is a catalytic subunit of PI3K, a target of Ras activation, and promotes cell growth, survival, and cytoskeleton reorganization.	6%–8%	10%	[7,13,51,52]
EGFR	Epidermal growth factor receptor	7p12	Oncogene that is a receptor tyrosine kinase in the ErbB family and involved in cell proliferation, apoptosis, invasion, angiogenesis, and metastasis.	N/A	10%	[7,53–57]

Abbreviation: N/A, not applicable.

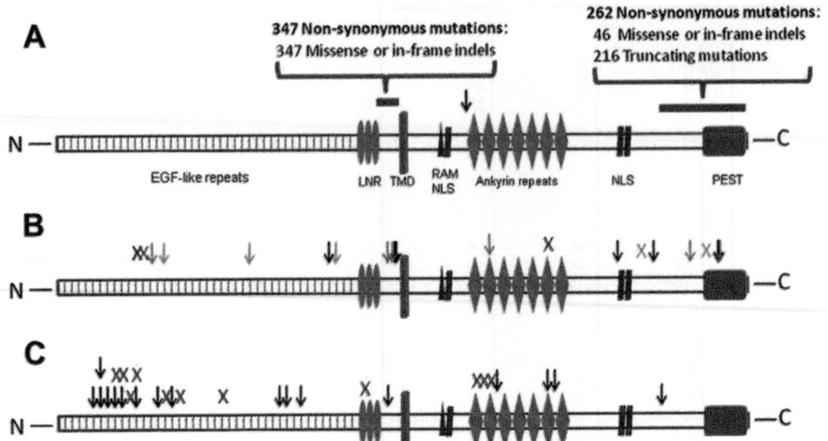

Fig. 2. Mutations in *NOTCH1* noted in Agrawal and colleagues.[7] (*A*) Previously observed *NOTCH1* mutations in hematopoietic malignancies. Red bars represent previously described mutation hot spots (amino acids 1575 to 1630 and 2250–2550). (*B*) Previously observed *NOTCH1* mutations in solid tumors. Colored arrow (missense mutation) and *X* (truncating mutation) depict mutations found in different tumor types: Pink, breast cancer; black, glioma; blue, lung cancer; green, pancreatic adenocarcinoma; red, esophageal squamous cell carcinoma; purple, tongue squamous cell carcinoma. (*C*) Mutations in *NOTCH1* in HNSCC observed in this study. Black arrow indicates missense mutation, and red *X* indicates truncating mutation. EGF, epidermal growth factor; LNR, Lin12-Notch repeats; NLS, nuclear localization signal; PEST, proline, glutamic acid, serine/threonine-rich motifs; RAM, recombination signal-binding protein 1 for J-k association module; TMD, transmembrane domain. (*From* Agrawal N, Frederick MJ, Pickering CR, et al. Exome sequencing of head and neck squamous cell carcinoma reveals inactivating mutations in NOTCH1. Science 2011:333;1154; with permission.)

inactive state.[48] Ras downstream effector pathways include Raf. Activated Raf phosphorylates MEK, which in turn activates ERK. The Raf/MEK/ERK pathway is involved in the regulation of cell proliferation, differentiation, and survival.[49,50]

PIK3CA Mutations were identified in the oncogene *PIK3CA* in 6% to 8% of tumors.[7,13] Previous studies have found rates of *PIK3CA* mutation as high as 20%.[51] *PIK3CA*, which encodes the catalytic subunit p110alpha of the PI3K heterodimer, activates the AKT/mTOR pathway and promotes cell growth, cell survival, transformation, and drug resistance.[52]

EGF receptor The EGF receptor (EGFR) is a receptor tyrosine kinase that belongs to the ErbB family of cell surface receptors and is involved in cellular proliferation, apoptosis, invasion, angiogenesis, and metastasis via the MAPK, AKT, ERK and JAK/STAT pathways.[53–55] Focal amplification of 7p, which contains the *EGFR* gene, was found in approximately 10% of samples by copy number analysis.[7] Dysfunction of the EGFR pathway has been described in 80% to 90% of HNSCC, with overexpression of EGFR being the most common cause of dysregulation.[54,56,57]

Comparative Genomic Hybridization

Variations in chromosomal structure, including inversions, deletions, translocations, or gains or losses of entire chromosomal segments, are common in the development and progression of HNSCC.[58] Resultant DNA copy number alterations may change gene expression and function, resulting in tumor development.

The most commonly described chromosomal aberrations in HNSCC include the following[4,7,59–62]:

- Gains in 1q, 3q, 5p, 7p, 8q, 9q, 11q, 14q, and 18p
- Losses in 3p, 4p, 4q, 5q, 8p, 9p, 10p, 11q, 13q, 17p, 18q, and 21q

Many of these genomic gains and losses were originally detected using loss of heterozygosity analysis or traditional cytogenetic techniques, such as karyotype analysis. However, karyotype analysis is technically challenging to perform in solid tumors and, furthermore, does not allow detection of submicroscopic losses or rearrangements.[63]

CGH permits the efficient analysis of the entire genome for DNA copy number variation

However, the minimum size of a detectable segment in standard CGH is 3 to 5 Mb,[64] which limits the detection of smaller alterations and makes identification of specific candidate genes difficult. More recently, microarray-based assays, or array CGH, have been developed to overcome the pitfalls of karyotype and standard CGH-based analyses. Array CGH, which uses bacterial artificial chromosome (BAC) arrays, allows for the high-throughput analysis of DNA copy number variations throughout the whole genome and allows high-resolution mapping of these changes directly onto genomic sequence.[2,59] The resolution of array CGH platforms continues to improve to submegabase levels, so that variations ranging from gene-size aberrations to entire chromosomal arms may now be detected.[65] Of note, whole-genome analysis of copy number variation can also be assessed using newer single-nucleotide polymorphism array platforms, which have the additional advantage of being able to detect the loss of heterozygosity.[66] However, to date, most whole-genome studies of copy number variation in HNSCC have used BAC-based array CGH (**Table 2**).

Array CGH has been used in several studies to identify candidate pathways and genes in HNSCC tumorigenesis

Sparano and colleagues[67] identified 22 amplified and 17 deleted genes in at least 25% of oral SCC. Snijders and colleagues[68] used array CGH to identify several common regions of chromosomal amplification containing genes involved in integrin signaling, adhesion, migration, and survival pathways in oral SCC. They also found dysregulation of the Hedgehog and Notch pathways. In another study, array CGH was used to identify a novel gene possibly involved in oral SCC tumorigenesis. Two neighboring regions on chromosome 8q were found to be amplified, one of which harbored a novel putative oncogene, *LRP12*. Overexpression of *LRP12*, but not of two flanking genes, was then confirmed using reverse transcription–polymerase chain reaction (RT-PCR).[69]

Array CGH has been used to attempt to delineate differences in the molecular and clinical characteristics of tumors

Smeets and colleagues[70] used array CGH to compare HPV-positive and HPV-negative tumors. The two subsets of tumors were found to harbor different genomic gains and losses, although both tumor types shared some genetic changes. This finding provides evidence of differences in the genetic alterations observed in HPV-positive compared with HPV-negative tumors.

Associations between clinical outcomes and specific structural variations have also been identified. A study using standard CGH in HNSCC identified significant associations between a gain of 3q25 to 3q27 and a loss of 22q with reduced disease-specific

Table 2
Selected studies using standard or array comparative genomic hybridization in HNSCC

Author, Year	Methodology	Cohort	Findings
Snijders et al,[68] 2005	In-house HumArray2.0 (UCSF)	89 oral SCC	Identified 9 recurrent amplified regions <3 Mb, which contained genes involved in integrin signaling, adhesion, migration, survival, Hedgehog, and Notch pathways, which were amplified and overexpressed.
Garnis et al,[69] 2004	In-house BAC array	22 oral SCC	Identified 5.3 Mb region of common amplification at 8q22 containing 16 known genes. Gene expression analysis revealed overexpression of LRP12, a novel putative oncogene.
Smeets et al,[70] 2006	In-house BAC array	12 oral SCC, 12 oropharynx SCC	Compared HPV-positive and HPV-negative tumors. Four regions of gains or losses were unique to HPV-negative tumors. Seven regions of gains or losses were altered at high frequency in both tumor subsets.
Ashman et al,[71] 2003	Standard CGH	10 oral or oropharynx SCC, 35 other HNSCC	Gain of 3q25–q27 and loss of 22q were associated with reduced disease-specific survival. Gains of 17q and 20q, loss of 19p and 22q, and amplification of 11q13 were associated with reduced disease-free survival.
Ambatipudi et al,[72] 2011	Human Genome CGH Microarray 105K (Agilent)	60 oral SCC	Gain of 11q22.1–q22.2 and losses of 17p13.3 and 11q23–q25 were associated with earlier loco-regional recurrence and shorter overall survival.
Uchida et al,[73] 2011	MacArray Karyo 4K (Macrogen)	50 oral SCC	Loss of a 0.2 Mb region at 3p26.3 was associated with reduced disease-specific survival.
Sugahara et al,[74] 2011	Human Genome CGH Microarray 44 K (Agilent)	54 oral SCC (22 with cervical LN metastasis, 32 without cervical LN metastasis)	Compared tumors that had or had not metastasized to the cervical lymph nodes. Two distinct regions of amplification at 11q13 were associated with cervical metastasis.
van den Broek et al,[76] 2007	Standard CGH	34 oral or oropharynx SCC, 6 other HNSCC	Compared chemoradiotherapy-sensitive and resistant tumors. Gains of 3q11-q13, 3q21-q26.1, and 6q22-q27 and losses of 3p11-pter and 4p11-pter were associated with chemoradiotherapy resistance.

Abbreviations: BAC, bacterial artificial chromosome; LN, lymph node; Mb, megabase.

survival and a gain of 17q and 20q and a deletion of 19p and 22q with reduced disease-free survival.[71] A more recent study conducted array CGH in advanced-stage oral SCC and found that a gain of region 11q22.1-q22.2 and losses of 17p13.3 and 11q23-q25 were significantly associated with earlier locoregional recurrence and shorter overall survival.[72] Uchida and colleagues[73] found that a loss of 3p26.3 was significantly associated with poorer disease-specific survival. Another study demonstrated an association between amplification at 2 distinct regions of 11q13 and metastases to the cervical lymph nodes.[74]

CGH has also been used to predict differences in response to treatment

Although such studies have not yet been performed using array-based approaches. Akervall and colleagues[75] demonstrated that cisplatin-resistant cell lines had higher rates of chromosomal gains and losses compared with cisplatin-sensitive cell lines. Another study used standard CGH to compare chemoradiotherapy-resistant primary HNSCC tumors with sensitive tumors. Both groups had similar total numbers of genetic changes, but high-level DNA amplifications were more frequent in the resistant tumors. Several specific chromosomal gains and losses were significantly associated with resistance to treatment. Such genomic profiles may be useful as predictors of resistance to chemoradiotherapy.[76]

EPIGENETIC ALTERATIONS

Epigenetic regulation of gene expression occurs through several mechanisms, including DNA methylation, histone modification, and RNA interference by microRNA and small interfering RNA. Promoter methylation in particular is thought to play a role in the carcinogenesis of many human cancers.[77] Regions rich in cytosine-guanine dinucleotides, known as CpG islands, exist throughout the genome, typically within or upstream of promoter regions. CpG islands are found in up to half of all human genes.[78] Methylation occurs at the 5′ carbon of the cytosine ring, which results in the recruitment of methyl-CpG binding domain proteins and histone deacetylases that inhibit binding of RNA polymerase. Gene expression is, thereby, silenced, even if the DNA coding sequence remains unchanged.[79]

Epigenetic regulation of several genes, such as *CDKN2A*, *CDH1*, *MGMT*, and *DAPK1*, has been demonstrated in HNSCC.[78,80] However, most studies to date in HNSCC have analyzed the methylation status of individual genes previously implicated in carcinogenesis. Several techniques have been used to evaluate genome-wide methylation, including restriction landmark genomic scanning (RLGS), methylation-specific restriction enzyme (MSRE) analysis, and arbitrarily primed PCR.[59,78]

The first genome-wide analysis of promoter methylation in HNSCC used RLGS, which uses gel electrophoresis to determine methylation status (**Table 3**). This study analyzed 1300 CpG islands in 13 matched primary and metastatic HNSCC tumors. Global hypermethylation was found in the metastatic tumors compared with primary tumors.[81] Adrien and colleagues[82] performed the first study using array-based technology. MSRE analysis was used to assess more than 12 000 CpG sites in 37 HNSCC tumors. Unsupervised hierarchical clustering yielded 3 distinct DNA methylation profiles among the tumors, although no correlations between methylation profiles and tumor or patient characteristics were identified.

Several methylation microarray platforms are now commercially available. Such technologies permit the rapid assessment of global methylation and the identification of specific epigenetically regulated genes. One study identified a candidate gene family that may be involved in carcinogenesis by querying more than 27,000 CpG sites in 24 oropharyngeal tumors and matched normal tissues. They identified 958 loci that

Table 3
Selected studies of genome-wide methylation status in HNSCC

Author, Year	Methodology	Numbers of CpG Sites, Genes Analyzed	Cohort	Findings
Smiraglia et al,[81] 2003	RLGS	1293, N/A	13 matched primary tumor and cervical LN metastasis (12 oral or oropharynx SCC, 1 other HNSCC)	Found global hypermethylation in metastatic LNs compared with primary tumors. However, different loci were methylated in LNs compared with primary tumors.
Adrien et al,[82] 2006	MRSE analysis	12,288, N/A	6 oral SCC, 17 oropharynx SCC, 13 other HNSCC	Identified 3 distinct methylation profiles. No associations found between methylation profile and tumor or patient characteristics.
Lleras et al,[83] 2011	Infinium HumanMethylation27 BeadChip (Illumina Inc, San Diego, CA)	27,578, 14,495	24 oropharynx SCC, 24 matched normal mucosa	Identified 958 loci that were differentially methylated between tumors and normal tissue. Many of these loci on chromosome 19 were associated with Kruppel-type zinc finger protein genes. Gene expression analysis verified decreased expression of these genes.
Langevin et al,[84] 2012	Infinium HumanMethylation27 BeadChip (Illumina Inc, San Diego, CA)	27,578, 14,495	39 oral SCC, 35 oropharynx SCC, 18 other HNSCC, 92 cancer-free controls	Evaluated DNA from peripheral blood. Identified a methylation profile of 6 CpG loci that differentiated between patients with HNSCC and controls.
Poage et al,[85] 2012	Infinium HumanMethylation27 BeadChip (Illumina Inc, San Diego, CA)	27,578, 14,495	46 oral SCC, 15 oropharynx SCC, 15 other HNSCC	Hypermethylation at 2 specific CpG sites, associated with the genes *TAP1* and *ALDH3A1*, was associated with decreased overall survival.

Abbreviations: LN, lymph node; MSRE, methylation-specific restriction enzyme; N/A, not available; RLGS, restriction landmark genomic scanning.

were differentially methylated between tumors and normal tissues. Several of these loci were located on chromosome 19 and were associated with Kruppel-type zinc finger protein genes. Further analysis of these genes with quantitative RT-PCR confirmed decreased gene expression, although the clinical relevance of these changes in gene expression was not assessed.[83]

Methylation arrays have also been used to generate methylation profiles that may be used as biomarkers for disease or prognosis. One study identified a methylation profile of 6 CpG loci that differentiated patients with HNSCC from those without cancer.[84] Poage and colleagues[85] found that promoter hypermethylation at 2 specific CpG sites, associated with the genes *TAP1* and *ALDH3A1*, was significantly correlated with decreased overall survival. This study not only identified 2 genes for possible therapeutic intervention but also delineated a methylation profile that may serve as a biomarker of more aggressive disease. Therefore, methylation profiles using DNA obtained from minimally invasive methods may eventually be used in the clinical setting for diagnostic and screening purposes.

ALTERED GENE EXPRESSION PROFILES

Although sometimes used for gene discovery, gene expression arrays are most commonly used to establish expression profiles to serve as biomarkers that may distinguish tumors from normal or premalignant samples, identify subgroups of tumors, or predict clinical behavior.[3,4,59]

Several studies have identified gene expression profiles that differ between normal mucosa, premalignant lesions, and invasive carcinoma (**Table 4**). Data demonstrate that premalignant and malignant lesions cluster together, apart from normal mucosa, supporting the notion that altered patterns of gene expression most often occur before the development of malignancy.[86,87] Multiple groups have established specific gene panels that may be used to distinguish normal tissues from malignant lesions. For example, one study established a signature of 25 genes that can differentiate between oral SCC tumors and normal specimens. This signature achieved 96% predictive accuracy on a cross-validation study and an average of 87% accuracy on 3 independent validation sets.[88] Other studies in oral SCC have defined gene sets to distinguish oral leukoplakia from invasive carcinoma. Kondoh and colleagues[89] identified 11 genes that distinguished oral SCC from leukoplakia with greater than 97% accuracy. Another group identified a panel of 9 genes that differentiated normal mucosa, oral leukoplakia, and invasive carcinoma.[62] The results of each of these studies differ, likely because of differences in patient selection, tumor heterogeneity, and the use of different microarray platforms. However, their findings demonstrate the possibility that expression profiles may eventually be used as biomarkers in the clinical setting to assist in diagnosis or disease monitoring.

Data from expression arrays have also been used to classify tumors based on their molecular characteristics. For example, Chung and colleagues[6] identified four subtypes of HNSCC, each with a distinct gene expression pattern and different recurrence-free survival rates. Several groups have also identified differences in gene expression between HPV-positive and HPV-negative tumors. One study found differential expression of 347 genes in HPV-positive compared with HPV-negative tumors. Of note, some of the differentially expressed genes, including *CCND1* and *TYMS*, play roles in sensitivity to cisplatin and fluorouracil, whereas another gene, *RBBP4*, plays a role in sensitivity to radiation.[90] The results of these studies may, therefore, elucidate some of the molecular mechanisms of HPV-related tumorigenesis and response to therapy and may help guide therapeutic decision making.

Table 4
Selected studies using gene expression arrays in HNSCC

Author, Year	Array Platform	Number of Genes Analyzed	Cohort	Findings
Ziober et al,[88] 2006	Affymetrix U133A (Affymetrix Inc, Santa Clara, CA)	14,500	13 oral SCC, 13 matched normal mucosa	Identified a panel of 25 genes that differentiated between oral SCC and controls with 96% predictive accuracy on cross-validation and an average of 87% accuracy on 3 independent validation sets
Kondoh et al,[89] 2007	IntelliGene HS Human Expression CHIP (TaKaRa, Japan)	16,600	5 oral SCC, 5 leukoplakia	Identified a panel of 11 genes that differentiated oral SCC from leukoplakia with >97% accuracy
Liu et al,[62] 2011	Oligo GEArray Human Cancer Microarray (SuperArray, Frederick, MD)	440	3 oral SCC, 3 leukoplakia, 3 normal mucosa	Identified a panel of 9 genes that differentiated between normal mucosa, oral leukoplakia, and invasive carcinoma
Lohavanichbutr et al,[90] 2009	GeneChip Human Genome U133 Plus 2.0 (Affymetrix Inc, Santa Clara, CA)	39,000	88 oral SCC, 31 oropharynx SCC, 35 normal mucosa	Compared HPV-positive and HPV-negative tumors. Found differential expression of 347 genes, including *CCND1*, *TYMS*, and *RBBP4*, which play roles in sensitivity to chemotherapy and radiation
Nguyen et al,[91] 2007	GeneChip Human Genome U133 Plus 2.0 (Affymetrix Inc, Santa Clara, CA)	39,000	30 oral SCC (13 with cervical LN metastasis, 17 without cervical LN metastasis)	Compared primary tumors that had or had not metastasized to the cervical LNs. Identified a panel of 8 genes that could predict LN metastasis with 92.3% accuracy
Roepman et al,[92] 2005	Human Array-Ready Oligo set (Qiagen, Valencia, CA)	21,329	82 oral or oropharynx SCC (45 with cervical LN metastasis, 37 without cervical LN metastasis)	Compared primary tumors that had or had not metastasized to the cervical LNs Identified a panel of 102 genes that could predict LN metastasis with 86% accuracy
Zhou et al,[93] 2006	GeneChip Human Genome U133 Plus 2.0 (Affymetrix Inc, Santa Clara, CA)	39,000	25 oral tongue SCC (11 with cervical LN metastasis, 14 without cervical LN metastasis)	Compared primary tumors that had or had not metastasized to the cervical LNs. Also compared tumors that did or did not have extracapsular spread. Identified 2 panels of 3 genes each that could predict nodal metastasis or extracapsular spread with 100% sensitivity and specificity
Dumur et al,[94] 2009	GeneChip Human Genome U133 Plus 2.0 (Affymetrix Inc, Santa Clara, CA)	39,000	8 oral or oropharynx SCC, 6 other HNSCC	Compared tumors that were sensitive or resistant to radiation Identified a panel of 142 genes that could predict treatment response with >93% accuracy

Several studies have identified specific gene expression profiles that may predict disease progression and clinical outcomes. Two studies analyzed the gene expression profiles of primary tumors that had or had not metastasized to the cervical lymph nodes. The first study identified a panel of 8 genes with predictive accuracy of 92.3%,[91] and the second identified a panel of 102 genes with 86.0% accuracy.[92] Another study looked specifically at primary oral tongue SCC tumors in patients with cervical lymph node metastases, extracapsular spread, or both. They identified distinct gene panels of 3 genes each that could predict either nodal metastasis or extracapsular spread with 100% sensitivity and specificity by analysis of the primary tumor.[93]

Attempts have also been made to define expression profiles that can predict the response to chemotherapy or radiation. A small prospective study of 14 patients with HNSCC found differential expression in 142 genes between tumors that were responsive or resistant to radiation therapy with or without chemotherapy. The gene panel showed greater than 93% accuracy for the prediction of treatment response.[94]

IMPLICATIONS FOR THERAPY

The biologic complexity of HNSCC has become even more apparent with advances in our understanding of cancer genomics. The disease represents a heterogeneous collection of tumors in which multiple genes and pathways are altered. As evident in this review, aberrations may occur via a combination of genetic and epigenetic mechanisms affecting any number of genes and pathways. More sophisticated analyses of the pathways implicated in HNSCC tumorigenesis are, therefore, critical in the development of new targeted therapies and individualized medicine.

Knowledge gleaned from recent genomic studies offers new promise for the treatment of HNSCC. In particular, several therapies are currently being evaluated that target some of the genes mutated by whole-exome sequencing.[7,13]

Gene therapies aimed at restoring wild-type *TP53* have shown promise in the treatment of patients with HNSCC. Wild-type *TP53* is incorporated into adenoviral vectors and injected into the tumor, resulting in expression of normal p53 protein within tumors.[95,96] ONYX-015, another adenoviral-based therapy that has oncolytic effects specifically in cells lacking functional p53, has recently been approved for use in China.[96]

Targeting *NOTCH1* for therapeutic intervention is complicated by the fact that the gene may have either tumor suppressor or oncogenic functions depending on the cellular context. Several gamma-secretase inhibitors (GSI) block proteolytic activation of NOTCH1.[32,97] GSIs are currently being evaluated in human trials for the treatment of T-cell acute lymphoblastic leukemia and breast cancers.[98,99] However, successful inhibition of *NOTCH1* oncogenic activity at one site may result in the loss of its tumor suppressor function at another site. A phase III trial of GSIs for the treatment of Alzheimer disease was recently halted because of an elevated incidence of skin cancer in treated patients, possibly through adverse effects on squamous epithelial differentiation.[100] Further investigation into the functions of *NOTCH1* in different cell types is, therefore, necessary for the development of new targeted treatments.

Several therapies targeted against *HRAS* have been studied. Farnesyltransferase inhibitors (FTI) prevent localization of Ras proteins to the cell membrane, thereby preventing signal transduction. FTIs have shown some antitumor effect in early clinical trials in several cancers, including multiple myeloma, lung cancer, and some leukemias.[101] In addition, the use of antisense oligonucleotides directed against *HRAS* mRNA has been studied in solid tumors.[102,103] However, a phase II clinical trial in pancreatic adenocarcinoma showed no additional benefit of the antisense compound beyond standard therapy.[104] Overall, strategies to inhibit Ras signaling have shown limited efficacy in clinical trials, possibly because of secondary alterations in upstream and downstream Ras pathway effectors.[105]

Therapies directed against *PI3KCA* and its downstream effectors have also been investigated. The addition of PI3K pathway inhibitors to standard therapy is being studied as an approach to overcoming resistance to conventional chemoradiotherapy. The PI3K inhibitor PX-866 is now in phase I and II trials in individual combinations with docetaxel or cetuximab for the treatment of HNSCC.[106,107] PI3K has many downstream effectors, including Akt and mTOR, which may be targeted. The mTOR inhibitor rapamycin, an immunosuppressant approved by the Food and Drug Administration, is in phase I trials for patients with treatment-naïve advanced HNSCC,[108] whereas an Akt inhibitor, MK2206, is currently in phase II trials for treatment of recurrent and metastatic HNSCC.[109]

Lastly, therapeutic targeting of *CDKN2A* is limited by the challenge of restoring tumor suppressor activity. Therefore, strategies are instead aimed at inhibiting downstream targets that have been rendered overactive, such as CDKs. The results of phase II and III clinical trials of several first-generation CDK inhibitors have been disappointing, but several second-generation CDK inhibitors, which are thought to be more potent, are in advanced preclinical or clinical trials.[110]

The authors have reviewed several genomic signatures, at the levels of DNA sequence, methylation, and gene expression, which may serve as potential biomarkers in HNSCC. Specific tumor profiles may be used in the clinical setting for confirming diagnoses, predicting prognosis, tracking recurrence, or monitoring therapeutic response. Detection of these biomarkers in readily available sources like saliva or peripheral blood may be of particular value for early detection or disease surveillance.

FUTURE GOALS FOR GENOMICS STUDIES

The advent of genomic technologies discussed in this review has resulted in the rapid generation of knowledge in our understanding of HNSCC. Genome-wide studies have identified aberrant genes and pathways that may play an active role in tumorigenesis as well as potential biomarkers that may serve as indicators of disease state. However, these studies have thus far been largely descriptive, and much remains unknown about the specific molecular mechanisms underlying tumor formation and progression. Furthermore, because of the discrepancies between studies in tumor characteristics and treatments, it is difficult to draw consistent, wide-ranging conclusions. The quality of available clinical data is also widely variable. More standardized, prospective collection of specimens and of clinical data is necessary to identify associations between specific genetic alterations and prognosis or other clinical outcomes.

Other genomic tools include next-generation sequencing of the whole genome and RNA (RNA-seq). As noted earlier, NGS detects base substitutions, insertion/deletions, and chromosomal inversions or translocations. NGS can, therefore, be used to identify chromosomal variations with very high resolution and is a useful adjunct to conventional or array CGH. RNA-seq will permit direct analysis of the complete transcriptome and will greatly increase the resolution of gene expression data beyond the limits of available expression microarrays. Data obtained from RNA-seq can also be integrated with data from other platforms to give insight into gene expression in the context of known mutations, DNA copy number alterations, or other genomic aberrations. RNA-seq can also be used to detect alternative splicing isoforms and fusion transcripts.[9]

Genomic tools offer insight into the many genetic and epigenetic changes occurring in a single tumor. Emphasis will increasingly be placed on integrated pathway analysis, resulting in a better understanding of the complex interactions that occur within tumor cells. In addition, the integration of multiple platforms, such as gene expression profiling, methylation arrays, or array CGH experiments, will allow us to answer increasingly sophisticated questions regarding the molecular underpinnings of HNSCC.

Ultimately, the goals of these investigations are to provide new tools to be used for diagnosis or disease monitoring and to uncover new targets for therapeutic intervention. Further research may help to ultimately realize the possibilities of targeted therapies and personalized medicine.

SUMMARY

The advent of genomic technologies has greatly advanced our knowledge of the molecular changes underlying HNSCC. Technologies including next-generation sequencing and array-based platforms have provided us with new insight into the genes and pathways that may be altered in this disease. These innovations offer new targets for therapeutic intervention and new options for diagnosis and surveillance of the disease. However, as underscored by the findings outlined in this review, HNSCC is a complex and heterogeneous disease that we are only beginning to understand. It is hoped that genomic approaches will continue to support the development of diagnostic or prognostic indicators and targeted therapies for our patients.

REFERENCES

1. Califano J, Westra WH, Meininger G, et al. Genetic progression and clonal relationship of recurrent premalignant head and neck lesions. Clin Cancer Res 2000;6:347.
2. Pinkel D, Albertson DG. Array comparative genomic hybridization and its applications in cancer. Nat Genet 2005;37(Suppl):S11.
3. Weber BL. Cancer genomics. Cancer Cell 2002;1:37.
4. Ha PK, Chang SS, Glazer CA, et al. Molecular techniques and genetic alterations in head and neck cancer. Oral Oncol 2009;45:335.
5. Leemans CR, Braakhuis BJ, Brakenhoff RH. The molecular biology of head and neck cancer. Nat Rev Cancer 2011;11:9.
6. Chung CH, Parker JS, Karaca G, et al. Molecular classification of head and neck squamous cell carcinomas using patterns of gene expression. Cancer Cell 2004;5:489.
7. Agrawal N, Frederick MJ, Pickering CR, et al. Exome sequencing of head and neck squamous cell carcinoma reveals inactivating mutations in NOTCH1. Science 2011;333:1154.
8. Mardis ER. Next-generation DNA sequencing methods. Annu Rev Genomics Hum Genet 2008;9:387.
9. Mardis ER, Wilson RK. Cancer genome sequencing: a review. Hum Mol Genet 2009;18:R163.
10. Ross JS, Cronin M. Whole cancer genome sequencing by next-generation methods. Am J Clin Pathol 2011;136:527.
11. Choi M, Scholl UI, Ji W, et al. Genetic diagnosis by whole exome capture and massively parallel DNA sequencing. Proc Natl Acad Sci U S A 2009;106:19096.
12. Clark MJ, Chen R, Lam HY, et al. Performance comparison of exome DNA sequencing technologies. Nat Biotechnol 2011;29:908.

13. Stransky N, Egloff AM, Tward AD, et al. The mutational landscape of head and neck squamous cell carcinoma. Science 2011;333:1157.
14. Poeta ML, Manola J, Goldwasser MA, et al. TP53 mutations and survival in squamous-cell carcinoma of the head and neck. N Engl J Med 2007;357:2552.
15. Brennan JA, Boyle JO, Koch WM, et al. Association between cigarette smoking and mutation of the p53 gene in squamous-cell carcinoma of the head and neck. N Engl J Med 1995;332:712.
16. Hollstein M, Sidransky D, Vogelstein B, et al. p53 mutations in human cancers. Science 1991;253:49.
17. Nigro JM, Baker SJ, Preisinger AC, et al. Mutations in the p53 gene occur in diverse human tumour types. Nature 1989;342:705.
18. Boyle JO, Hakim J, Koch W, et al. The incidence of p53 mutations increases with progression of head and neck cancer. Cancer Res 1993;53:4477.
19. el-Naggar AK, Lai S, Luna MA, et al. Sequential p53 mutation analysis of pre-invasive and invasive head and neck squamous carcinoma. Int J Cancer 1995;64:196.
20. el-Deiry WS, Harper JW, O'Connor PM, et al. WAF1/CIP1 is induced in p53-mediated G1 arrest and apoptosis. Cancer Res 1994;54:1169.
21. Haupt S, Berger M, Goldberg Z, et al. Apoptosis - the p53 network. J Cell Sci 2003;116:4077.
22. Ganly I, Soutar DS, Brown R, et al. p53 alterations in recurrent squamous cell cancer of the head and neck refractory to radiotherapy. Br J Cancer 2000;82:392.
23. Koch WM, Brennan JA, Zahurak M, et al. p53 mutation and locoregional treatment failure in head and neck squamous cell carcinoma. J Natl Cancer Inst 1996;88:1580.
24. Alsner J, Sorensen SB, Overgaard J. TP53 mutation is related to poor prognosis after radiotherapy, but not surgery, in squamous cell carcinoma of the head and neck. Radiother Oncol 2001;59:179.
25. Skinner HD, Sandulache VC, Ow TJ, et al. TP53 disruptive mutations lead to head and neck cancer treatment failure through inhibition of radiation-induced senescence. Clin Cancer Res 2011;18:290.
26. Temam S, Flahault A, Perie S, et al. p53 gene status as a predictor of tumor response to induction chemotherapy of patients with locoregionally advanced squamous cell carcinomas of the head and neck. J Clin Oncol 2000;18:385.
27. Cabelguenne A, Blons H, de Waziers I, et al. p53 alterations predict tumor response to neoadjuvant chemotherapy in head and neck squamous cell carcinoma: a prospective series. J Clin Oncol 2000;18:1465.
28. Bolos V, Grego-Bessa J, de la Pompa JL. Notch signaling in development and cancer. Endocr Rev 2007;28:339.
29. Durinck S, Ho C, Wang NJ, et al. Temporal dissection of tumorigenesis in primary cancers. Cancer Discov 2011;1:137.
30. Wang NJ, Sanborn Z, Arnett KL, et al. Loss-of-function mutations in Notch receptors in cutaneous and lung squamous cell carcinoma. Proc Natl Acad Sci U S A 2011;108:17761.
31. Klinakis A, Lobry C, Abdel-Wahab O, et al. A novel tumour-suppressor function for the Notch pathway in myeloid leukaemia. Nature 2011;473:230.
32. Grabher C, von Boehmer H, Look AT. Notch 1 activation in the molecular pathogenesis of T-cell acute lymphoblastic leukaemia. Nat Rev Cancer 2006;6:347.
33. Baldus CD, Thibaut J, Goekbuget N, et al. Prognostic implications of NOTCH1 and FBXW7 mutations in adult acute T-lymphoblastic leukemia. Haematologica 2009;94:1383.

34. Reed AL, Califano J, Cairns P, et al. High frequency of p16 (CDKN2/MTS-1/INK4A) inactivation in head and neck squamous cell carcinoma. Cancer Res 1996;56:3630.
35. Ohta S, Uemura H, Matsui Y, et al. Alterations of p16 and p14ARF genes and their 9p21 locus in oral squamous cell carcinoma. Oral Surg Oral Med Oral Pathol Oral Radiol Endod 2009;107:81.
36. Merlo A, Herman JG, Mao L, et al. 5' CpG island methylation is associated with transcriptional silencing of the tumour suppressor p16/CDKN2/MTS1 in human cancers. Nat Med 1995;1:686.
37. Chen PL, Scully P, Shew JY, et al. Phosphorylation of the retinoblastoma gene product is modulated during the cell cycle and cellular differentiation. Cell 1989;58:1193.
38. Lukas J, Parry D, Aagaard L, et al. Retinoblastoma-protein-dependent cell-cycle inhibition by the tumour suppressor p16. Nature 1995;375:503.
39. Mihara K, Cao XR, Yen A, et al. Cell cycle-dependent regulation of phosphorylation of the human retinoblastoma gene product. Science 1989;246:1300.
40. Califano J, van der Riet P, Westra W, et al. Genetic progression model for head and neck cancer: implications for field cancerization. Cancer Res 1996;56:2488.
41. Nishikawa Y, Miyazaki T, Nakashiro K, et al. Human FAT1 cadherin controls cell migration and invasion of oral squamous cell carcinoma through the localization of beta-catenin. Oncol Rep 2011;26:587.
42. Nakaya K, Yamagata HD, Arita N, et al. Identification of homozygous deletions of tumor suppressor gene FAT in oral cancer using CGH-array. Oncogene 2007;26:5300.
43. Okami K, Wu L, Riggins G, et al. Analysis of PTEN/MMAC1 alterations in aerodigestive tract tumors. Cancer Res 1998;58:509.
44. Saranath D, Chang SE, Bhoite LT, et al. High frequency mutation in codons 12 and 61 of H-ras oncogene in chewing tobacco-related human oral carcinoma in India. Br J Cancer 1991;63:573.
45. Sathyan KM, Nalinakumari KR, Kannan S. H-Ras mutation modulates the expression of major cell cycle regulatory proteins and disease prognosis in oral carcinoma. Mod Pathol 2007;20:1141.
46. Xu J, Gimenez-Conti IB, Cunningham JE, et al. Alterations of p53, cyclin D1, Rb, and H-ras in human oral carcinomas related to tobacco use. Cancer 1998;83:204.
47. Murugan AK, Munirajan AK, Tsuchida N. Ras oncogenes in oral cancer: the past 20 years. Oral Oncol 2012;48:383.
48. Bos JL. ras oncogenes in human cancer: a review. Cancer Res 1989;49:4682.
49. Castellano E, Downward J. Role of RAS in the regulation of PI 3-kinase. Curr Top Microbiol Immunol 2010;346:143.
50. Giehl K. Oncogenic Ras in tumour progression and metastasis. Biol Chem 2005;386:193.
51. Murugan AK, Hong NT, Fukui Y, et al. Oncogenic mutations of the PIK3CA gene in head and neck squamous cell carcinomas. Int J Oncol 2008;32:101.
52. Hennessy BT, Smith DL, Ram PT, et al. Exploiting the PI3K/AKT pathway for cancer drug discovery. Nat Rev Drug Discov 2005;4:988.
53. Hynes NE, Lane HA. ERBB receptors and cancer: the complexity of targeted inhibitors. Nat Rev Cancer 2005;5:341.
54. Kalyankrishna S, Grandis JR. Epidermal growth factor receptor biology in head and neck cancer. J Clin Oncol 2006;24:2666.
55. Rogers SJ, Harrington KJ, Rhys-Evans P, et al. Biological significance of c-erbB family oncogenes in head and neck cancer. Cancer Metastasis Rev 2005;24:47.

56. Ibrahim SO, Vasstrand EN, Liavaag PG, et al. Expression of c-erbB proto-oncogene family members in squamous cell carcinoma of the head and neck. Anticancer Res 1997;17:4539.
57. Rodrigo JP, Ramos S, Lazo PS, et al. Amplification of ERBB oncogenes in squamous cell carcinomas of the head and neck. Eur J Cancer 1996;32A:2004.
58. Cassidy LD, Venkitaraman AR. Genome instability mechanisms and the structure of cancer genomes. Curr Opin Genet Dev 2012;22:10.
59. Viet CT, Schmidt BL. Understanding oral cancer in the genome era. Head Neck 2010;32:1246.
60. Jin C, Jin Y, Wennerberg J, et al. Cytogenetic abnormalities in 106 oral squamous cell carcinomas. Cancer Genet Cytogenet 2006;164:44.
61. Uchida K, Oga A, Okafuji M, et al. Molecular cytogenetic analysis of oral squamous cell carcinomas by comparative genomic hybridization, spectral karyotyping, and fluorescence in situ hybridization. Cancer Genet Cytogenet 2006; 167:109.
62. Liu W, Zheng W, Xie J, et al. Identification of genes related to carcinogenesis of oral leukoplakia by oligo cancer microarray analysis. Oncol Rep 2011;26:265.
63. Vissers LE, de Vries BB, Osoegawa K, et al. Array-based comparative genomic hybridization for the genome wide detection of submicroscopic chromosomal abnormalities. Am J Hum Genet 2003;73:1261.
64. Gebhart E. Comparative genomic hybridization (CGH): ten years of substantial progress in human solid tumor molecular cytogenetics. Cytogenet Genome Res 2004;104:352.
65. Baldwin C, Garnis C, Zhang L, et al. Multiple microalterations detected at high frequency in oral cancer. Cancer Res 2005;65:7561.
66. Curtis C, Lynch AG, Dunning MJ, et al. The pitfalls of platform comparison: DNA copy number array technologies assessed. BMC Genomics 2009;10:588.
67. Sparano A, Quesnelle KM, Kumar MS, et al. Genome-wide profiling of oral squamous cell carcinoma by array-based comparative genomic hybridization. Laryngoscope 2006;116:735.
68. Snijders AM, Schmidt BL, Fridlyand J, et al. Rare amplicons implicate frequent deregulation of cell fate specification pathways in oral squamous cell carcinoma. Oncogene 2005;24:4232.
69. Garnis C, Coe BP, Zhang L, et al. Overexpression of LRP12, a gene contained within an 8q22 amplicon identified by high-resolution array CGH analysis of oral squamous cell carcinomas. Oncogene 2004;23:2582.
70. Smeets SJ, Braakhuis BJ, Abbas S, et al. Genome-wide DNA copy number alterations in head and neck squamous cell carcinomas with or without oncogene-expressing human papillomavirus. Oncogene 2006;25:2558.
71. Ashman JN, Patmore HS, Condon LT, et al. Prognostic value of genomic alterations in head and neck squamous cell carcinoma detected by comparative genomic hybridisation. Br J Cancer 2003;89:864.
72. Ambatipudi S, Gerstung M, Gowda R, et al. Genomic profiling of advanced-stage oral cancers reveals chromosome 11q alterations as markers of poor clinical outcome. PLoS One 2011;6:e17250.
73. Uchida K, Oga A, Nakao M, et al. Loss of 3p26.3 is an independent prognostic factor in patients with oral squamous cell carcinoma. Oncol Rep 2011;26:463.
74. Sugahara K, Michikawa Y, Ishikawa K, et al. Combination effects of distinct cores in 11q13 amplification region on cervical lymph node metastasis of oral squamous cell carcinoma. Int J Oncol 2011;39:761.

75. Akervall J, Guo X, Qian CN, et al. Genetic and expression profiles of squamous cell carcinoma of the head and neck correlate with cisplatin sensitivity and resistance in cell lines and patients. Clin Cancer Res 2004;10:8204.
76. van den Broek GB, Wreesmann VB, van den Brekel MW, et al. Genetic abnormalities associated with chemoradiation resistance of head and neck squamous cell carcinoma. Clin Cancer Res 2007;13:4386.
77. Herman JG, Baylin SB. Gene silencing in cancer in association with promoter hypermethylation. N Engl J Med 2003;349:2042.
78. Ha PK, Califano JA. Promoter methylation and inactivation of tumour-suppressor genes in oral squamous-cell carcinoma. Lancet Oncol 2006;7:77.
79. Kulis M, Esteller M. DNA methylation and cancer. Adv Genet 2010;70:27.
80. Shaw R. The epigenetics of oral cancer. Int J Oral Maxillofac Surg 2006;35:101.
81. Smiraglia DJ, Smith LT, Lang JC, et al. Differential targets of CpG island hypermethylation in primary and metastatic head and neck squamous cell carcinoma (HNSCC). J Med Genet 2003;40:25.
82. Adrien LR, Schlecht NF, Kawachi N, et al. Classification of DNA methylation patterns in tumor cell genomes using a CpG island microarray. Cytogenet Genome Res 2006;114:16.
83. Lleras RA, Adrien LR, Smith RV, et al. Hypermethylation of a cluster of Kruppel-type zinc finger protein genes on chromosome 19q13 in oropharyngeal squamous cell carcinoma. Am J Pathol 1965;178:2011.
84. Langevin SM, Koestler DC, Christensen BC, et al. Peripheral blood DNA methylation profiles are indicative of head and neck squamous cell carcinoma: an epigenome-wide association study. Epigenetics 2012;7:291.
85. Poage GM, Butler RA, Houseman EA, et al. Identification of an epigenetic profile classifier that is associated with survival in head and neck cancer. Cancer Res 2012;72:2728.
86. Ha PK, Benoit NE, Yochem R, et al. A transcriptional progression model for head and neck cancer. Clin Cancer Res 2003;9:3058.
87. Mendez E, Cheng C, Farwell DG, et al. Transcriptional expression profiles of oral squamous cell carcinomas. Cancer 2002;95:1482.
88. Ziober AF, Patel KR, Alawi F, et al. Identification of a gene signature for rapid screening of oral squamous cell carcinoma. Clin Cancer Res 2006;12:5960.
89. Kondoh N, Ohkura S, Arai M, et al. Gene expression signatures that can discriminate oral leukoplakia subtypes and squamous cell carcinoma. Oral Oncol 2007;43:455.
90. Lohavanichbutr P, Houck J, Fan W, et al. Genome wide gene expression profiles of HPV-positive and HPV-negative oropharyngeal cancer: potential implications for treatment choices. Arch Otolaryngol Head Neck Surg 2009;135:180.
91. Nguyen ST, Hasegawa S, Tsuda H, et al. Identification of a predictive gene expression signature of cervical lymph node metastasis in oral squamous cell carcinoma. Cancer Sci 2007;98:740.
92. Roepman P, Wessels LF, Kettelarij N, et al. An expression profile for diagnosis of lymph node metastases from primary head and neck squamous cell carcinomas. Nat Genet 2005;37:182.
93. Zhou X, Temam S, Oh M, et al. Global expression-based classification of lymph node metastasis and extracapsular spread of oral tongue squamous cell carcinoma. Neoplasia 2006;8:925.
94. Dumur CI, Ladd AC, Wright HV, et al. Genes involved in radiation therapy response in head and neck cancers. Laryngoscope 2009;119:91.

95. Ganly I, Kirn D, Eckhardt G, et al. A phase I study of Onyx-015, an E1B attenuated adenovirus, administered intratumorally to patients with recurrent head and neck cancer. Clin Cancer Res 2000;6:798.
96. Nemunaitis J, Nemunaitis J. Head and neck cancer: response to p53-based therapeutics. Head Neck 2011;33:131.
97. Fortini ME. Gamma-secretase-mediated proteolysis in cell-surface-receptor signalling. Nat Rev Mol Cell Biol 2002;3:673.
98. Merck. A Notch Signalling Pathway Inhibitor for Patients With T-cell Acute Lymphoblastic Leukemia/Lymphoma (ALL). ClinicalTrials.gov. Bethesda (MD): National Library of Medicine (US). Available from: http://www.clinicaltrials.gov/ct2/show/NCT00100152 NLM Identifier: NCT00100152. Accessed May 13, 2013.
99. Loyola University; Merck. Study Of MK-0752 In Combination With Tamoxifen Or Letrozole to Treat Early Stage Breast Cancer. ClinicalTrials.gov. Bethesda (MD): National Library of Medicine (US). Available from: http://www.clinicaltrials.gov/ct2/show/NCT00756717 NLM Identifier: NCT00756717. Accessed May 13, 2013.
100. Extance A. Alzheimer's failure raises questions about disease-modifying strategies. Nat Rev Drug Discov 2010;9:749.
101. Blum R, Kloog Y. Tailoring Ras-pathway–inhibitor combinations for cancer therapy. Drug Resist Updat 2005;8:369.
102. Adjei AA, Dy GK, Erlichman C, et al. A phase I trial of ISIS 2503, an antisense inhibitor of H-ras, in combination with gemcitabine in patients with advanced cancer. Clin Cancer Res 2003;9:115.
103. Cunningham CC, Holmlund JT, Geary RS, et al. A Phase I trial of H-ras antisense oligonucleotide ISIS 2503 administered as a continuous intravenous infusion in patients with advanced carcinoma. Cancer 2001;92:1265.
104. Alberts SR, Schroeder M, Erlichman C, et al. Gemcitabine and ISIS-2503 for patients with locally advanced or metastatic pancreatic adenocarcinoma: a North Central Cancer Treatment Group phase II trial. J Clin Oncol 2004;22:4944.
105. Downward J. Targeting RAS signalling pathways in cancer therapy. Nat Rev Cancer 2003;3:11.
106. Oncothyreon Inc. Study of PX-866 and Docetaxel in Solid Tumors. ClinicalTrials.gov. Bethesda (MD): National Library of Medicine (US); 2000. Available from: http://www.clinicaltrials.gov/ct2/show/NCT01204099. NLM Identifier: NCT01204099. Accessed May 13th, 2013.
107. Oncothyreon Inc. Phase 1 and 2 Study of PX-866 and Cetuximab. ClinicalTrials.gov. Bethesda (MD): National Library of Medicine (US). Available from: http://www.clinicaltrials.gov/ct2/show/NCT01252628 NLM Identifier NCT01252628. Accessed May 13th, 2013.
108. National Institute of Dental and Craniofacial Research. Rapamycin Therapy in Head and Neck Squamous Cell Carcinoma. ClinicalTrials.gov. Bethesda (MD): National Library of Medicine (US). Available from: http://www.clinicaltrials.gov/ct2/show/NCT01195922 NLM Identifier: NCT01195922. Accessed May 13th, 2013.
109. National Cancer Institute. Akt Inhibitor MK2206 in Treating Patients With Recurrent or Metastatic Head and Neck Cancer. ClinicalTrials.gov. Bethesda (MD): National Library of Medicine (US). Available from: http://www.clinicaltrials.gov/ct2/show/NCT01349933 NLM Identifier: NCT01349933. Accessed May 13th, 2013.
110. Malumbres M, Pevarello P, Barbacid M, et al. CDK inhibitors in cancer therapy: what is next? Trends Pharmacol Sci 2008;29:16.

Why Otolaryngologists Need to be Aware of Fanconi Anemia

Jiahui Lin[a], David I. Kutler, MD[b,*]

KEYWORDS

• Fanconi anemia • Squamous cell carcinoma • Head and neck

KEY POINTS

- Fanconi anemia (FA) is an autosomal recessive caretaker gene disorder with a heterogeneous clinical presentation, although most commonly presenting with bone marrow failure and physical growth defects. Patients with FA have a propensity to squamous cell carcinomas, particularly in the head and neck and the anogenital regions, and should a young patient (ie, <40 years) present with such a cancer, FA should be considered.
- Although hematopoietic stem cell transplantation is the only curative therapy for the hematologic manifestations of FA, it may increase the risk of FA-associated head and neck squamous cell carcinoma (HNSCC), increasing the already high 500-fold baseline risk.
- FA-associated HNSCC is most commonly found in the oral cavity, and surgical resection is considered to be the standard treatment. Because of the chromosomal fragility of patients with FA, radiation therapy and chemotherapy can cause major toxicities and morbidity compared with other patients with HNSCC and can be recommended only in highly selected cases. If at all possible, FA-associated HNSCC should be referred to major centers for management.
- In any patient with HNSCC without a known diagnosis of FA (particularly younger patients) who experience abnormality severe toxicity to radiation therapy and especially chemotherapy, it is critically important that a work-up for FA be considered.
- Fanconi Anemia Research Fund, Inc. (www.faconi.org) is a rich resource for patients, families, and clinicians dealing with this disease.

INTRODUCTION TO FANCONI ANEMIA

Fanconi anemia (FA) is a rare disorder inherited in an autosomal recessive fashion, with an estimated incidence of 1:360,000 births.[1] In certain populations, such as Ashkenazi Jews, Spanish gypsies, and black South Africans, the carrier frequency

[a] Weill Cornell Medical College, New York, NY, USA; [b] Division of Head and Neck Surgery, Department of Otolaryngology-Head and Neck Surgery, Weill Cornell Medical Center, New York Presbyterian Hospital, 1305 York Avenue, 5th Floor, New York, NY 10065, USA
* Corresponding author.
E-mail address: dik2002@med.cornell.edu

Otolaryngol Clin N Am 46 (2013) 567–577
http://dx.doi.org/10.1016/j.otc.2013.04.002
oto.theclinics.com
0030-6665/13/$ – see front matter

Abbreviations: Maximizing Outcomes of Rehabilitation	
AML	acute myeloid leukemia
FA	Fanconi anemia
GVHD	graft versus host disease
HNSCC	head and neck squamous cell carcinoma
HPV	human papillomavirus
MDS	myelodysplastic syndrome

is believed to be as high as 1:100.[2–4] It is the most common form of inherited aplastic anemia, a syndrome characterized by pancytopenia and hypocellular bone marrow.[5,6] FA is one of many caretaker gene disorders, which also includes Bloom syndrome and ataxia-telangiectasia.[7]

Since FA was first described by the Swiss physician Dr Guido Fanconi in 1927, more than 2000 cases have been reported, with the disease affecting slightly more males than females at a ratio of 1.1 to 1.2 to 1.[8,9] Clinical features of FA include growth retardation, learning disability, bone marrow failure, and cancer. Pancytopenia and bone marrow hypocellularity usually do not appear until 5 to 10 years of age, both of which develop over time and progressively become more severe.[5] Bone marrow failure, the most common presentation of FA, has a cumulative incidence of 90% by the age of 40 years.[10] Congenital physical malformations affect 60% to 75% of patients and include abnormalities of the bone, heart, eyes, kidneys, and gonads.[8,11] Hyperpigmentation of the skin as café-au-lait spots, varying from 1 to 12 cm in diameter, occurs in approximately 25% of patients, with generalized hyperpigmentation in 50% to 65% of patients.[5,12] Central nervous system, gastrointestinal, hepatic, gynecologic, fertility, endocrine, and hearing defects may also occur in FA. However, FA is a heterogeneous disease and can present without any physical manifestations. Therefore, lack of physical findings does not preclude a diagnosis of FA, and a work-up for FA should be considered for patients with head and neck squamous cell carcinoma (HNSCC) presenting at an unusually young age.

FA Risk for Cancers

Patients with FA are also at a 500-fold increased risk for developing acute myeloid leukemia (AML) and at a nearly 5000-fold increased risk for developing myelodysplastic syndrome (MDS).[8,13,14] The incidence of head and neck cancer in this patient population has also been shown to be increased by 500-fold to 700-fold compared with the general population.[13,15,16]

Genes Implicated in FA

At least 15 genes have been implicated in FA that are responsible for the various complementation groups (A-C, D1, D2, E-G, I, J, L-P).[11] Mutations in *FANCA*, *FANCC*, and *FANCG* are the most common, involved in 60%, 14%, and 10% of cases, respectively.[8] These FA genes have been identified as cancer susceptibility genes involved in various aspects of DNA repair, DNA stabilization, and modification of downstream proteins. The FA proteins A, B, C, E, F, G, L, and M make up the FA core complex, a nuclear E3 ubiquitin ligase complex that mediates the monoubiquitination of FANCD2 and FANCI after DNA damage.[8,17] Any mutation or loss of a component of the FA core complex results in failure of monoubiquitination. *FANCD1* has since been identified as *BRCA2*, *FANCG* as *XRCC9*, *FANCJ* as *BACH1/BRIP1*, *FANCN* as *PALB2*, *FANCO* as *RAD51 C*, and *FANCP* as *SLX4*.[8,18–20] All mutations in FA genes are inherited in an autosomal recessive manner, with the exception of *FANCB*, which is an X-linked gene.[21] The FA proteins play an important role in DNA repair, and many of them interact in other DNA repair pathways. Defects in any of these proteins result in increased chromosomal fragility.

Clinical Diagnosis of FA

Most cases of FA are diagnosed between the ages of 6 and 9 years, although some diagnoses may be delayed until adulthood, with malignancies such as HNSCC as the primary clinical manifestation.[22] Diagnosis of FA is made by culturing the patient's cells with a DNA cross-linking agent, such as diepoxybutane or mitomycin C. Detection of chromosomal fragility or aberrations, in addition to common clinical manifestations, points to a diagnosis of FA.[11] Other diagnostic tools include cell-cycle analysis and the FANCD2 protein monoubiquitination assay.[11,17] The latter method takes advantage of the fact that monoubiquitination of the FANCD2 protein is normal in other bone marrow failure syndromes.[23] However, this assay is only useful for patients with mutations in the monoubiquitination pathway, including the FA core complex; downstream mutations are not detected. Because of the various shortcomings of these more traditional methods, germline genetic testing may soon become the standard for FA diagnosis in the near future, especially as several clinics now offer this service.[11]

Because of its rarity and variable phenotypic expression, FA may be underdiagnosed. Clinical manifestations of FA resemble other bone marrow failure syndromes, such as dyskeratosis congenital, Shwachman-Diamond syndrome, and Diamond-Blackfan anemia.[11,24] Furthermore, earlier detection of the disease typically improves outcome, because the hematologic manifestations would otherwise progress with time. Physicians are then also able to provide cancer surveillance and earlier treatment of malignancies. Therefore, it is important to test patients for FA who present at unusually young age with MDS, primary AML, or cancers of the head and neck, cervix, breast, or anogenital tract.

SOLID TUMORS IN PATIENTS WITH FA

Patients with FA are known to have an increased risk of developing solid, nonhematologic tumors. Kaplan and colleagues[25] postulated that defective DNA repair and immunodeficiency are key players in the development of such tumors in these patients. Solid tumors appear at a median age of 26 years in those with FA.[26] In studies of the International Fanconi Anemia Registry and German Fanconi Anemia Registry, the cumulative incidence of developing solid tumors with FA is around 30% by the fourth decade of life.[10,13] Such malignancies are predominantly located in the head and neck, followed by the anogenital region, although cancers of the skin, brain, breast, and liver also occur.

FA-associated HNSCC

Patients with FA have a significantly higher risk of developing head and neck cancers, and most occur in the oral cavity. In a study of the International Fanconi Anemia Registry, patients had a 500-fold increase in the incidence of HNSCC, with a cumulative incidence rate of 14% by the age of 40 years.[15] Patients who develop FA-associated HNSCC tend to be female at a 2:1 ratio, with a median age at diagnosis of 31 years. According to the Surveillance Epidemiology and End Results national cancer registry, HNSCC incidence in the general population by age 40 years is only 0.038%, with a median age at presentation of 53 years.[27] However, this increased cumulative incidence in FA is considered an underestimation of risk, as many patients with FA have other complications of the disease earlier in life.

Oral cavity cancers are the most common FA-associated HNSCC, representing 68% of the head and neck cancers diagnosed in patients with FA. Tongue cancer is the most common subsite identified, followed in frequency by tumors in the larynx (11%), oropharynx (11%), and hypopharynx (5%).[15] Similarly, in a review of the literature, Lustig and colleagues[28] found the proportion of tongue carcinomas among FA-associated HNSCC to be 52%. In the general HNSCC population, the proportion of oral cavity cancer among HNSCC is only 27%.[27]

In addition, patients with FA often present with multiple primary tumors. Sixty-three percent of patients with FA who had HNSCC developed multiple malignancies, including 1 patient who developed a total of 4 primary tumors.[15] Locations for a second primary squamous cell carcinoma were distributed equally among anal, cervical, vulvar, and head and neck regions.

Environmental factors, including tobacco and alcohol, play a key role in the development of HNSCC in the general population. Although the use of alcohol and tobacco in a typical population with HNSCC has been reported to be as high as 75% to 85%, only 16% of patients with FA with HNSCC had a history of such factors.[15,29] Therefore, in young patients with HNSCC without a history of environmental triggers, particularly in those with other hematologic abnormalities, FA should be considered in the diagnosis. In a review of the literature, 22% of patients with FA who developed solid tumors were diagnosed with FA only after discovery of their cancer.[13]

FA and Human Papillomavirus

Because of the affinity of FA-associated squamous cell carcinoma to localize in the body's mucous membranes, associations between HNSCC and human papillomavirus (HPV) have also been explored, although this link is still considered controversial. In a study by Kutler and colleagues,[30] HPV DNA was detected in 83% of FA HNSCC, compared with only 36% of control non-FA HNSCC, and HPV16 was the type most frequently detected. Spardy and colleagues[31] showed that HPV16 E7 oncoprotein is able to trigger the FA pathway, and expression of HPV16 in FA-deficient cells increases chromosomal instability. However, a study of 21 squamous cell carcinomas primarily from European patients with FA found HPV DNA in only 10% of their tumor samples and none in their HNSCC samples.[32] In further work from this group on 4 cell lines derived from FA HNSCC, no HPV DNA could be detected although mutations in *TP53* (as typical for non-FA HNSCC) were found.[33] Kutler and colleagues,[30] on the other hand, detected no *TP53* mutations in their samples. Although these 2 groups are in conflict with one another, *TP53* can be inactivated by either mutation or the HPV E7 oncoprotein and consequently the carcinogenic processes proposed by each group are both plausible. Thus, the benefits of using prophylactic HPV vaccinations against development of squamous cell carcinoma in patients with FA remain uncertain.

THERAPEUTIC OPTIONS IN FA

Because of the high risk of developing HNSCC and the early age of onset in the FA population, screening of the oral cavity in patients with FA by should begin by the ages of 10 to 12 years (**Fig. 1**).[24] Surveillance should be performed by a professional experienced in head and neck cancer detection every 6 months, including physical examination and fiberoptic evaluation of the hypopharynx, nasopharynx, oropharynx, and larynx. Appearance of other potentially malignant lesions, such as lichen planus, leukoplakia, and erythroplakia, should also be noted and biopsied as appropriate, and any patient with such lesions should be evaluated even more frequently. Frequent

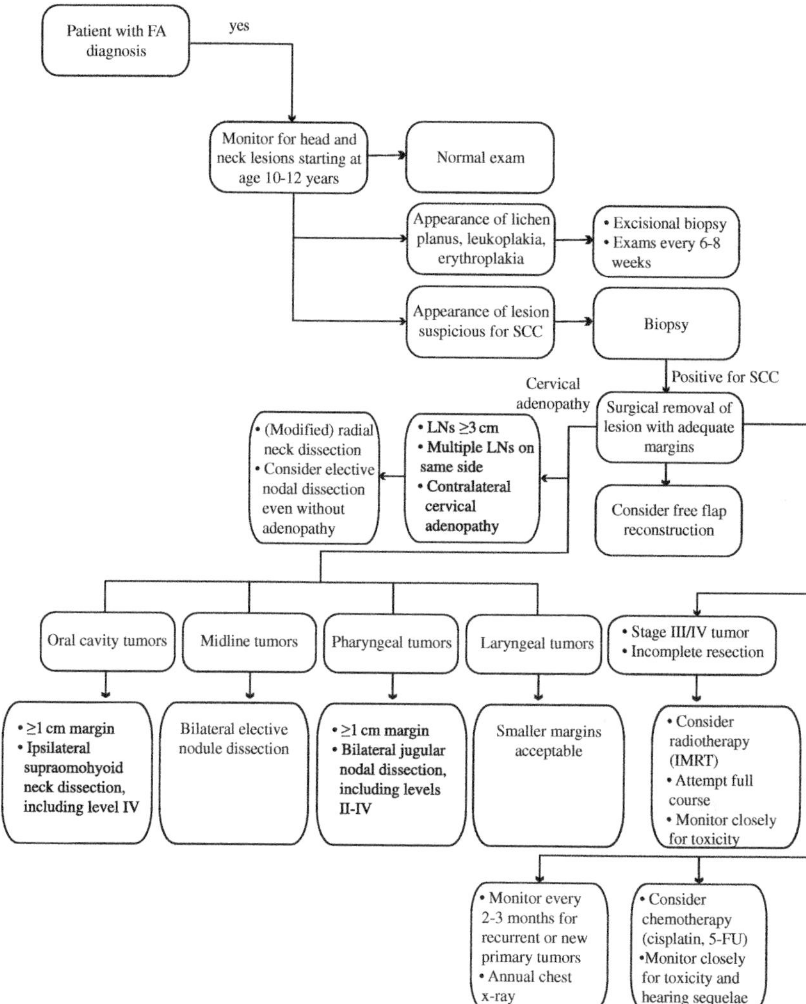

Fig. 1. Screening and treatment of HNSCC in patients with FA. 5-FU, 5-fluorouracil; IMRT, intensity modulated radiation thetherapy; LN, lymph node; SCC, squamous cell carcinoma.

surveillance in patients with FA may improve outcome or reduce the need for more aggressive treatment.

Surgical Excision

The treatment of oral cavity cancer in patients with FA is similar to that for the general HNSCC population, with surgery being the preferred primary therapy.[24,28] Most frequently, radical surgical excision with negative margins is required. A neck dissection is necessary if there is a risk of lymph node metastases. Extensive radical surgery is sometimes required to remove high stage cancers, and microvascular free-flap reconstruction may be needed.[15] Although such complex surgeries requiring microvascular free-flap reconstructions are uncommon among patients with FA, they have been tolerated without significant mortality or morbidity and should be considered when developing a treatment plan.[34–36] Perioperatively, patients with FA must be closely monitored for bone marrow failure, and the possibility of blood and platelet transfusions must be kept in mind both preoperatively and postoperatively.[15,24] Postoperative complications may also occur, the most common being hematomas and wound infections. In a study of the International Fanconi Anemia Registry, 26% of patients suffered postoperative complications, but most patients tolerated the procedure well with low long-term morbidity.[15]

Radiation Therapy

Radiation therapy has been used successfully in patients with FA, but these patients have a significantly increased complication rate compared with the general HNSCC population. The most common complications of radiation include high-grade mucositis, dysphagia, and hematologic complications (**Table 1**).[37] Several patients with FA undergoing radiation therapy have experienced severe systemic complications, such as bone marrow failure and sepsis, requiring termination of radiation therapy; several deaths as a result of these severe radiation complications have also been reported.[15,28,38] Radiation therapy is therefore advised with caution and should be administered by physicians with extensive experience in treating head and neck cancer. Chemotherapy is not commonly used for patients with FA primarily because of the even higher rates of complications and toxicity.[15,28] In any HNSCC patient without a known FA diagnosis (particularly younger patients) who experience abnormally severe toxicity to radiation therapy and especially chemotherapy, it is critically important that a work-up for FA be considered.

Although 5-year survival rates improve with adjuvant radiotherapy for patients with more advanced stage III and IV HNSCC,[39] radiotherapy for FA-associated HNSCC must only be used in selected cases and be individually tailored to the specific patient. Because of the nature of this disorder, patients are more susceptible to toxicities from both adjuvant therapies. High-grade mucositis, for example, has been reported in 75% of patients with FA treated with radiation therapy, compared with 34% to 57% in the general HNSCC population.[37,40] Blood cell counts must also be monitored closely if radiation therapy is chosen, because patients with FA are at an increased

Table 1
Risks and complications of HNSCC therapy in patients with FA

Treatment Modality	Risks/Complications (Frequency in International Fanconi Anemia Registry Population)
Surgery only (n = 17)	Wound infection (11%) Aspiration pneumonia (5%)
Extensive reconstruction (n = 17)	Hematoma (40%)
Radiation therapy (n = 12, all treated with radiotherapy)	High-grade mucositis (75%) Dysphagia (67%) Cytopenia (50%) Sepsis (33%) Hemorrhage (25%) Dermatitis (16%) Esophageal stenosis (16%) Tracheal stenosis (8%) Recurrent pneumonia (8%)
Chemotherapy (n = 17)[a]	Aplastic anemia Organ failure

[a] Insufficient literature data to calculate frequency.

risk for developing pancytopenia. For HNSCC in patients with FA, radiation therapy using longer duration treatment courses with lower dose per fraction (150–180 cGy) may maximize the treatment effect and decrease complications.[37] Patients should also be monitored closely for signs of infection and for cytopenia both during and after radiotherapy. New research has suggested that the use of organ-specific radioprotectors might benefit patients with FA who are undergoing radiotherapy but are not yet available for clinical use.[41]

Chemotherapy

Although radiation therapy has been used successfully in many patients with FA with HNSCC, use of chemotherapy in patients with FA has resulted in major complications leading to interruption or termination of therapy.[37] Chemotherapy protocols typically use cisplatin, a cross-linking agent, to which FA cells are particularly sensitive.[15] Conventional chemotherapy may cause irreversible aplastic anemia and organ damage in patients with FA, and extreme care should be taken to monitor these patients if attempting to use this treatment modality. Several patients have successfully received targeted agents, such as cetuximab, with only minimal complications, but reports of patients receiving these drugs are limited.

CLINICAL OUTCOMES/COMPLICATIONS/CONCERNS IN FA

There seems to be 2 groups of patients with FA who develop HNSCC: those with more severe FA genetic mutations, earlier FA symptoms, and malignancies; and those with milder FA mutations, delayed/milder FA symptoms, and later malignancies.[28] Those who have milder mutations are often able to live to an age at which their risk for cancer becomes the limiting factor. Median patient survival with FA from the International Fanconi Anemia Registry was 24 years from diagnosis.[10] Survival after development of HNSCC, however, was much lower. Of these patients, median time to recurrence was 16 months, with a median follow-up period of surviving patients of 29 months. Overall survival for patients with FA with HNSCC at 2 years was 49%, compared with non-FA HNSCC 2-year survival of 70%.[15,27]

Genotype as a Predictor of Prognosis

Associations between genotype and patient outcome have been studied and may be a predictor of prognosis. Patients with mutations in *FANCD1/BRCA2* have the shortest survival time and develop cancer at an earlier age, with a 70% cumulative incidence of leukemia by 10 years of age and 83% cumulative incidence of solid tumors by age 6.7 years.[42] A case series of 3 patients with this genotype reported that all 3 patients developed MDS/AML as well as multiple solid tumors.[43] The risk of developing any malignancy for those with the *FANCD1/BRCA2* genotype was 66-fold compared with other complementation groups. Wagner and colleagues[44] advise that testing for *BRCA2* mutations should be considered if the complementation group cannot be assigned, because of the increased risk of solid tumors in patients with this genotype. More recently, the *FANCN* genotype has been linked to *PALB2*, whose gene product is crucial to the homologous recombination function of *BRCA2*. Similar to the *FAND1/BRCA2* genotype, all patients with this genotype have developed cancers early in life, many by the age of 2 years, pointing to the severity of the FANCN mutation.[45,46] Those with mutations in *FANCA*, on the other hand, had the longest survival rate, with a median of 40 years after diagnosis.[14] This is also the most common genotype found in the FA population.[10,16] One of the more recently discovered FA genotypes, *FANCP/SLX4*, has also been linked to a milder phenotype.[20]

Hematopoietic Stem Cell Transplantation

Although hematopoietic stem cell transplantation (HSCT) is the only curative option for hematologic manifestations of FA, it may be associated with an increased risk of cancer development. In patients with FA who have undergone HSCT, the median age for development of HNSCC is 18 years, typically approximately 10 years after transplantation. Their non-HSCT-treated FA counterparts, on the other hand, developed HNSCC at a median age of 30 to 33 years.[14,15,47] Studies of various FA cohorts have shown that post-HSCT patients have a 3.8-fold to 4.4-fold higher risk of developing solid tumors than their nontransplanted counterparts.[14,16,48] In a review of the literature, most solid tumors post-HSCT were located in the oral cavity.[14] Rosenberg and colleagues[48] calculated that the cause-specific hazard rates of squamous cell carcinoma over time increased from 4.7% by 10 years post-HSCT to 24% by 15 years post-HSCT. Furthermore, a study by Jansisyanont and colleagues[49] found that 5 of 6 patients with FA who developed squamous cell carcinoma after bone marrow transplant were female, contrary to the overall ratio of males to females with FA of 1.1 to 1.2.

Graft Versus Host Disease

A common complication of HSCT is graft versus host disease (GVHD) to various degrees.[50] Chronic GVHD has also been associated with the development of squamous cell carcinoma and other solid tumors; severe acute GVHD is also a risk factor.[48,51] In a study of patients with undergoing HSCT, the cumulative incidence of HNSCC in those who developed chronic GVHD reached 53% by 15 years after transplant.[50] More recently, HSCT conditioning regimens have incorporated less cyclophosphamide, irradiation, and T-cell depletion by using fludarabine.[52,53] Although this method has been shown to decrease GVHD in patients with FA, studies have yet to show the effects of such a treatment for reducing the risk of HNSCC.

SUMMARY

FA is a heterogeneous syndrome that requires multidisciplinary coordination to screen and care for these typically young patients. Although hematologic complications are the most common manifestation of this disease, cancers, especially of the head and neck, are also prominent. The chromosomal fragility of patients with FA necessitates careful planning of therapy and monitoring, and awareness of this rare disorder is crucial to recognizing it in the clinic. Translational research into various aspects of care will shed new light on minimizing treatment complications for these patients. In the meantime, screening young patients diagnosed with HNSCC for FA and appropriate treatment of HNSCC diagnosed in FA patients remain priorities.

REFERENCES

1. Swift M. Fanconi's anaemia in the genetics of neoplasia. Nature 1971;230(5293):370–3.
2. Kutler DI, Auerbach AD. Fanconi anemia in Ashkenazi Jews. Fam Cancer 2004;3(3–4):241–8.
3. Callen E, Casado JA, Tischkowitz MD, et al. A common founder mutation in FANCA underlies the world's highest prevalence of Fanconi anemia in Gypsy families from Spain. Blood 2005;105(5):1946–9.

4. Morgan NV, Essop F, Demuth I, et al. A common Fanconi anemia mutation in black populations of sub-Saharan Africa. Blood 2005;105(9):3542–4.
5. Segel GB, Halterman MW, Lichtman MA. Aplastic anemia: acquired and inherited. In: Prchal JT, Kaushansky K, Lichtman MA, et al, editors. Williams hematology, vol. 89. New York: McGraw-Hill; 2010. p. 112–3.
6. Young NS. Aplastic anemia, myelodysplasia, and related bone marrow failure syndromes. In: Longo DL, Fauci AS, Kasper DL, et al, editors. Harrison's principles of internal medicine. 18th edition. New York: McGraw-Hill; 2012. Available at: http://www.accessmedicine.com/content.aspx?aID=9118038.
7. Joenje H, Patel KJ. The emerging genetic and molecular basis of Fanconi anaemia. Nat Rev Genet 2001;2(6):446–57.
8. Shimamura A, Alter BP. Pathophysiology and management of inherited bone marrow failure syndromes. Blood Rev 2010;24(3):101–22.
9. Rosenberg PS, Greene MH, Alter BP. Cancer incidence in persons with Fanconi anemia. Blood 2003;101(3):822–6.
10. Kutler DI, Singh B, Satagopan J, et al. A 20-year perspective on the International Fanconi Anemia Registry (IFAR). Blood 2003;101(4):1249–56.
11. Alter BP, Kupfer G. Fanconi Anemia. In: Pagon RA, Bird TD, Dolan CR, et al, editors. GeneReviewsTM. Seattle (WA): University of Washington; 1993. Available at: http://www.ncbi.nih.gov/book/NBK1401. Accessed July 31, 2012.
12. Tekin M, Bodurtha JN, Riccardi VM. Cafe au lait spots: the pediatrician's perspective. Pediatr Rev 2001;22(3):82–90.
13. Alter BP, Greene MH, Velazquez I, et al. Cancer in Fanconi anemia. Blood 2003; 101(5):2072.
14. Alter BP, Giri N, Savage SA, et al. Malignancies and survival patterns in the National Cancer Institute inherited bone marrow failure syndromes cohort study. Br J Haematol 2010;150(2):179–88.
15. Kutler DI, Auerbach AD, Satagopan J, et al. High incidence of head and neck squamous cell carcinoma in patients with Fanconi anemia. Arch Otolaryngol Head Neck Surg 2003;129(1):106–12.
16. Rosenberg PS, Alter BP, Ebell W. Cancer risks in Fanconi anemia: findings from the German Fanconi Anemia Registry. Haematologica 2008;93(4):511–7.
17. Soulier J. Fanconi anemia. Hematology Am Soc Hematol Educ Program 2011; 2011:492–7.
18. Parikh S, Bessler M. Recent insights into inherited bone marrow failure syndromes. Curr Opin Pediatr 2012;24(1):23–32.
19. Vaz F, Hanenberg H, Schuster B, et al. Mutation of the RAD51C gene in a Fanconi anemia-like disorder. Nat Genet 2010;42(5):406–9.
20. Kim Y, Lach FP, Desetty R, et al. Mutations of the SLX4 gene in Fanconi anemia. Nat Genet 2011;43(2):142–6.
21. Meetei AR, Levitus M, Xue Y, et al. X-linked inheritance of Fanconi anemia complementation group B. Nat Genet 2004;36(11):1219–24.
22. Alter BP. Inherited bone marrow failure syndromes. In: Nathan DG, Orkin SH, Ginsburg D, et al, editors. Nathan and Oski's hematology of infancy and childhood. Philadelphia: WB Saunders; 2003. p. 280.
23. Shimamura A, Montes de Oca R, Svenson JL, et al. A novel diagnostic screen for defects in the Fanconi anemia pathway. Blood 2002;100(13):4649–54.
24. Eiler ME, Frohnmayer D, Frohnmayer L, et al, editors. Fanconi anemia: guidelines for diagnosis and management. 3rd edition. Eugene (OR): Fanconi Anemia Research Fund; 2008. Available at: http://www.fanconi.org.

25. Kaplan MJ, Sabio H, Wanebo HJ, et al. Squamous cell carcinoma in the immunosuppressed patient: Fanconi's anemia. Laryngoscope 1985;95(7 Pt 1):771–5.
26. Alter BP. Fanconi's anemia, transplantation, and cancer. Pediatr Transplant 2005;9(Suppl 7):81–6.
27. Ries LA, Eisner MP, Kosary CL, et al. SEER cancer statistics review, 1973-1999. Bethesda (MD): 2002.
28. Lustig JP, Lugassy G, Neder A, et al. Head and neck carcinoma in Fanconi's anaemia–report of a case and review of the literature. Eur J Cancer B Oral Oncol 1995;31B(1):68–72.
29. Hashibe M, Brennan P, Benhamou S, et al. Alcohol drinking in never users of tobacco, cigarette smoking in never drinkers, and the risk of head and neck cancer: pooled analysis in the International Head and Neck Cancer Epidemiology Consortium. J Natl Cancer Inst 2007;99(10):777–89.
30. Kutler DI, Wreesmann VB, Goberdhan A, et al. Human papillomavirus DNA and p53 polymorphisms in squamous cell carcinomas from Fanconi anemia patients. J Natl Cancer Inst 2003;95(22):1718–21.
31. Spardy N, Duensing A, Charles D, et al. The human papillomavirus type 16 E7 oncoprotein activates the Fanconi anemia (FA) pathway and causes accelerated chromosomal instability in FA cells. J Virol 2007;81(23):13265–70.
32. van Zeeburg HJ, Snijders PJ, Wu T, et al. Clinical and molecular characteristics of squamous cell carcinomas from Fanconi anemia patients. J Natl Cancer Inst 2008;100(22):1649–53.
33. van Zeeburg HJ, Snijders PJ, Pals G, et al. Generation and molecular characterization of head and neck squamous cell lines of fanconi anemia patients. Cancer Res 2005;65(4):1271–6.
34. Chao JW, Cohen BD, Rohde CH, et al. Free fibular flap reconstruction of the mandible in a patient with Fanconi anemia. Plast Reconstr Surg 2010;125(2): 61e–3e.
35. Alkaabi M, Regan PJ, Kelly J, et al. Double paddle free fibular flap for reconstruction of the composite facial tumour in patient with Fanconi's anaemia. J Plast Reconstr Aesthet Surg 2009;62(11):471–3.
36. Kaplan KA, Reiffel AJ, Kutler DI, et al. Sequential second free flap for head and neck reconstruction in a patient with fanconi anemia and metachronous squamous cell carcinoma. Plast Reconstr Surg 2011;128(1):18e–9e.
37. Birkeland AC, Auerbach AD, Sanborn E, et al. Postoperative clinical radiosensitivity in patients with fanconi anemia and head and neck squamous cell carcinoma. Arch Otolaryngol Head Neck Surg 2011;137(9):930–4.
38. Bremer M, Schindler D, Gross M, et al. Fanconi's anemia and clinical radiosensitivity report on two adult patients with locally advanced solid tumors treated by radiotherapy. Strahlenther Onkol 2003;179(11):748–53.
39. Lavaf A, Genden EM, Cesaretti JA, et al. Adjuvant radiotherapy improves overall survival for patients with lymph node-positive head and neck squamous cell carcinoma. Cancer 2008;112(3):535–43.
40. Trotti A, Bellm LA, Epstein JB, et al. Mucositis incidence, severity and associated outcomes in patients with head and neck cancer receiving radiotherapy with or without chemotherapy: a systematic literature review. Radiother Oncol 2003;66(3):253–62.
41. Bernard ME, Kim H, Berhane H, et al. GS-nitroxide (JP4-039)-mediated radioprotection of human Fanconi anemia cell lines. Radiat Res 2011;176(5):603–12.
42. Alter BP, Rosenberg PS, Brody LC. Clinical and molecular features associated with biallelic mutations in FANCD1/BRCA2. J Med Genet 2007;44(1):1–9.

43. Myers K, Davies SM, Harris RE, et al. The clinical phenotype of children with Fanconi anemia caused by biallelic FANCD1/BRCA2 mutations. Pediatr Blood Cancer 2012;58(3):462–5.
44. Wagner JE, Tolar J, Levran O, et al. Germline mutations in BRCA2: shared genetic susceptibility to breast cancer, early onset leukemia, and Fanconi anemia. Blood 2004;103(8):3226–9.
45. Xia B, Dorsman JC, Ameziane N, et al. Fanconi anemia is associated with a defect in the BRCA2 partner PALB2. Nat Genet 2007;39(2):159–61.
46. Reid S, Schindler D, Hanenberg H, et al. Biallelic mutations in PALB2 cause Fanconi anemia subtype FA-N and predispose to childhood cancer. Nat Genet 2007;39(2):162–4.
47. Masserot C, Peffault de Latour R, Rocha V, et al. Head and neck squamous cell carcinoma in 13 patients with Fanconi anemia after hematopoietic stem cell transplantation. Cancer 2008;113(12):3315–22.
48. Rosenberg PS, Socie G, Alter BP, et al. Risk of head and neck squamous cell cancer and death in patients with Fanconi anemia who did and did not receive transplants. Blood 2005;105(1):67–73.
49. Jansisyanont P, Pazoki A, Ord RA. Squamous cell carcinoma of the tongue after bone marrow transplantation in a patient with Fanconi's anemia. J Oral Maxillofac Surg 2000;58(12):1454–7.
50. Guardiola P, Socie G, Li X, et al. Acute graft-versus-host disease in patients with Fanconi anemia or acquired aplastic anemia undergoing bone marrow transplantation from HLA-identical sibling donors: risk factors and influence on outcome. Blood 2004;103(1):73–7.
51. Socie G, Devergie A, Girinski T, et al. Transplantation for Fanconi's anaemia: long-term follow-up of fifty patients transplanted from a sibling donor after low-dose cyclophosphamide and thoraco-abdominal irradiation for conditioning. Br J Haematol 1998;103(1):249–55.
52. Shimada A, Takahashi Y, Muramatsu H, et al. Excellent outcome of allogeneic bone marrow transplantation for Fanconi anemia using fludarabine-based reduced-intensity conditioning regimen. Int J Hematol 2012;95(6):675–9.
53. de la Fuente J, Reiss S, McCloy M, et al. Non-TBI stem cell transplantation protocol for Fanconi anaemia using HLA-compatible sibling and unrelated donors. Bone Marrow Transplant 2003;32(7):653–6.

Evaluation and Therapy

Oral Premalignancy

The Roles of Early Detection and Chemoprevention

Jean-Philippe Foy, MD[a], Chloé Bertolus, MD, PhD[a], William N. William Jr, MD[b], Pierre Saintigny, MD, PhD[b,*]

KEYWORDS

- Head and neck cancer • Chemoprevention
- Head and neck squamous cell carcinoma • Oral squamous cell carcinoma
- Potentially malignant disorder • Biomarkers of risk • Loss of heterozygocity

KEY POINTS

- Premalignancy and chemoprevention studies in head and neck cancer typically focus on the oral cavity.
- Avoiding or cessation of alcohol and smoking, early detection of potentially malignant disorders (PMD) or cancer, and early detection of recurrent and/or second primary tumor form the basis of prevention of oral cancer.
- Oral leukoplakia represents the most frequent PMD.
- Clinical and pathologic parameters are poor predictors of oral cancer development.
- Despite disappointing results of extensive evaluation of retinoids for chemoprevention in the secondary or tertiary prevention setting, analysis of the tissue prospectively collected in those trials allowed identification of molecular biomarkers of risk to develop oral cancer, loss of heterozygosity being the most validated one.
- Improving risk assessment and identification of new targets for chemoprevention represent the main challenges in this field.

INTRODUCTION

Head and neck cancer is the fifth most common cancer worldwide.[1] Males are more affected than females. The incidence is high in some regions of Europe, Hong Kong, India, and Brazil and among African Americans in the Unites States. In the United States, 52,000 Americans develop head and neck cancer annually and 11,500 die from the disease.[2] Most premalignancy and chemoprevention studies have focused

[a] Department of Maxillofacial Surgery, Pitié-Salpêtrière Hospital, 47-83 boulevard de l' Hôpital, Paris 75013, France; [b] Department of Thoracic/Head & Neck Medical Oncology, The University of Texas MD Anderson Cancer Center, 1515 Holcombe Boulevard, Unit 0421, Houston, TX 77030, USA

* Corresponding author.
E-mail address: psaintig@mdanderson.org

Otolaryngol Clin N Am 46 (2013) 579–597
http://dx.doi.org/10.1016/j.otc.2013.04.010
oto.theclinics.com
0030-6665/13/$ – see front matter

Key Abbreviations for Oral Premalignancy	
COX2	Cyclooxygenase-2
EGCG	Epigallocatevhin-3-gallate
EPOC	Erlotinib for Prevention of Oral Cancer
EUROSCAN	The European Study on Chemoprevention with Vitamin A and N-Acetylcysteine
GWAS	Genome-wide association studies
HNSCC	Head and neck squamous cell carcinoma
LOH	Loss of heterozygocity
NSND	Non-smoker non-drinker
OL	Oral leukoplakia
OSCC	Oral squamous cell carcinoma
PMDs	Potentially malignant disorders
SNPs	Single nucleotide polymorphisms
SPTs	Second primary tumors
TKI	Tyrosine kinase inhibitor

on head and neck squamous cell carcinoma (HNSCC) of the oral cavity. The primary risk factors associated with HNSCC cancer include tobacco use and alcohol consumption, with a dose-response relationship and synergistic effect.[3] Betel nut chewing in Asia is an independent risk factor.[4–7] A subgroup of nonsmoker-nondrinker (NSND) patients has been identified: (1) young to middle-aged men with oropharyngeal cancer associated with human papilloma virus infection, and (2) young women with oral tongue cancer, or elderly women with gingival/buccal cancer with no clear etiologic factor.[8–10]

Field cancerization and multistep carcinogenesis form the biologic basis of chemoprevention. The concept of field cancerization refers to the effects of chronic exposure to tobacco and alcohol in patients with or without cancer, with progressive onset of molecular alterations in initially histologically and clinically normal epithelia.[11] It is supported by the identification of similar genetic alterations in matched dysplastic and malignant lesions from the oral cavity.[12] The lateral migration of genetically altered cells through the oral mucosa can form multiple lesions, a phenomenon called clonal cancerization.[13] In other cases, genetic alterations found in dysplastic lesions were not found in matched cancer, providing some evidence that multifocal disease can arise from the development of several genetically altered clones from different initiating events. Finally, the frequent development of synchronous or metachronous second or multiple primaries in the head and neck and/or the lung also supports the concept of field cancerization.[14] The use of molecular markers, such as DNA methylation of individual genes or global gene expression changes, has validated the concept of field cancerization.[15–17]

Califano and colleagues[18] proposed a “Vogelgram” for HNSCC, which linked histologic changes to specific molecular alterations. They proposed that the accumulation of genetic events drives the transformation of squamous mucosa of the head and neck. Histologically, changes occur from normal to hyperkeratosis; hyperplasia; mild, moderate, and severe dysplasia; and carcinoma in situ before becoming invasive carcinoma. Molecular alterations in epithelial cells precede histologic changes. Clinically, the mucosa may appear normal, or appear grossly abnormal with the findings of leukoplakia, erythroplakia, leukoerythroplakia, or lichen planus. Lesions appearing with these characteristics or submucous fibrosis, palatal lesions in reverse smokers, or other less common findings are referred to as potentially malignant disorders (PMDs).[19]

PRIMARY, SECONDARY, AND TERTIARY PREVENTION FOR ORAL SQUAMOUS CELL CARCINOMA

Primary prevention of HNSCC refers to the prevention of cancer by avoiding known carcinogens (**Table 1**).[20] Secondary cancer prevention includes early detection of cancer through screening programs in a population at risk and asymptomatic, as well as prevention of the transformation of PMDs.[21] Tertiary cancer prevention refers to the prevention and early detection of second primary tumors (SPTs) in individuals who have been treated for cancer.[14] Individuals with tobacco and/or smoking history and normal-appearing mucosa, patients with PMDs, and patients who have been treated for HNSCC and at risk for recurrent disease and SPT have increasing risks of developing HNSCC.

Primary Cancer Prevention

Quitting tobacco smoking and alcohol reduces the risk of developing HNSCC. It has been reported that the benefit of smoking cessation is great and can be realized in a relatively short period of time. For example, those who have stopped smoking for 1 to 4 years have a 30% lower risk for developing HNSCC than those who continue smoking. The risk of HNSCC decreases to that of never smokers for those who have quit smoking for 20 years or more. Cessation of alcohol is also associated with a reversal of HNSCC risk after quitting for 20 years or more.[22]

Secondary Cancer Prevention

Diagnostic delay is a recognized challenge in the population of patients diagnosed with oral squamous cell carcinoma (OSCC) and includes patient delay, limited accessibility to the health care system, and health care provider delay.[23] Diagnostic delay has been shown as a risk factor for tumor growth.[24] Diagnostic delays have been associated with decreased survival in some recent studies.[25] Therefore, increased public awareness of early symptoms of PMDs, as well as education of health care providers about these lesions should improve early detection, increase cure rates, and decrease treatment-related morbidity.[23]

Screening for OSCC

Recommendations regarding screening for OSCC have been recently published.[26] Screening by means of examination can detect PMDs and malignant lesions[27]; however, clinical features alone cannot reliably distinguish between malignant and benign or premalignant lesions and the clinician cannot always accurately predict the risk of malignant transformation on the basis of routine biopsy.[28–30] Only one randomized clinical trial has evaluated the effect of screening by means of visual and tactile examination on oral cancer mortality in India.[31]

Table 1
Approaches for primary, secondary, and tertiary prevention of oral cancer

	Definition
Primary prevention	Avoiding known carcinogens
Secondary prevention	Early detection of cancer Prevention of the transformation of potentially malignant disorders
Tertiary prevention	Prevention of second primary tumors or recurrence Early detection of second primary tumors or recurrence

Between 1996 and 2004, of the 96,517 eligible participants in the intervention group, 87,655 (91%) were screened at least once, 53,312 (55%) were screened twice, and 29,102 (30%) were screened 3 times. Of the 5145 individuals who screened positive, 3218 (63%) complied only with referral; 95,356 eligible participants in the control group received standard care. The mortality rate was not significantly different in the intervention group compared with the control group when considering the overall population. Interestingly, men who used tobacco and/or alcohol who underwent screening had a significant mortality rate decrease (hazard ratio 0.57, 95% confidence interval [CI]: 0.35–0.93). This suggests that visual and tactile examination in a high-risk population may improve survival; however, this observation came from a subgroup analysis and needs further validation in a prospective study. Also, the applicability of these findings in Western countries remains to be demonstrated.

Commercially available visualization devices based on tissue reflectance (ViziLite and ViziLite Plus Aila Inc, Colins, CO) and autofluorescence (VELscope, DenMat Holdings LLC, Santa Maria, CA) have been evaluated but there is insufficient evidence that they improve the detection of PMDs beyond that of a conventional visual and tactile examination, and their use can be associated with an increased risk of false-positive findings.[26] In patients with clinically suspicious lesions, the Oral CDx Brush Test (CDx Diagnostics, Suffern, NY) can detect transepithelial cytology of disaggregated cells; however, in these cases, immediate biopsy is indicated, which makes the relevance of this test questionable. The American Dental Association Council on Scientific Affairs recommends that clinicians remain alert for signs of potential malignancy when performing a routine visual and tactile examination in dental patients, especially those with a history of smoking and heavy alcohol use.[26] The expert review panel also recommended that further research is needed to develop reliable, cost-effective screening tests.

Tertiary Prevention

Regular posttreatment follow-up is highly recommended in patients after curative treatment of HNSCC by the National Comprehensive Cancer Network in order to detect the following:

1. Recurrence
2. A second primary cancer in the head and neck or lung
3. Complications of treatment

Another major goal should also include smoking and alcohol cessation. In patients with a smoking history of 20 pack-years or more, the use of low-dose helical computed tomography scanning of the lung can be discussed for screening of a second primary tumor in the lung.[32]

NATURAL HISTORY AND TREATMENT OF ORAL LEUKOPLAKIA, THE MOST FREQUENT PREMALIGNANCY DISEASE

Oral leukoplakia (OL) is clinically defined as a white patch or plaque on the oral mucosa that cannot be removed by scraping and cannot be classified clinically or microscopically as another disease entity. It encompasses a wide variety of histologic findings from hyperkeratosis to hyperplasia and various grades of dysplasia. Three classifications have been proposed to describe the degree of dysplasia.[33–35] To increase the likelihood of agreement between pathologists, a 2-class classification has been recently proposed that will need to be evaluated prospectively[36]:

1. No/questionable/mild: low risk
2. Moderate/severe: high risk

Liu and colleagues[37] studied the usefulness of the binary system of grading dysplasia by reviewing retrospectively 218 Chinese cases of OL with a median follow-up period of 5.3 years. High-risk OL had a hazard ratio of 4.6 (95% CI: 2.36–8.84) to develop OSCC and was an independent risk factor of transformation. The risk was particularly high during the first 2 to 3 years of follow-up.

The natural history of OL remains poorly understood.[28] OL can remain for many years without changing, can regress spontaneously or after cessation of tobacco or alcohol use, and can transform to invasive SCC. The reported rate of malignant transformation has been low in community-based studies in developing countries (0.06% per year) and higher in observational studies in Western countries involving patients followed in hospital-based academic centers (1%–5% per year). Most the studies in the United States found a rate of malignant transformation between 17% and 24% during periods of up to 30 years.[38–40]

No consensus is available for the treatment of OL.[41] Various surgical techniques, including scalpel excision, cryosurgery, and laser surgery, have been reported; however, no prospective studies are available to compare the efficacy and morbidities of treatments, or to test whether excision versus observation decreases the risk of recurrence or the risk of malignant transformation.[42] Kuribayashi and colleagues[43] reported an OL recurrence rate of 15.1% with 2.0% of the patients developing OSCC after scalpel excision. Recurrence occurs more often in patients with positive or close resection margins, and in patients with gingival leukoplakia. When a complete excision of OL is not feasible, cryosurgery is an option.[44] Laser obliteration has been proposed as an alternative to scalpel excision of premalignant lesions.[45] The duration of the interval that the lesion has been present and the size of the lesion are 2 additional factors associated with recurrence and transformation.[46] Recurrence and malignant transformation rates of 29.3% and 1.2%, respectively, have been reported after laser surgery.[47] Laser treatment provides good hemostasis, preservation of oral function, satisfactory wound healing, and can be done repeatedly under local anesthesia, but is associated with delayed epithelial healing. It is important to note that the main disadvantage of cryosurgery and laser surgery is that obliteration of the lesion by these means precludes histologic evaluation of the entire specimen as opposed to a true excision. Therefore, in the case of laser obliteration, the pretreatment biopsy provides only a representative sample of the entire lesion.

The main challenge of surgical excision remains the multifocal nature of "field cancerization" and the notion that normal-appearing mucosa may also have the potential for malignant transformation. To reduce the rate of margins positive for dysplasia and the risk of recurrence and malignant transformation, the use of vital tissue staining is suggested by some investigators.[47] In patients with multiple malignant and premalignant lesions, the use of photodynamic therapy has also been proposed. Grant and colleagues[48] pioneered the method in a small series of patients. In a large series of patients with oral dysplasia from the United Kingdom, a complete response was observed in 81.0% of patients, a partial response or stable disease was observed in 8.0% and 3.4% of patients, respectively, and malignant transformation was observed in 7.5%, with a mean follow-up of 7.3 years.[49] Zhang and colleagues[50] suggested the use of biomarkers (loss of heterozygosity [LOH]) to guide surgical resection of low-grade dysplasia and reduce the risk of transformation, and some investigators propose an association of resection and chemoprevention.[51]

Several studies have shown tobacco cessation was associated with decreased incidence and resolution of OLs.[52–54] Although it is tempting to believe that alcohol and/or tobacco cessation is associated with a decreased risk of malignant transformation, no evidence is available. Patient follow-up strategies are discussed elsewhere but have not been prospectively evaluated.[41] A clinician survey has indicated follow-up regimens of 6 monthly for lesions without dysplasia, 3 monthly for mild/moderate dysplasia, and monthly for severe dysplasia/carcinoma in situ.[42,55] The degree of dysplasia and the anatomic site were the 2 factors influencing the follow-up schema.

CLINICAL, PATHOLOGIC, AND MOLECULAR MARKERS FOR RISK ASSESSMENT

Most of the work in predictive biomarkers has been done in patients with PMDs of the oral cavity, the most frequent being OL (**Table 2**).[19,28,36,41] Clinical factors associated with malignant transformation of OL are the following[28]:

- Female gender
- Long duration of leukoplakia
- Patient age
- Never smokers
- Size greater than 200 mm^2
- Nonhomogeneous type
- Location on the lateral and ventral tongue, floor of mouth, and retromolar trigone and soft palate sites

However, the presence of dysplasia is often the criterion that influences clinical management of OLs. The challenges are that OL without dysplasia may still progress to cancer, that a high interobserver- and intraobserver discordance rate has been reported in the evaluation of dysplasia, that the degree of dysplasia has not always been associated with increased cancer risk, and that OL may be reversible even when dysplasia is identified, irrespective of environmental factors.[36]

Inconsistencies in the value of clinical and pathologic factors to predict the risk of malignant transformation of OL led to the development of biomarkers. However there have been several challenges to biomarker development, including the low prevalence of OL in Western countries, the fact that many lesions are not biopsied, and the rate of malignant transformation per year is generally low, which requires long follow-up periods to be able to derive any conclusion.[55] Chemoprevention studies with retinoids allowed unique prospective collections of biospecimens that led to biomarker development.[56]

Table 2
Clinical, pathologic, and molecular markers of risk to develop oral cancer in patients with oral leukoplakia

Clinical	Pathologic	Biomarkers
Female gender	Degree of dysplasia	LOH
Long duration of leukoplakia		Chromosomal instability or aneuploidy
Older patients		
Never smokers		DeltaNp63 expression
Size >200 mm^2		Podoplanin
Nonhomogeneous type		EGFR expression and gene copy number
Lateral and ventral tongue		
Floor of mouth, and retromolar/ soft palate sites		Gene expression profiles
		Constitutional genetic variations

LOH at various sites is the only molecular marker that has been validated prospectively and appears in bold.

Abbreviations: EGFR, epidermal growth factor receptor; LOH, loss of heterozygosity.

Biomarkers: LOH

The most robust and validated biomarkers were described in LOH studies performed by Mao and colleagues[57] in 1996. OL harboring LOH at 3p14 and/or 9p21 were associated with a risk of developing invasive cancer in 37%, compared with only 6% in lesions without LOH at 3p14 and/or 9p21. These findings were subsequently validated by larger retrospective studies from 2 independent groups.[58–60] OLs at former cancer sites with LOH at 3p and/or 9p were associated with a higher risk of development of invasive cancer (72% at 5 years) compared with leukoplakias without LOH (6% at 5 years).[61]

The presence of LOH at the histologically negative margins of resection in patients with surgically treated HNSCC was a marker of risk of recurrence.[62] Lee and colleagues[40] have shown that the most predictive factors of risk of cancer are the following:

- Degree of dysplasia
- Previous cancer history
- Three of the 5 biomarkers assessed:
  1. Chromosomal polysomy
  2. p53 protein expression
  3. LOH at 3p or 9p

A recent study prospectively validated LOH profiles as risk predictors of progression in a prospective cohort of 296 patients with primary mild/moderate oral dysplasia. High-risk lesions (3p and/or 9p LOH) had a 22.6-fold increase in risk compared with low-risk lesions (3p and/or 9p retention). Addition of another 2 markers (loci on 4q/17p) further improved risk prediction, with 5-year progression rates of 3.1%, 16.3%, and 63.1% for the low-risk, intermediate-risk, and high-risk lesions, respectively.[63]

Biomarkers Beyond LOH

TP63 is involved in the stem cell biology of stratified squamous epithelium, and is a marker of SCC commonly used in clinical practice; the deltaNp63 isoform has oncogenic properties.[64] Podoplanin was shown to promote invasion in different cancer types, and was shown to be associated with poor prognosis in OSCC.[65] We reported that overexpression of podoplanin and deltaNp63 were prevalent in OL and associated with a higher risk to develop OSCC.[64,66] We also reported increased epidermal growth factor receptor (*EGFR*) gene copy number in 41% of OLs, and showed a strong association with the risk of developing OSCC in patients with OLs overexpressing EGFR.[67] In the same cohort of patients, we showed that the vast majority of the genes associated with a high risk or low risk to develop OSCC are upregulated or downregulated in HNSCC versus normal mucosa, respectively.[68] A 25-gene signature improved our prediction of OSCC development over clinical and pathologic biomarkers, including the degree of dysplasia and the expression of deltaNp63 and podoplanin. Validation of those biomarkers in other cohorts of patients is pending.[55] Other markers, such as DNA content and DNA instability, have shown some potential for risk assessment as well, and are reviewed elsewhere.[55,69,70]

Molecular Epidemiology: Genetic Polymorphisms

Molecular epidemiologic studies have identified genetic polymorphisms associated with the risk of HNSCC. Most of studied genes are related to single nucleotide polymorphisms (SNPs) in genes involved in cell cycle control and alcohol and more general metabolism.[71] Recent genome-wide association studies (GWAS) have identified variants in the nicotinic acetylcholine receptor associated with nicotine dependence and lung cancer risk.[72–74] Interestingly, one variant was shown to be associated with the risk of HNSCC and esophagus cancer in women but not in men.[75] This finding was replicated in the International Head and Neck Cancer Epidemiology (INHANCE) consortium cohorts.[76] A particular situation is Fanconi anemia, which represents a population at higher risk of developing HNSCC in the absence of other risk factors.[77] Wu and colleagues[78] identified 6 chromosomal SNPs and 7 mitochondrial SNPs significantly associated with risk of SPT/recurrence from a panel of 9645 SNPs representing 998 cancer-related genes with risk of SPT/recurrence. These studies underscore the potential of incorporating germ-line genetic variation data with clinical and risk factor data in constructing prediction models for clinical outcomes, but will require further validation in independent cohort of patients.

CHEMOPREVENTION: RATIONALE AND RESULTS

Chemoprevention refers to the use of natural or synthetic products to arrest or reverse the process of malignant transformation. The rationale that led to the development of chemoprevention is the failure of conventional therapies, including surgery, radiation, and chemotherapy, to prevent recurrence in a significant number of patients, and the risk of SPT. Systemic administration of chemopreventive agents aims to address the challenge associated with the field cancerization. Different classes of agents have been evaluated so far, including natural products that may act through various mechanisms (green tea), and more targeted agents, such as retinoid receptors ligands, selective cyclooxygenase inhibitors, p53-targeted agents, peroxisome activator receptor gamma (PPARγ) agonists, and EGFR inhibitors.

RETINOIDS

Retinoids are naturally occurring and synthetic vitamin A (retinol) metabolites and analogues that bind to retinoid receptors of the RAR and RXR types, and promote cell differentiation and decrease proliferation and apoptosis. The loss of nuclear RARβ has been described as an early event observed in premalignant dysplastic lesions,[79] which suggested that targeting the retinoid signaling pathway could have merit as a chemopreventive strategy. This led to the extensive evaluation of retinoids in chemoprevention that helped to prove the principle of chemoprevention of oral cancer. However, the toxicity of the retinoids and the rapid reversal of their beneficial effects after stopping these agents prevented them from being considered as a standard of care. However, significant advances in cancer risk assessment were achieved from correlative studies of clinical specimens obtained through these efforts.[56]

Retinoids for OL (Secondary Prevention)

Limitations of most of the studies of retinoids for OL is that the primary end point focused on OL clinical and/or histologic response, which only marginally correlates with long-term oral cancer-free survival,[80] and molecular abnormalities may still persist despite disappearance of the lesion with the chemopreventive agent.[81]

In 1986, Hong and colleagues[82] reported the first double-blind, placebo-controlled trial of high-dose 13-cis retinoic acid (13cRA) (1–2 mg/kg per day for 3 months) in this setting. The clinical response rate and rate of histologic improvement were 67% and 54%, respectively, in the retinoid arm and 10% in the placebo arm. However, mucocutaneous adverse events and hypertriglyceridemia were frequent and severe, requiring dose reductions in half of patients, and more than half of the patients experienced a relapse within 3 months of treatment cessation.

Lippman and colleagues[83] conducted a phase IIb maintenance trial following induction retinoid therapy. In this study, patients with OL were treated with 13cRA 1.5 mg/kg per day for 3 months (induction phase), followed by either low-dose 13cRA (0.5 mg/kg per day) or beta-carotene for 9 months in individuals not experiencing progression of the lesion (maintenance phase). Consistent with the previous trials, 55% and 43% of the patients had a clinical and pathologic response, respectively, to the induction therapy. After the maintenance phase, further clinical response was observed. Severity of adverse events was lower during the maintenance phase, with a more favorable toxicity profile in the beta-carotene arm. However, on long-term follow-up, the incidence of in situ or invasive carcinoma was not different between the 13cRA and beta-carotene groups.[38]

The follow-up trial consisted of 13cRA (0.5 mg/kg per day for 1 year followed by 0.25 mg/kg per day orally for 2 years) versus vitamin A (retinyl palmitate 25,000 IU per day) plus beta-carotene (50 mg per day) for 3 years.[80] During the conduct of the study, data became available with regards to the increased lung cancer incidence and mortality associated with beta-carotene in other ongoing chemoprevention studies.[84,85] As a result, the experimental arm was modified to vitamin A single agent. Vitamin A single agent was associated with a lower 3-month clinical response rate (20%) compared with beta-carotene plus vitamin A (32.5%) and 13cRA (48.1%). The 5-year oral cancer-free survival was similar across the treatment groups (78%–84%), and clinical response at 3 months was only marginally correlated with long-term oral cancer-free survival. This was one of the largest and longest-term studies in OL ever conducted, and it brought into question whether the use of clinical response is a valid end point in trials of PMD oral premalignant lesions. Prevention of OSCC development has been recently considered as a more meaningful end point than clinical or histologic response of the oral premalignant lesions.[86]

Fenretinide is a synthetic retinoid with a more favorable toxicity profile.[87–90] In a randomized study including 170 patients with resected oral premalignant lesions, Chiesa and colleagues[91] demonstrated that, compared with observation, treatment with fenretinide for 12 months was associated with a significant reduction in the risk of relapse 19 months after randomization. The drug was well tolerated. Unfortunately, the trial had to be stopped prematurely because of slow accrual.

Retinoids to Prevent SPTs (Tertiary Prevention)

In 1990, Hong and colleagues[92] reported the results of a randomized trial of 13cRA (50–100 mg/m^2 per day) versus placebo for 12 months in patients with stage I to IV HNSCC who completed definitive therapy showing a lower incidence of SPT compared with placebo.[93] Unfortunately, a large, multicenter, phase III, placebo-controlled trial of 13cRA for 3 years that enrolled 1190 patients with stage I or II HNSCC who completed definitive treatment failed to confirm the results originally reported by Khuri and colleagues.[94] Subsequent analysis of SNPs in the RXRA gene in 450 patients from this trial[95] revealed that more than 70% of patients had the rs3118570 allele and this SNP was associated a 3.33-fold increased risk of developing a second primary. Interestingly, this locus also identified individuals who received benefit from chemoprevention with a significant 38% reduced risk (95% CI, 0.43–0.90), suggesting that a pharmacogenetic approach could help select patients for 13-cRA chemoprevention.

The European Study on Chemoprevention with Vitamin A and N-Acetylcysteine (EUROSCAN) randomized 2592 patients with treated lung (40%) or head and neck (60%) malignancies to receive no intervention, retinyl palmitate, N-acetylcysteine, or both in a 2 × 2 factorial design. Unfortunately, the EUROSCAN failed to show a benefit from either N-acetylcysteine or retinyl palmitate in terms of survival, event-free survival, or second primary tumor rates.[96] Bairati and colleagues[97] randomized 540 patients with stage I or II HNSCC treated with radiation therapy to receive alpha-tocopherol plus beta-carotene versus placebo for 3 years. After enrollment of 156 patients, beta-carotene supplementation was discontinued, given the increased risk of lung cancers observed in other ongoing chemoprevention studies.[84,85] The remaining patients received alpha-tocopherol or placebo. After a median follow-up of 52 months, there was a higher rate of SPTs during the alpha-tocopherol supplementation period, but a lower rate after supplementation was discontinued. After 8 years of follow-up, the proportion of patients free of SPTs was similar between the groups.[97]

CYCLOOXYGENASE INHIBITORS

Cyclooxygenase-2 (COX2) has been shown to be frequently overexpressed in oral dysplasias and HNSCC.[98,99] Preclinical evidence suggests that COX2 inhibitors may have chemopreventive activity.[100,101]

Mulshine and colleagues[102] randomized 57 patients with oral premalignant lesions to receive placebo or a 0.1% oral rinse solution of ketorolac for 30 days. There were no significant differences in either clinical or histologic response. Papadimitrakopoulou and colleagues[103] conducted a pilot, randomized study of celecoxib in individuals with OL. Patients were treated with placebo or celecoxib 100 mg twice daily or 200 mg twice daily for 12 weeks during the blinded phase of the study. Celecoxib was well tolerated, but there were no differences in the response rates among the groups. Those disappointing results and the cardiovascular toxicities observed with COX2 inhibitors in chemoprevention studies of colonic polyps[104] have decreased the enthusiasm for further evaluation of these drugs for HNSCC prevention.

GREEN TEA POLYPHENOLS

The polyphenol (−)-epigallocatechin-3-gallate (EGCG) is the most abundant antioxidant present in green tea extract. Multiple signaling pathways are modulated by EGCG, including inhibition of receptor tyrosine kinases and their downstream pathways, inhibition of NF-kappa-B, and activation of the p53 pathway.[105] Studies evaluating EGCG in the prevention setting have used different preparations with varying amounts of EGCG and other potentially active ingredients. Therefore, results from these studies should be interpreted carefully.

Li and colleagues[106] reported the first placebo-controlled, randomized study of green tea in 59 patients with oral premalignant lesions. Patients assigned to the experimental arm received 760 mg of mixed tea capsules orally four times per day and 10% of mixed tea ointment topically (EGCG content not known). There was a favorable clinical response rate in the experimental arm (37.9%) compared to placebo (10%).

Recently, Tsao and colleagues[107] conducted a placebo-controlled, phase II study of 3 different doses of green tea extract for 12 weeks in 41 patients with OL. Each 350-mg green tea extract capsule contained 13.2% of EGCG. The dose levels were 500 mg/m^2 versus 750 mg/m^2 versus 1000 mg/m^2 3 times per day. The higher doses of the drug were associated with insomnia and nervousness. The response rates in the 2 higher-dose arms combined (58.8%) were significantly better than in the 500 mg/m^2 arm (36.4%), and placebo (18.2%), suggesting a dose-response effect; however, no differences in oral cancer–free survival was observed. This study supports the evaluation of green tea extracts in longer-term trials. Different formulations of green tea extracts[108] and combination with other agents (eg, EGFR inhibitors)[109] are being developed.

P53-TARGETED AGENTS

TP53 inactivating mutations are seen in 47% to 62% of HNSCC and are the most frequent somatic mutations.[110,111] Attempts at restoring p53 function in premalignant lesions, or targeting p53 mutant premalignant cells have been described. ONYX-015 is an attenuated adenovirus cytotoxic to cells with dysfunctional p53-dependant signaling pathways.

Rudin and colleagues[112] enrolled 22 patients with dysplastic lesions of the oral mucosa in a study of a mouthwash of ONYX-015. Histologic resolution of dysplasia occurred in 37% of the patients, but most of the responses were short-lived and baseline p53 expression did not predict for response to ONYX-015.

Li and colleagues[113] evaluated the effects of multipoint intraepithelial injections of a recombinant human adenovirus-p53 in 22 patients with dysplastic OL. After treatment, 100% of the lesions demonstrated positive staining for p53 protein expression, mainly located in the basal and spinous layer of the epithelium. After 24 months of follow-up, 22.7% of the patients had a complete response, 50.0% of the patients had a 20.0% to 70.0% reduction in the size of the OL, 18.2% had stable lesions, and 9.1% developed invasive cancer. Although those results are encouraging, the topical delivery of these agents may not address the remaining mucosa at risk.

THIAZOLIDINEDIONES

Following binding of the ligand to the receptor, PPARγ heterodimerizes with RXR and the complex binds to response elements of target genes. PPARγ agonists have been shown to promote terminal differentiation, inhibition of proliferation, and stimulation of apoptosis in cancer cell lines in vitro. In preclinical animal models, the thiazolidinediones pioglitazone[114] or troglitazone[115] decreased the tongue carcinoma multiplicity and incidence, respectively, compared with placebo. Diabetic patients treated with thiazolidinediones had a reduced incidence of lung[116] and head and neck[117] cancers in retrospective epidemiologic studies, when compared with diabetic patients receiving alternative oral hypoglycemic agents. In a randomized, placebo-controlled, phase II study including 43 patients with OL, treatment with pioglitazone daily for 3 months led to a higher clinical and/or histologic response rate compared with placebo (68% vs 0, respectively).[118] This trial formed the basis for a larger, ongoing, multicenter, phase IIb study of pioglitazone versus placebo in patients with oral premalignant lesions.

EGFR INHIBITORS

The concept of reverse migration, that is, importing agents, targets, and study designs to personalize interventions, and concepts developed in advanced cancer to the setting of cancer prevention, has been recently proposed.[119] The evaluation of EGFR inhibitors for chemoprevention is a good example of the reverse migration concept, given the efficacy of cetuximab-based therapies in locally advanced and metastatic disease.[120] EGFR is overexpressed in malignant, premalignant, and normal-appearing tissues from patients with HNSCC. EGFR expression increases progressively with increasing degree of dysplasia and is markedly elevated in more than 90% of HNSCC.[121,122] We have reported that increased EGFR gene copy number in OLs was frequent and associated with an increased risk of developing OSCC.[67] Erlotinib has been shown to decrease the incidence of OSCC in a chemically induced mouse model.[123] The use of EGFR tyrosine kinase inhibitor (TKI) in the chemoprevention setting is currently being evaluated in the multicenter, Erlotinib for Prevention of Oral Cancer (EPOC) trial activated in 2006, which has completed accrual recently. Patients with OL (with or without a prior history of OSCC) are first evaluated for the presence of LOH that have been shown to be associated with a high risk to develop OSCC.[57,58,61] All patients are followed for development of OSCC, but only the molecularly defined high-risk patients are randomized to receive placebo or erlotinib 150 mg orally daily for 1 year. Unlike most previous studies in oral premalignant lesions, the primary end point of this trial is incidence of OSCC. EPOC is an example of more efficient clinical trial designs for cancer prevention. Because it focuses on a high-risk population based on a molecular profile, it allows for a smaller trial (n = 150 total patients) that is sufficiently powered to detect a possible effect of erlotinib in preventing the development of invasive cancer. Results are eagerly awaited.

SUMMARY

The mutational etiology of HNSCC is diverse and few targetable mutations have been identified, further emphasizing the need to improve prevention strategies.[110,111] Studies of chemopreventive agents have not resulted in the development of an intervention that can be considered as standard of care, but have allowed for the identification of LOH as a biomarker of risk of disease progression. More work is needed to improve our understanding of the natural history of PMDs and to identify key molecular changes that render transformation irreversible. We are entering a new era of chemoprevention, using novel trial designs and agents, focusing on molecularly defined high-risk cohorts, and supported by improved preclinical models.[124] This will hopefully lead to effective strategies to reduce the incidence, morbidity, and mortality from head and neck cancers in the near future.

REFERENCES

1. Parkin DM, Bray F, Ferlay J, et al. Global cancer statistics, 2002. CA Cancer J Clin 2005;55:74–108.
2. Siegel R, Naishadham D, Jemal A. Cancer statistics, 2012. CA Cancer J Clin 2012;62:10–29.
3. Sankaranarayanan R, Masuyer E, Swaminathan R, et al. Head and neck cancer: a global perspective on epidemiology and prognosis. Anticancer Res 1998;18:4779–86.
4. Jeng JH, Chang MC, Hahn LJ. Role of areca nut in betel quid-associated chemical carcinogenesis: current awareness and future perspectives. Oral Oncol 2001;37:477–92.
5. Lee KW, Kuo WR, Tsai SM, et al. Different impact from betel quid, alcohol and cigarette: risk factors for pharyngeal and laryngeal cancer. Int J Cancer 2005;117:831–6.
6. Goldenberg D, Lee J, Koch WM, et al. Habitual risk factors for head and neck cancer. Otolaryngol Head Neck Surg 2004;131:986–93.
7. Thomas SJ, Bain CJ, Battistutta D, et al. Betel quid not containing tobacco and oral cancer: a report on a case-control study in Papua New Guinea and a meta-analysis of current evidence. Int J Cancer 2007;120:1318–23.
8. Dahlstrom KR, Little JA, Zafereo ME, et al. Squamous cell carcinoma of the head and neck in never smoker-never drinkers: a descriptive epidemiologic study. Head Neck 2008;30:75–84.
9. Marur S, D'Souza G, Westra WH, et al. HPV-associated head and neck cancer: a virus-related cancer epidemic. Lancet Oncol 2010;11:781–9.

10. Bertolus C, Goudot P, Gessain A, et al. Clinical relevance of systematic human papillomavirus (HPV) diagnosis in oral squamous cell carcinoma. Infect Agent Cancer 2012;7:13.
11. Slaughter DP, Southwick HW, Smejkal W. Field cancerization in oral stratified squamous epithelium; clinical implications of multicentric origin. Cancer 1953; 6:963–8.
12. Partridge M, Emilion G, Pateromichelakis S, et al. Field cancerisation of the oral cavity: comparison of the spectrum of molecular alterations in cases presenting with both dysplastic and malignant lesions. Oral Oncol 1997;33:332–7.
13. Partridge M, Pateromichelakis S, Phillips E, et al. Profiling clonality and progression in multiple premalignant and malignant oral lesions identifies a subgroup of cases with a distinct presentation of squamous cell carcinoma. Clin Cancer Res 2001;7:1860–6.
14. Strong MS, Incze J, Vaughan CW. Field cancerization in the aerodigestive tract—its etiology, manifestation, and significance. J Otolaryngol 1984;13:1–6.
15. Bhutani M, Pathak AK, Fan YH, et al. Oral epithelium as a surrogate tissue for assessing smoking-induced molecular alterations in the lungs. Cancer Prev Res (Phila) 2008;1:39–44.
16. Belinsky SA, Klinge DM, Dekker JD, et al. Gene promoter methylation in plasma and sputum increases with lung cancer risk. Clin Cancer Res 2005;11:6505–11.
17. Gower AC, Steiling K, Brothers JF 2nd, et al. Transcriptomic studies of the airway field of injury associated with smoking-related lung disease. Proc Am Thorac Soc 2011;8:173–9.
18. Califano J, van der Riet P, Westra W, et al. Genetic progression model for head and neck cancer: implications for field cancerization. Cancer Res 1996;56:2488–92.
19. Warnakulasuriya S, Johnson NW, van der Waal I. Nomenclature and classification of potentially malignant disorders of the oral mucosa. J Oral Pathol Med 2007;36:575–80.
20. Blackburn EH. Highlighting the science of cancer prevention. Cancer Prev Res (Phila) 2010;3:393.
21. Smith RA, Cokkinides V, Brawley OW. Cancer screening in the United States, 2012: a review of current American Cancer Society guidelines and current issues in cancer screening. CA Cancer J Clin 2012;62(2):129–42.
22. Marron M, Boffetta P, Zhang ZF, et al. Cessation of alcohol drinking, tobacco smoking and the reversal of head and neck cancer risk. Int J Epidemiol 2010; 39:182–96.
23. Gomez I, Warnakulasuriya S, Varela-Centelles PI, et al. Is early diagnosis of oral cancer a feasible objective? Who is to blame for diagnostic delay? Oral Dis 2010;16:333–42.
24. Gomez I, Seoane J, Varela-Centelles P, et al. Is diagnostic delay related to advanced-stage oral cancer? A meta-analysis. Eur J Oral Sci 2009;117:541–6.
25. Peacock ZS, Pogrel MA, Schmidt BL. Exploring the reasons for delay in treatment of oral cancer. J Am Dent Assoc 2008;139:1346–52.
26. Rethman MP, Carpenter W, Cohen EE, et al. Evidence-based clinical recommendations regarding screening for oral squamous cell carcinomas. J Am Dent Assoc 2010;141:509–20.
27. Brocklehurst P, Kujan O, Glenny AM, et al. Screening programmes for the early detection and prevention of oral cancer. Cochrane Database Syst Rev 2010;(11):CD004150.
28. Napier SS, Speight PM. Natural history of potentially malignant oral lesions and conditions: an overview of the literature. J Oral Pathol Med 2008;37:1–10.

29. Kujan O, Oliver RJ, Khattab A, et al. Evaluation of a new binary system of grading oral epithelial dysplasia for prediction of malignant transformation. Oral Oncol 2006;42:987–93.
30. Mehanna HM, Rattay T, Smith J, et al. Treatment and follow-up of oral dysplasia—a systematic review and meta-analysis. Head Neck 2009;31: 1600–9.
31. Sankaranarayanan R, Ramadas K, Thomas G, et al. Effect of screening on oral cancer mortality in Kerala, India: a cluster-randomised controlled trial. Lancet 2005;365:1927–33.
32. Aberle DR, Adams AM, Berg CD, et al. Reduced lung-cancer mortality with low-dose computed tomographic screening. N Engl J Med 2011;365:395–409.
33. Barnes L, Eveson JW, Reichart P, et al, editors. World Health Organization classification of tumours: pathology and genetics of head and neck tumours. International Agency for Research on Cancer (IARC). Lyon (France): IARC Press; 2005. p. 177–80.
34. Hellquist H, Cardesa A, Gale N, et al. Criteria for grading in the Ljubljana classification of epithelial hyperplastic laryngeal lesions. A study by members of the Working Group on Epithelial Hyperplastic Laryngeal Lesions of the European Society of Pathology. Histopathology 1999;34:226–33.
35. Kuffer R, Lombardi T. Premalignant lesions of the oral mucosa. A discussion about the place of oral intraepithelial neoplasia (OIN). Oral Oncol 2002;38: 125–30.
36. Warnakulasuriya S, Reibel J, Bouquot J, et al. Oral epithelial dysplasia classification systems: predictive value, utility, weaknesses and scope for improvement. J Oral Pathol Med 2008;37:127–33.
37. Liu W, Wang YF, Zhou HW, et al. Malignant transformation of oral leukoplakia: a retrospective cohort study of 218 Chinese patients. BMC Cancer 2010;10:685.
38. Papadimitrakopoulou VA, Hong WK, Lee JS, et al. Low-dose isotretinoin versus beta-carotene to prevent oral carcinogenesis: long-term follow-up. J Natl Cancer Inst 1997;89:257–8.
39. Silverman S Jr, Gorsky M, Lozada F. Oral leukoplakia and malignant transformation. A follow-up study of 257 patients. Cancer 1984;53:563–8.
40. Lee JJ, Hong WK, Hittelman WN, et al. Predicting cancer development in oral leukoplakia: ten years of translational research. Clin Cancer Res 2000;6: 1702–10.
41. Lodi G, Porter S. Management of potentially malignant disorders: evidence and critique. J Oral Pathol Med 2008;37:63–9.
42. Marley JJ, Linden GJ, Cowan CG, et al. A comparison of the management of potentially malignant oral mucosal lesions by oral medicine practitioners and oral and maxillofacial surgeons in the UK. J Oral Pathol Med 1998;27:489–95.
43. Kuribayashi Y, Tsushima F, Sato M, et al. Recurrence patterns of oral leukoplakia after curative surgical resection: important factors that predict the risk of recurrence and malignancy. J Oral Pathol Med 2012;41:682–8.
44. Hausamen JE. The basis, technique and indication for cryosurgery in tumours of the oral cavity and face. J Maxillofac Surg 1975;3:41–9.
45. Flynn MB, White M, Tabah RJ. Use of carbon dioxide laser for the treatment of premalignant lesions of the oral mucosa. J Surg Oncol 1988;37:232–4.
46. Chiesa F, Boracchi P, Tradati N, et al. Risk of preneoplastic and neoplastic events in operated oral leukoplakias. Eur J Cancer B Oral Oncol 1993;29B:23–8.
47. Ishii J, Fujita K, Komori T. Laser surgery as a treatment for oral leukoplakia. Oral Oncol 2003;39:759–69.

48. Grant WE, Hopper C, Speight PM, et al. Photodynamic therapy of malignant and premalignant lesions in patients with 'field cancerization' of the oral cavity. J Laryngol Otol 1993;107:1140–5.
49. Jerjes W, Upile T, Hamdoon Z, et al. Photodynamic therapy outcome for oral dysplasia. Lasers Surg Med 2011;43:192–9.
50. Zhang L, Poh CF, Lam WL, et al. Impact of localized treatment in reducing risk of progression of low-grade oral dysplasia: molecular evidence of incomplete resection. Oral Oncol 2001;37:505–12.
51. De Palo G, Veronesi U, Marubini E, et al. Controlled clinical trials with fenretinide in breast cancer, basal cell carcinoma and oral leukoplakia. J Cell Biochem Suppl 1995;22:11–7.
52. Gupta PC, Murti PR, Bhonsle RB, et al. Effect of cessation of tobacco use on the incidence of oral mucosal lesions in a 10-yr follow-up study of 12,212 users. Oral Dis 1995;1:54–8.
53. Roed-Petersen B. Effect on oral leukoplakia of reducing or ceasing tobacco smoking. Acta Derm Venereol 1982;62:164–7.
54. Martin GC, Brown JP, Eifler CW, et al. Oral leukoplakia status six weeks after cessation of smokeless tobacco use. J Am Dent Assoc 1999;130:945–54.
55. Nankivell P, Mehanna H. Oral dysplasia: biomarkers, treatment, and follow-up. Curr Oncol Rep 2011;13:145–52.
56. William WN Jr. Oral premalignant lesions: any progress with systemic therapies? Curr Opin Oncol 2012;24:205–10.
57. Mao L, Lee JS, Fan YH, et al. Frequent microsatellite alterations at chromosomes 9p21 and 3p14 in oral premalignant lesions and their value in cancer risk assessment. Nat Med 1996;2:682–5.
58. Rosin MP, Cheng X, Poh C, et al. Use of allelic loss to predict malignant risk for low-grade oral epithelial dysplasia. Clin Cancer Res 2000;6:357–62.
59. Partridge M, Emilion G, Pateromichelakis S, et al. Allelic imbalance at chromosomal loci implicated in the pathogenesis of oral precancer, cumulative loss and its relationship with progression to cancer. Oral Oncol 1998;34:77–83.
60. Partridge M, Pateromichelakis S, Phillips E, et al. A case-control study confirms that microsatellite assay can identify patients at risk of developing oral squamous cell carcinoma within a field of cancerization. Cancer Res 2000;60: 3893–8.
61. Rosin MP, Lam WL, Poh C, et al. 3p14 and 9p21 loss is a simple tool for predicting second oral malignancy at previously treated oral cancer sites. Cancer Res 2002;62:6447–50.
62. Sardi I, Franchi A, Ferriero G, et al. Prediction of recurrence by microsatellite analysis in head and neck cancer. Genes Chromosomes Cancer 2000;29: 201–6.
63. Zhang L, Poh CF, Williams M, et al. Loss of heterozygosity (LOH) profiles–validated risk predictors for progression to oral cancer. Cancer Prev Res (Phila) 2012;5:1081–9.
64. Saintigny P, El-Naggar AK, Papadimitrakopoulou V, et al. DeltaNp63 overexpression, alone and in combination with other biomarkers, predicts the development of oral cancer in patients with leukoplakia. Clin Cancer Res 2009;15:6284–91.
65. Yuan P, Temam S, El-Naggar A, et al. Overexpression of podoplanin in oral cancer and its association with poor clinical outcome. Cancer 2006;107:563–9.
66. Kawaguchi H, El-Naggar AK, Papadimitrakopoulou V, et al. Podoplanin: a novel marker for oral cancer risk in patients with oral premalignancy. J Clin Oncol 2008;26:354–60.

67. Taoudi Benchekroun M, Saintigny P, Thomas SM, et al. Epidermal growth factor receptor expression and gene copy number in the risk of oral cancer. Cancer Prev Res (Phila) 2010;3:800–9.
68. Saintigny P, Zhang L, Fan YH, et al. Gene expression profiling predicts the development of oral cancer. Cancer Prev Res (Phila) 2011;4:218–29.
69. Hogmo A, Munck-Wikland E, Kuylenstierna R, et al. Nuclear DNA content and p53 immunostaining in metachronous preneoplastic lesions and subsequent carcinomas of the oral cavity. Head Neck 1996;18:433–40.
70. Bergshoeff VE, Hopman AH, Zwijnenberg IR, et al. Chromosome instability in resection margins predicts recurrence of oral squamous cell carcinoma. J Pathol 2008;215:347–8.
71. Cadoni G, Boccia S, Petrelli L, et al. A review of genetic epidemiology of head and neck cancer related to polymorphisms in metabolic genes, cell cycle control and alcohol metabolism. Acta Otorhinolaryngol Ital 2012;32:1–11.
72. Hung RJ, McKay JD, Gaborieau V, et al. A susceptibility locus for lung cancer maps to nicotinic acetylcholine receptor subunit genes on 15q25. Nature 2008;452:633–7.
73. Thorgeirsson TE, Geller F, Sulem P, et al. A variant associated with nicotine dependence, lung cancer and peripheral arterial disease. Nature 2008;452:638–42.
74. Amos CI, Wu X, Broderick P, et al. Genome-wide association scan of tag SNPs identifies a susceptibility locus for lung cancer at 15q25.1. Nat Genet 2008;40:616–22.
75. Lips EH, Gaborieau V, McKay JD, et al. Association between a 15q25 gene variant, smoking quantity and tobacco-related cancers among 17 000 individuals. Int J Epidemiol 2010;39:563–77.
76. Chen D, Truong T, Gaborieau V, et al. A sex-specific association between a 15q25 variant and upper aerodigestive tract cancers. Cancer Epidemiol Biomarkers Prev 2011;20:658–64.
77. Kutler DI, Singh B, Satagopan J, et al. A 20-year perspective on the International Fanconi Anemia Registry (IFAR). Blood 2003;101:1249–56.
78. Wu X, Spitz MR, Lee JJ, et al. Novel susceptibility loci for second primary tumors/recurrence in head and neck cancer patients: large-scale evaluation of genetic variants. Cancer Prev Res (Phila) 2009;2:617–24.
79. Xu XC, Ro JY, Lee JS, et al. Differential expression of nuclear retinoid receptors in normal, premalignant, and malignant head and neck tissues. Cancer Res 1994;54:3580–7.
80. Papadimitrakopoulou VA, Lee JJ, William WN Jr, et al. Randomized trial of 13-cis retinoic acid compared with retinyl palmitate with or without beta-carotene in oral premalignancy. J Clin Oncol 2009;27:599–604.
81. Mao L, El-Naggar AK, Papadimitrakopoulou V, et al. Phenotype and genotype of advanced premalignant head and neck lesions after chemopreventive therapy. J Natl Cancer Inst 1998;90:1545–51.
82. Hong WK, Endicott J, Itri LM, et al. 13-cis-retinoic acid in the treatment of oral leukoplakia. N Engl J Med 1986;315:1501–5.
83. Lippman SM, Batsakis JG, Toth BB, et al. Comparison of low-dose isotretinoin with beta carotene to prevent oral carcinogenesis. N Engl J Med 1993;328:15–20.
84. The effect of vitamin E and beta carotene on the incidence of lung cancer and other cancers in male smokers. The Alpha-Tocopherol, Beta Carotene Cancer Prevention Study Group. N Engl J Med 1994;330:1029–35.

85. Omenn GS, Goodman GE, Thornquist MD, et al. Effects of a combination of beta carotene and vitamin A on lung cancer and cardiovascular disease. N Engl J Med 1996;334:1150–5.
86. William WN Jr, Heymach JV, Kim ES, et al. Molecular targets for cancer chemoprevention. Nat Rev Drug Discov 2009;8:213–25.
87. Clifford JL, Menter DG, Wang M, et al. Retinoid receptor-dependent and -independent effects of N-(4-hydroxyphenyl)retinamide in F9 embryonal carcinoma cells. Cancer Res 1999;59:14–8.
88. Clifford JL, Sabichi AL, Zou C, et al. Effects of novel phenylretinamides on cell growth and apoptosis in bladder cancer. Cancer Epidemiol Biomarkers Prev 2001;10:391–5.
89. Sun SY, Yue P, Kelloff GJ, et al. Identification of retinamides that are more potent than N-(4-hydroxyphenyl)retinamide in inhibiting growth and inducing apoptosis of human head and neck and lung cancer cells. Cancer Epidemiol Biomarkers Prev 2001;10:595–601.
90. Ponzoni M, Bocca P, Chiesa V, et al. Differential effects of N-(4-hydroxyphenyl) retinamide and retinoic acid on neuroblastoma cells: apoptosis versus differentiation. Cancer Res 1995;55:853–61.
91. Chiesa F, Tradati N, Grigolato R, et al. Randomized trial of fenretinide (4-HPR) to prevent recurrences, new localizations and carcinomas in patients operated on for oral leukoplakia: long-term results. Int J Cancer 2005;115:625–9.
92. Hong WK, Lippman SM, Itri LM, et al. Prevention of second primary tumors with isotretinoin in squamous-cell carcinoma of the head and neck. N Engl J Med 1990;323:795–801.
93. Benner SE, Pajak TF, Lippman SM, et al. Prevention of second primary tumors with isotretinoin in patients with squamous cell carcinoma of the head and neck: long-term follow-up. J Natl Cancer Inst 1994;86:140–1.
94. Khuri FR, Lee JJ, Lippman SM, et al. Randomized phase III trial of low-dose isotretinoin for prevention of second primary tumors in stage I and II head and neck cancer patients. J Natl Cancer Inst 2006;98:441–50.
95. Lee JJ, Wu X, Hildebrandt MA, et al. Global assessment of genetic variation influencing response to retinoid chemoprevention in head and neck cancer patients. Cancer Prev Res (Phila) 2011;4:185–93.
96. van Zandwijk N, Dalesio O, Pastorino U, et al. EUROSCAN, a randomized trial of vitamin A and N-acetylcysteine in patients with head and neck cancer or lung cancer. For the European Organization for Research and Treatment of Cancer Head and Neck and Lung Cancer Cooperative Groups. J Natl Cancer Inst 2000;92:977–86.
97. Bairati I, Meyer F, Gelinas M, et al. A randomized trial of antioxidant vitamins to prevent second primary cancers in head and neck cancer patients. J Natl Cancer Inst 2005;97:481–8.
98. Nathan CO, Leskov IL, Lin M, et al. COX-2 expression in dysplasia of the head and neck: correlation with eIF4E. Cancer 2001;92:1888–95.
99. Saba NF, Choi M, Muller S, et al. Role of cyclooxygenase-2 in tumor progression and survival of head and neck squamous cell carcinoma. Cancer Prev Res (Phila) 2009;2:823–9.
100. Lyons JG, Patel V, Roue NC, et al. Snail up-regulates proinflammatory mediators and inhibits differentiation in oral keratinocytes. Cancer Res 2008;68:4525–30.
101. Tanaka T, Nishikawa A, Mori Y, et al. Inhibitory effects of non-steroidal anti-inflammatory drugs, piroxicam and indomethacin on 4-nitroquinoline 1-oxide-induced tongue carcinogenesis in male ACI/N rats. Cancer Lett 1989;48:177–82.

102. Mulshine JL, Atkinson JC, Greer RO, et al. Randomized, double-blind, placebo-controlled phase IIb trial of the cyclooxygenase inhibitor ketorolac as an oral rinse in oropharyngeal leukoplakia. Clin Cancer Res 2004;10:1565–73.
103. Papadimitrakopoulou VA, William WN Jr, Dannenberg AJ, et al. Pilot randomized phase II study of celecoxib in oral premalignant lesions. Clin Cancer Res 2008; 14:2095–101.
104. Bertagnolli MM. Chemoprevention of colorectal cancer with cyclooxygenase-2 inhibitors: two steps forward, one step back. Lancet Oncol 2007;8: 439–43.
105. Kim JW, Amin AR, Shin DM. Chemoprevention of head and neck cancer with green tea polyphenols. Cancer Prev Res (Phila) 2010;3:900–9.
106. Li N, Sun Z, Han C, et al. The chemopreventive effects of tea on human oral precancerous mucosa lesions. Proc Soc Exp Biol Med 1999;220:218–24.
107. Tsao AS, Liu D, Martin J, et al. Phase II randomized, placebo-controlled trial of green tea extract in patients with high-risk oral premalignant lesions. Cancer Prev Res (Phila) 2009;2:931–41.
108. Siddiqui IA, Adhami VM, Bharali DJ, et al. Introducing nanochemoprevention as a novel approach for cancer control: proof of principle with green tea polyphenol epigallocatechin-3-gallate. Cancer Res 2009;69:1712–6.
109. Zhang X, Zhang H, Tighiouart M, et al. Synergistic inhibition of head and neck tumor growth by green tea (−)-epigallocatechin-3-gallate and EGFR tyrosine kinase inhibitor. Int J Cancer 2008;123:1005–14.
110. Agrawal N, Frederick MJ, Pickering CR, et al. Exome sequencing of head and neck squamous cell carcinoma reveals inactivating mutations in NOTCH1. Science 2011;333:1154–7.
111. Stransky N, Egloff AM, Tward AD, et al. The mutational landscape of head and neck squamous cell carcinoma. Science 2011;333:1157–60.
112. Rudin CM, Cohen EE, Papadimitrakopoulou VA, et al. An attenuated adenovirus, ONYX-015, as mouthwash therapy for premalignant oral dysplasia. J Clin Oncol 2003;21:4546–52.
113. Li Y, Li LJ, Zhang ST, et al. In vitro and clinical studies of gene therapy with recombinant human adenovirus-p53 injection for oral leukoplakia. Clin Cancer Res 2009;15:6724–31.
114. Suzuki R, Kohno H, Suzui M, et al. An animal model for the rapid induction of tongue neoplasms in human c-Ha-ras proto-oncogene transgenic rats by 4-nitroquinoline 1-oxide: its potential use for preclinical chemoprevention studies. Carcinogenesis 2006;27:619–30.
115. Yoshida K, Hirose Y, Tanaka T, et al. Inhibitory effects of troglitazone, a peroxisome proliferator-activated receptor gamma ligand, in rat tongue carcinogenesis initiated with 4-nitroquinoline 1-oxide. Cancer Sci 2003;94:365–71.
116. Govindarajan R, Ratnasinghe L, Simmons DL, et al. Thiazolidinediones and the risk of lung, prostate, and colon cancer in patients with diabetes. J Clin Oncol 2007;25:1476–81.
117. Govindarajan R, Siegel ER, Simmons DL, et al. Thiazolidinedione (TZD) exposure and risk of squamous cell carcinoma of head and neck (SCCHN) (2007 ASCO Annual Meeting Proceedings Part I). J Clin Oncol 2007;25 [abstract 1511].
118. Rhodus N, Rohrer M, Pambuccian S, et al. Phase IIa Chemoprevention Clinical Trial of Pioglitazone for Oral Leukoplakia. J Dent Res 2011;90(A) [abstract 945].
119. Gold KA, Kim ES, Lee JJ, et al. The BATTLE to personalize lung cancer prevention through reverse migration. Cancer Prev Res (Phila) 2011;4:962–72.

120. William WN Jr, Kim ES, Herbst RS. Cetuximab therapy for patients with advanced squamous cell carcinomas of the head and neck. Nat Clin Pract Oncol 2009;6:132–3.
121. Grandis JR, Tweardy DJ. Elevated levels of transforming growth factor alpha and epidermal growth factor receptor messenger RNA are early markers of carcinogenesis in head and neck cancer. Cancer Res 1993;53:3579–84.
122. Temam S, Kawaguchi H, El-Naggar AK, et al. Epidermal growth factor receptor copy number alterations correlate with poor clinical outcome in patients with head and neck squamous cancer. J Clin Oncol 2007;25:2164–70.
123. Leeman-Neill RJ, Seethala RR, Singh SV, et al. Inhibition of EGFR-STAT3 signaling with erlotinib prevents carcinogenesis in a chemically-induced mouse model of oral squamous cell carcinoma. Cancer Prev Res (Phila) 2011;4:230–7.
124. Lu SL, Herrington H, Wang XJ. Mouse models for human head and neck squamous cell carcinomas. Head Neck 2006;28:945–54.

Evaluation and Staging of Squamous Cell Carcinoma of the Oral Cavity and Oropharynx

Limitations Despite Technological Breakthroughs

Mark E. Zafereo, MD

KEYWORDS

- Squamous cell carcinoma oral cavity • Squamous cell carcinoma oropharynx
- Evaluation • Diagnosis • Staging • Prognosis • Sentinel lymph node biopsy
- Human papillomavirus • Smoking • PET

KEY POINTS

- Squamous cell carcinoma of the oral cavity (SCCOC) and squamous cell carcinoma of the oropharynx (SCCOP) represent two distinct disease entities.
- A clinical profile has emerged for the patient with an human papillomavirus (HPV)–associated SCCOP as typically a middle-aged, white male, without heavy tobacco history.
- The American Joint Committee on Cancer tumor, node, metastasis staging system has useful prognostic significance for SCCOC, but it does not include important prognostic histopathologic factors including tumor thickness, perineural invasion, lymphatic invasion, and extracapsular extension.
- Most patients with SCCOP in Western countries have HPV-associated tumors; tumor HPV status is one of the most important prognostic factors for these patients. Smoking status is emerging as an important prognostic factor for HPV-driven SCCOP, independent of tumor HPV status.
- For SCCOP, tumor HPV status and smoking status may have greater prognostic significance than traditional anatomic TNM staging; it is likely that future iterations of the AJCC TNM staging system will incorporate tumor HPV and/or p16 status, and perhaps smoking history.
- For patients with SCCOC with risk factors for occult lymph node metastases, the gold standard for treatment of the clinically node-negative neck remains an elective neck dissection. However, sentinel lymph node biopsy has been shown to be an effective clinical staging tool that may obviate an elective neck dissection in some patients.
- FDG-PET/CT imaging is useful in select patients with unknown primary squamous cell carcinoma of the head and neck (SCCHN), and in some patients with advanced SCCHN at high risk for distant metastases.

Disclosures: The author has no conflicts of interests to disclose.
Department of Head and Neck Surgery, MD Anderson Cancer Center, 1515 Holcombe Boulevard, Unit 1445, Houston, TX 77030, USA
E-mail address: mzafereo@mdanderson.org

Otolaryngol Clin N Am 46 (2013) 599–613
http://dx.doi.org/10.1016/j.otc.2013.04.011
oto.theclinics.com
0030-6665/13/$ – see front matter

Abbreviations	
FNA	Fine needle aspiration biopsy
FDG-PET/CT	Fluorodeoxyglucose positron emission tomography/computed tomography
HPV	Human papillomavirus
SCCOC	Squamous cell carcinoma of oral cavity
SCCOP	Squamous cell carcinoma of oropharynx
SNB	Sentinel lymph node biopsy
TROG	Trans Tasman Radiation Oncology Group

INTRODUCTION

As discussed elsewhere in this issue, it has become increasingly clear over the last several decades that squamous cell carcinoma (SCC) of the oral cavity (SCCOC) and SCC of the oropharynx (SCCOP) generally represent two different disease entities, with differing causes, prognosis, and response to treatment. The emergence and recognition of human papillomavirus (HPV) as the causative agent in most SCCOP over the last 2 decades necessitates separate discussion of SCCOC and SCCOP in terms of evaluation and staging. This article discusses evaluation and staging of these two distinct diseases, including a discussion of 2 novel diagnostic approaches: sentinel lymph node biopsy (SLNB) and fluorodeoxyglucose (FDG) positron emission tomography (PET)/computed tomography (CT) imaging.

DIAGNOSIS AND EVALUATION OF SCCOC

SCCOC generally presents with a painful oral lesion, although other presenting symptoms include a painful or bleeding ulcer, loose teeth or ill-fitting dentures, trismus (caused by pterygoid involvement), hypoesthesia (caused by perineural involvement), or otalgia (referred pain from the ninth and 10th cranial nerves). Evaluation of SCCOC should include a thorough history and physical examination, dental evaluation, and cross-sectional imaging (CT or magnetic resonance imaging [MRI]). Tissue biopsy, which can generally be performed with local anesthesia in the clinic, is essential to both confirm the suspected diagnosis and to provide prognostic information such as tumor thickness and perineural invasion, which further direct diagnostic evaluation and treatment. A good history should take into account the traditional risk factors for SCCOC (including tobacco, alcohol, and betel nut or pan chewing), family history, and a thorough dental history including a history of caries, extractions, and dentures. Multiple independent studies suggest that HPV does not often play a role in the pathogenesis of SCCOC, with an incidence of high-risk HPV type 16 identified in less than 3% of cases.[1,2]

A chest radiograph should routinely be performed to assess for distant metastases or second primary malignancies. CT scan is the typical cross-sectional imaging modality used for SCCOC, because it allows the best assessment of extent of both soft tissue and bony involvement. MRI may be used in conjunction or in place of CT, and can be beneficial in cases in which there is suspected perineural invasion along the inferior alveolar or greater palatine nerves, in cases in which dental amalgams result in CT artifact, and in cases in which better delineation of potential base of tongue invasion is desired.[3] Ultrasound with fine-needle aspiration (FNA) biopsy can be used to evaluate lymph nodes that are equivocal on cross-sectional imaging. The role of FDG-PET/CT in the initial evaluation and staging of SCCOC and SCCOP is discussed later.

DIAGNOSIS AND EVALUATION OF SCCOP

Considerations in the diagnosis and evaluation of SCCOP have changed over the last decade because of the emergence of HPV, which now may account for greater than 80% of SCCOP in Western countries.[4,5] A clinical profile has emerged for the patient with an HPV-associated SCCOP as typically a middle-aged, white male, without a heavy tobacco history.[6–9] Patients with HPV-associated SCCOP often present with a painless neck mass that is often cystic on cross-sectional imaging and can be easily confused and misdiagnosed as a second branchial cleft cyst (**Fig. 1**).[10,11] Often these patients are otherwise asymptomatic, with a small or occult tonsil or base of tongue painless tumor. Therefore, a middle-aged or elderly person who presents with a cystic neck mass in levels 2 or 3 of the neck should be considered an SCCOP until proved otherwise. Initial diagnostic evaluation of a middle-aged or elderly person with a cystic neck mass should include a thorough head and neck examination, focusing on the lymphoepithelial tissue of the tonsils and base of tongue; cross-sectional imaging; and FNA of the neck mass, with or without ultrasound guidance. If the all of these studies are negative for evidence of SCCOP, FNA biopsy may be repeated, or the patient may be taken to the operating room for an examination under anesthesia with panendoscopy and tonsillectomy. If an examination under anesthesia and frozen section analysis fail to reveal an SCCOP, an excisional biopsy of the neck mass may be performed. However, frozen section should be performed, and the surgeon should be prepared to complete the neck dissection if frozen section analysis of the neck mass confirms SCC.

Patients with SCCOP, or SCC found in a neck lymph node without obvious primary site of disease, should have the FNA or open biopsy specimen evaluated for HPV. In many academic centers, HPV testing is performed by a combination of p16 protein immunohistochemistry (highly sensitive, but not highly specific for HPV) and HPV DNA detection by in situ hybridization (highly specific, but not highly sensitive for HPV).[12] Polymerase chain reaction (PCR)–based amplification can be substituted

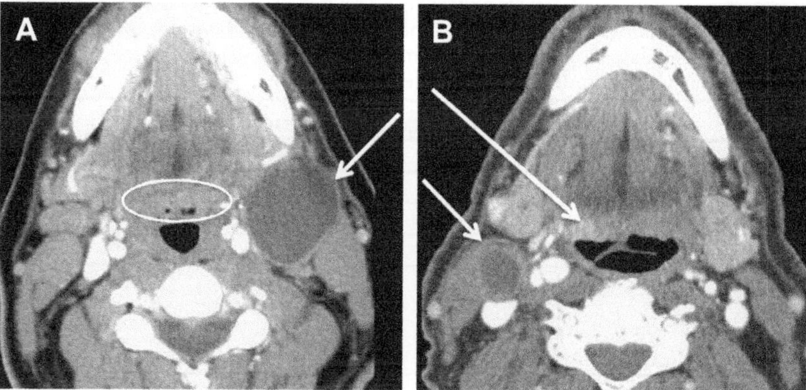

Fig. 1. Second branchial cleft cyst and an HPV-associated SCCOP. (*A*) Contrast-enhanced CT in a patient with a palpable asymptomatic left neck mass (*arrow*), which was later biopsy proved to be a branchial cleft cyst, with incidental prominent lymphoid tissue of the base of tongue (*circle*). (*B*) Contrast-enhanced CT in a patient with a palpable asymptomatic right neck mass (*arrows*). Enhancing lymphoid tissue in the right base of tongue was biopsied and proved to be HPV-positive SCCOP in a patient with a right level 2 cystic lymph node metastasis. (*From* Corey AS, Hudgins PA. Radiographic imaging of human papillomavirus related carcinomas of the oropharynx. Head Neck Pathol 2012;6:S38; with permission.)

for in situ hybridization as a method of HPV detection. In some cases, if there is strong and uniform p16 protein immunohistochemistry, the known presence of an oropharyngeal tumor, and typical HPV histomorphology, HPV confirmatory DNA detection with in situ hybridization or PCR-based amplification can be omitted.[12,13] Cytopathologic specimens from FNA in patients with a potential SCCOP should ideally be handled by a histopathology laboratory familiar with HPV testing techniques, because HPV testing often cannot be retrospectively performed from FNA smears.

PROGNOSTIC STAGING FOR SCCOC

The American Joint Committee on Cancer (AJCC) tumor, node, metastasis (TNM) staging system is a universally accepted, anatomically based clinical staging system for SCCOC (**Table 1** summarizes the most recent seventh edition guidelines published

Table 1
AJCC staging for SCCOC and SCCOP

Tumor (T) Stage SCCOC	Tumor (T) Stage SCCOP
T1: ≤2 cm	T1: ≤2 cm
T2: 2–4 cm	T2: 2–4 cm
T3: >4 cm	T3: >4 cm, or extension to lingual surface epiglottis
T4a: invades maxilla, mandible, extrinsic tongue muscles, maxillary sinus, or skin	T4a: invades larynx, extrinsic tongue muscles, medial pterygoid, hard palate, or mandible
T4b: invades masticator space, pterygoid plates, skull base; or encases carotid artery	T4b: invades lateral pterygoid muscle, pterygoid plates, lateral nasopharynx, skull base, or encases carotid artery

Lymph Node (N) Stage SCCOC and SCCOP

N0: no regional lymph node metastasis
N1: metastasis in a single ipsilateral lymph node, ≤3 cm in greatest dimension
N2a: metastasis in single ipsilateral lymph node, >3 cm but ≤6 cm in greatest dimension
N2b: metastases in multiple ipsilateral lymph nodes, none >6 cm in greatest dimension
N2c: metastases in bilateral or contralateral lymph nodes, none >6 cm in greatest dimension
N3: metastasis in a lymph node >6 cm in greatest dimension

Overall Stage SCCOC and SCCOP

Stage	T	N	M
0	Tis	N0	M0
I	T1	N0	M0
II	T2	N0	M0
III	T3	N0	M0
	T1	N1	M0
	T2	N1	M0
	T3	N1	M0
IVA	T4a	N0-N2	M0
	T1-T3	N2	M0
IVB	T4b	Any N	M0
	Any T	N3	M0
IVC	Any T	Any N	M1

From Edge SB, Byrd DR, Compton CC, et al, editors. AJCC cancer staging manual. 7th edition. Springer Science and Business Media, LLC; 2010. p. 21–101. Available at: www.springer.com; with permission.

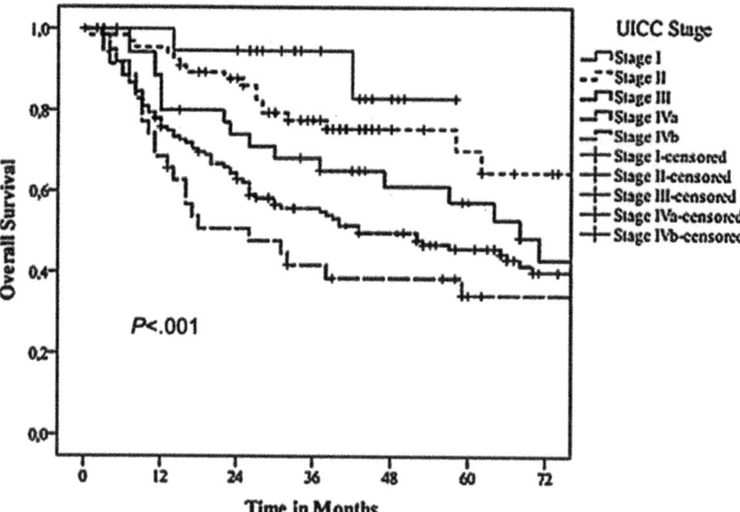

Fig. 2. SCCOC overall survival according to AJCC overall stage. UICC, Union for International Cancer Control. (*From* Kreppel M, Eich HT, Kubler A, et al. Prognostic value of the sixth edition of the UICC's TNM classification and stage grouping for oral cancer. J Surg Oncol 2010;102:447, with permission.)

in 2010).[14] Kreppel and colleagues[15] recently evaluated the sixth edition AJCC guidelines published in 2003, confirming that the T stage, N stage, and overall stage groupings remain good predictors of overall survival in patients with SCCOC (**Fig. 2**). Although the AJCC TNM staging system contains useful prognostic information for SCCOC, it does not include histopathologic features such as tumor thickness, perineural invasion, lymphatic invasion, and extracapsular extension, all of which have been shown to have prognostic significance and influence treatment outcomes for SCCOC.

Tumor thickness has long been shown to be a strong predictor for occult cervical lymph node involvement for SCCOC, and a recent meta-analysis by Huang and colleagues[16] supported an optimal tumor thickness cutoff point of 4 mm (negative predictive value of 96%) for determining the need for elective treatment of the neck. This 4-mm cutoff value has also previously been suggested by multiple single-institution studies.[17] Perineural invasion has been shown to be a significant independent predictor of local recurrence and overall survival, irrespective of tumor margin status.[18,19] Studies have also shown perineural invasion to be a significant prognostic indicator of regional metastases.[19–21] Lymphatic invasion is another poor prognostic marker for SCCOC, conferring a 5 times greater increased risk of recurrence within 3 years in a multivariate analysis by Fan and colleagues.[22] In addition, extracapsular lymph node disease extension has long been shown to be a poor prognostic feature for patients with all head and neck cancers, with an approximately 50% reduction in survival.[23]

PROGNOSTIC STAGING FOR SCCOP

TNM Staging

The most recent AJCC staging guidelines for SCCOP remain almost identical to those for SCCOC (see **Table 1**). Although there is subtle difference in characterization of advanced primary tumors (T3 and T4) related to invasion of adjacent structures, the early primary tumor (T1 and T2), regional lymph nodes (N), distant metastasis (M), and anatomic stage/prognostic groups for these two distinct diseases are the same. As discussed earlier, the staging system for SCCOC has been validated in the recent literature.[15] In contrast, recent literature has brought into question the staging system for SCCOP, which is still based on experience with SCCOP related to traditional tobacco and alcohol risk factors, and does not account for the improved outcomes of patients with HPV-positive tumors.

HPV Status

Greater than 80% of patients with SCCOP in Western countries may now have HPV-associated tumors.[4,24] A profile for these patients has become evident over the last decade, with HPV-associated SCCOP tumors often occurring in middle-aged white men with little or no tobacco history.[6–9] With the increasing incidence of HPV-associated SCCOP over the last several decades,[25] there has been a concomitant trend in these patients presenting with a more advanced stage of disease according to the AJCC staging guidelines, particularly because patients with HPV-associated SCCOP usually present with small primary tumors and are more likely to have multiple early lymph node metastases.

In the Trans Tasman Radiation Oncology Group (TROG) study of 185 patients with SCCOP, patients with p16-positive SCCOP:

- Had smaller primary tumors (T1-2 15% for p16 negative vs T1-2 37% for p16 positive; $P = .001$)
- Were more likely to have multiple or large metastatic lymph nodes (N2-3 65% for p16 negative vs N2-3 86% for p16 positive; $P = .001$)[26]

Additional prospective clinical trials of carcinomas of various head and neck sites by the Eastern Cooperative Oncology Group and the Danish Head and Neck Cancer Group have also shown that patients with HPV-positive or p16-positive carcinoma have more advanced nodal disease at presentation.[8,27] Notwithstanding that patients with HPV-associated tumors often present with more advanced nodal disease, patients with HPV-associated tumors also have consistently shown improved response to treatment and prognosis compared with patients with HPV-negative tumors.[7,8,26–28]

Smoking Status

In addition to HPV status, smoking status has emerged as a potentially important independent prognostic factor for patients with SCCOP. Smoking status has been shown to be a cofactor in the development of HPV-negative, but not HPV-positive, SCCOP.[29] Many patients with HPV-associated tumors have no tobacco exposure, or significantly less tobacco exposure, than patients with other mucosal upper aerodigestive tract SCCs. However, approximately 50% of patients with HPV-positive tumors may have some smoking history.[7,30] Several studies have indicated that tobacco exposure is associated with lower survival in patients with HPV-associated SCCOP.[31–33] Whether this occurs because of a different intrinsic tumor biology of HPV-positive tumors in smokers or is more related to the response of these tumors to therapy remains unanswered.

A recent study of patients with SCCOP treated in the RTOG 0129 trial (a randomized trial comparing accelerated-fractionation radiotherapy with standard-fractionation radiotherapy, each combined with cisplatin therapy, in patients with squamous cell carcinoma of the head and neck) specifically evaluated the interaction between tumor

HPV status and patient smoking status, finding tumor HPV status and tobacco smoking (≤10 or >10 pack-years) to be the two strongest independent determinants of overall and progression-free survival in patients with SCCOP.[7] Furthermore, patients were stratified into low-risk, intermediate-risk, and high-risk overall survival cohorts primarily based on these two independent risk factors, with 3-year overall survivals of 94%, 67%, and 42% for the low-risk, intermediate-risk, and high-risk groups, respectively (**Fig. 3**).[9] Nonsmokers with HPV-positive tumors were included in the low risk group, whereas smokers with HPV-negative tumors were included in the high-risk group. The intermediate group included smokers with HPV-positive tumors and higher nodal stage, as well as nonsmokers with HPV-negative tumors and lower tumor (T) stage. Therefore, although tumor HPV status and patient smoking status were the strongest prognostic factors in this risk stratification, traditional TNM anatomic staging factors helped define patients in the intermediate risk cohort.

A recent follow-up study on the RTOG trials 0129 and 9003 also confirmed tobacco exposure at diagnosis and during therapy as significant risk factors for oropharyngeal cancer progression and death, independent of tumor p16 status and treatment.[34] Risk of disease progression or death increased by 1% per pack-year or 2% per year of smoking in both trials. However, smoking status was not shown to significantly affect disease-free survival in a recent large retrospective review of patients with surgically treated HPV-associated SCCOP, with the investigators hypothesizing that smoking may be a more important prognostic factor for nonsurgical treatment protocols than for patients treated surgically.[35]

Survival Stratification

HPV status and smoking may better account for differences in survival than traditional pathologic risk factors and anatomic TNM staging. Overall AJCC TNM stage, nodal status, extracapsular extension, and perineural invasion have all been shown not to have significant prognostic value in studies of HPV-associated SCCOP.[35–37] A recent retrospective study by Dahlstrom and colleagues[6] highlights the disparity between the current TNM prognostic stratification and the clinical presentation and expected survival of patients presenting with SCCOP at one institution since 1995. This study compared the impact of clinical factors on survival for 1370 patients presenting between 1955 and 1994 with 632 patients presenting between 1995 and 2004. For the four earlier decades, traditional TNM anatomic staging variables accounted for most of the difference in survival stratification and accurately predicted survival. In contrast, smoking status and other HPV surrogates (eg, age and tumor site) provided the best risk stratification and survival differentiation for patients treated in the most recent decade.

In summary, patients with HPV-associated SCCOP (which now constitutes most patients with SCCOP) are commonly presenting with overall stage 4 disease because of more advanced nodal disease, but these patients have much better expected survival than their anatomic TNM stage would suggest. Furthermore, independent of HPV status, smoking status has been shown to significantly affect survival in patients with SCCOP. Because the current TNM anatomic staging system does not take tumor HPV status or patient smoking status into account, it may not provide an accurate prognostic stratification for most patients now presenting with SCCOP in Western countries. As these data are validated, it is possible that the staging system for SCCOP may soon incorporate tumor HPV status and perhaps even smoking status into the TNM staging system. In the meantime, clinicians should use the current data in the literature, in addition to TNM anatomic staging, to best educate patients with HPV-associated SCCOP with regard to their prognosis.

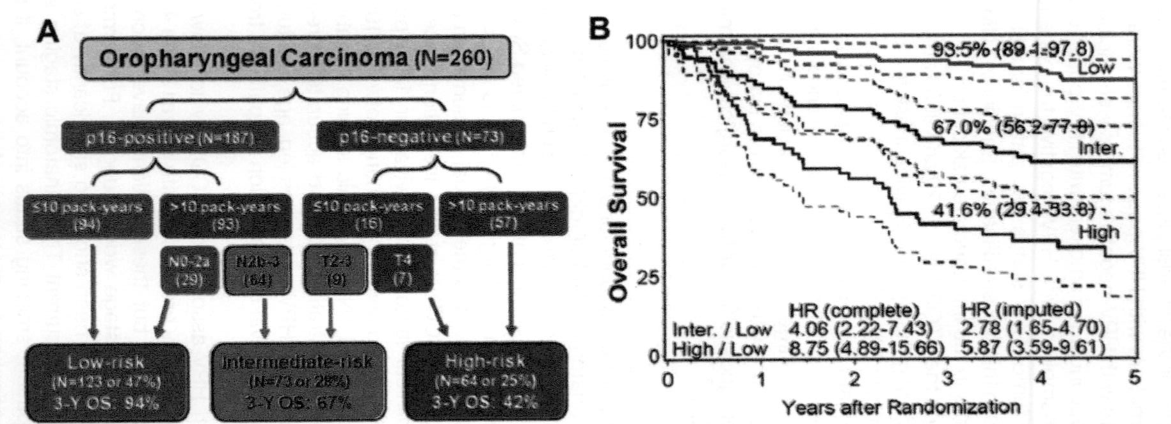

Fig. 3. Classification of oropharyngeal SCC patients from RTOG 0129 into risk-of-death categories by recursive partitioning analysis (*A*) and Kaplan-Meier estimates of overall survival according to these categories (*B*). OS, overall survival. (*From* Ang KK, Sturgis EM. Human papillomavirus as a marker of the natural history and response to therapy of head and neck squamous cell carcinoma. Semin Radiat Oncol 2012;22:138; with permission.)

NOVEL APPROACHES IN EVALUATION AND STAGING

Sentinel Lymph Node Biopsy

Lymph node involvement has long been known as one of the most important prognostic indicators guiding treatment of SCCOC.[38,39] Approximately 30% of clinically and radiographically negative necks may harbor occult lymph node metastases,[40–42] and therefore elective selective neck dissection has become the standard of care for many patients with SCCOC whose primary tumor depth of invasion places them at significant risk for occult lymph node metastases.[41,43] SNB has emerged over the last decade as a clinical staging tool to evaluate clinically negative necks in patients who would otherwise have undergone an elective selective neck dissection. Patients who have negative SNB undergo no further treatment of the neck, whereas patients with positive sentinel lymph nodes undergo a selective neck dissection. Although some centers have used SNB for select patients with SCCOP, most of the data for SNB come from studies of patients with SCCOC.

The clinical indications, techniques of the procedure, and histopathology protocols for SNB have recently been published in joint practice guidelines published by the European Association of Nuclear Medicine Oncology Committee and the European Sentinel Node Biopsy Trial Committee.[44] These guidelines suggest that SNB for SCCOC should be restricted to early stage tumors (T1 or T2), because larger tumors are technically difficult to inject accurately and would generally require a neck dissection for either access to the tumor or to prepare the regional blood vessels as donor vessels for microvascular reconstruction. In addition, because previous radiation or neck surgery can alter normal lymphatic drainage pathways and lead to unexpected patterns of lymphatic metastases, SNB is generally not recommended for patients with previous treatment of the neck. Pathology protocols for SNB include serial sectioning of lymph nodes and immunohistochemistry to detect micrometastases and isolated tumor cells with high sensitivity.

Over the last decade, SNB for SCCOC has been studied in more than 60 single-institution studies,[45] 2 European observational trials,[46,47] and a multiinstitutional clinical trial in the United States.[48] In a prospective multiinstitutional validation trial, Civantos and colleagues[48] showed a 96% negative predictive value when comparing a negative SNB with a negative selective neck dissection specimen. Long-term results from a Swiss observational trial reported an 89% negative predictive value for a negative SNB, with an ultimate 5-year neck control rate (including salvage surgery) of 96% in SNB-negative and 74% in SNB-positive patients. Disease-specific survival at 5 years was 96% in the node-negative group versus 77% in the node-positive cohort.[46] Reduced morbidity of SNB compared with selective neck dissection in terms of complication rates, shoulder function, and overall quality of life has been reported in several studies.[49,50] In addition, occult metastases (isolated tumor cells and micrometastases) identified through SNB have recently been shown to predict a significant decrease in disease-specific survival compared with sentinel node–negative patients.[51]

There have been several recent technological advances in SNB. Compared with dynamic planar lymphoscintigraphy, SPECT/CT offers the surgeon a three-dimensional preoperative image to identify sentinel lymph nodes in relation to surrounding structures, and SPECT/CT preoperative imaging may improve surgeon success in harvesting sentinel lymph nodes.[52] One traditional disadvantage of SNB has been the need for a 2-stage procedure in patients who have positive sentinel lymph nodes. However, intraoperative sentinel lymph node analysis by quantitative real-time reverse transcriptase PCR has recently shown promise in allowing lymph node evaluation for micrometastases in 30 minutes with approximately 95% concordance with final pathology.[53] Several other technologies under current investigation including a portable gamma camera may eventually contribute to real-time intraoperative three-dimensional nuclear imaging for detection of sentinel lymph nodes.[54,55] With development of reliable tumor-specific radiotracers in the future, a portable gamma camera may be able to direct identification and excision of lymph nodes containing occult tumor.[54,56]

SNB has shown efficacy in staging patients with SCCOC, providing selection of patients for elective neck dissection. However, elective neck dissection remains the gold standard for staging and treatment of the clinically negative neck. Clinical trials comparing recurrence and survival with SNB versus elective neck dissection are required before SNB may become a standard of care for patients with SCCOC. In the meantime, SNB for SCCOC continues to be studied in the context of ongoing clinical trials.[57]

FDG-PET/CT

Although the role of FDG-PET/CT has been established for posttreatment evaluation of persistent disease or recurrence, the role of FDG-PET/CT in the initial staging of SCCOC and SCCOP is less clear. FDG-PET/CT has been studied as a diagnostic tool in the initial evaluation and staging of SCCOC and SCCOP for various reasons including detection of unknown primary tumors, detection of nodal metastases not detectable with cross-sectional imaging, detection of distant metastases in patients with advanced local disease, radiotherapy planning, and prognostic value.

FDG-PET/CT can aid in the anatomic localization of unknown primary head and neck cancers, which are almost always found or presumed to be located in the lymphoid tissue of the tonsils or base of tongue. FDG-PET/CT has several important limitations in the diagnosis of unknown primary tumors.[58] The spatial resolution of FDG-PET is limited to 5 mm, so smaller lesions are often not detected. In addition, increased basal uptake of FDG in the lymphoid tissue of the head and neck (Waldeyer's ring), particularly in the tonsil, can also obscure detection of small primary lesions. An unknown primary tumor should not be diagnosed until after a thorough head and neck examination including manual palpation, flexible laryngoscopy, and cross-sectional imaging (either CT or MRI). It is important to bear in mind that, if a primary site of disease cannot be identified on physical examination or cross-sectional imaging, it is best to perform the FDG-PET/CT before an examination under anesthesia, because inflammation resulting from surgical biopsies can cause false-positive results and obscure detection of the site of disease on PET imaging. A recent prospective clinical trial evaluated FDG-PET/CT as an adjunct to diagnosis in patients with unknown primary SCCs.[59] In this small blinded study of 20 patients who were diagnosed with unknown primary SCCs after negative physical examination and cross-sectional imaging, FDG-PET/CT increased the detection of a primary site of disease during examination under anesthesia from 25% to 55% (P = .03).

Another potential use for FDG-PET/CT in the initial evaluation and staging of SCCOC and SCCOP is in the detection of unsuspected second primary metastases and distant metastases. Although FDG-PET/CT has shown a high sensitivity and specificity for diagnosing distant metastases, it has a lower positive predictive value (63% in a study of 349 head and neck patients), such that additional diagnostic imaging studies or procedures are required to rule out false-positive results.[58,60] Therefore, FDG-PET/CT should be reserved for patients with advanced locoregional disease who have a high pretreatment probability of distant metastases.

FDG-PET/CT has been studied as a diagnostic tool in the detection of occult lymph node metastases that are not otherwise detected on cross-sectional imaging (standard CT or MRI). Because the sensitivity and specificity of cross-sectional imaging in detecting lymph node metastases depend on the protocol of the imaging study and the expertise of the radiologist or surgeon reading the films, it can be difficult to extrapolate experience with cross-sectional imaging in the initial staging of SCCOC and SCCOP from one setting to another. Cross-sectional imaging is required in the initial evaluation of SCCOC and SCCOP for staging and treatment planning, and FDG-PET/CT has not consistently been shown to have increased sensitivity or specificity in localizing occult lymph node metastases compared with standard CT or MRI.[61] Furthermore, because of technical limitations of resolution (about 5 mm), FDG-PET/CT has been shown to be unreliable (detection rates between 0% and 30%) in localizing occult lymph node metastases in multiple studies.[62–64]

FDG-PET/CT has also been used in several centers for radiation therapy planning, where it has been variably shown to increase the precision of target volumes.[61] In addition, independent studies and a recent meta-analysis have suggested that patients with a high standard uptake value on FDG-PET/CT imaging have poorer disease-free and overall survival, indicating that FDG-PET/CT may have some prognostic value for patients with head and neck cancer.[65]

In summary, FDG-PET/CT has been studied as a clinical staging tool in the initial evaluation of patients with SCCOC and SCCOP for many reasons. Current data indicate 2 generally accepted clinical scenarios in which FDG-PET/CT may routinely be used. Patients with unknown primary SCCs of the head and neck that remain unknown after a thorough head and neck examination (including flexible laryngoscopy) and cross-sectional imaging (either CT or MRI) may benefit from FDG-PET/CT to direct surgical biopsies. In addition, patients with advanced local disease who are at high risk for distant metastases may benefit from FDG-PET/CT (or other whole-body distant metastatic work-up). FDG-PET/CT has not been shown to add value compared with cross-sectional imaging techniques in the evaluation of occult lymph node metastases. Other uses for FDG-PET/CT, such as radiotherapy planning and prognostic applications, are the focus of ongoing clinical studies.

REFERENCES

1. Liang XH, Lewis J, Foote R, et al. Prevalence and significance of human papillomavirus in oral tongue cancer: the Mayo Clinic experience. J Oral Maxillofac Surg 2008;66:1875–80.
2. Ha PK, Pai SI, Westra WH, et al. Real-time quantitative PCR demonstrates low prevalence of human papillomavirus type 16 in premalignant and malignant lesions of the oral cavity. Clin Cancer Res 2002;8(5):1203–9.
3. Cancer of the head and neck. In: Myers EN, Suen JY, Myers JN, et al, editors. Cancer of the oral cavity. Myers EN, Simental AA. Philadelphia: Elsevier; 2003. p. 289–90.
4. Attner P, Du J, Nasman A, et al. The role of human papilloma virus (HPV) in the increased incidence of base of tongue cancer. Int J Cancer 2010;126(12): 2879–84.
5. Nasman A, Attner P, Hammarstedt L, et al. Incidence of human papillomavirus (HPV) positive tonsillar carcinoma in Stockholm, Sweden: an epidemic of viral-induced carcinoma? Int J Cancer 2009;125:362–6.
6. Dahlstrom KR, Calzada G, Hanby JD, et al. An evolution in demographics, treatment, and outcomes of oropharyngeal cancer at a major cancer center: a staging system in need of repair. Cancer 2012. http://dx.doi.org/10.1002/cncr.27727.
7. Ang KK, Harris J, Wheeler R, et al. Human papillomavirus (HPV) and survival of patients with oropharyngeal cancer. N Engl J Med 2010;363:24–35.

8. Fakhry C, Westra WH, Li S, et al. Improved survival of patients with human papillomavirus-positive head and neck squamous cell carcinoma in a prospective clinical trial. J Natl Cancer Inst 2008;100:261–9.
9. Ang KK, Sturgis EM. Human papillomavirus as a marker of the natural history and response to therapy of head and neck squamous cell carcinoma. Semin Radiat Oncol 2012;22:128–42.
10. Corey AS, Hudgins PA. Radiographic imaging of human papillomavirus related carcinomas of the oropharynx. Head Neck Pathol 2012;6:S25–40.
11. Goldenberg D, Begum S, Westra WH, et al. Cystic lymph node metastasis in patients with head and neck cancer: an HPV-associated phenomenon. Head Neck 2008;30(7):898–903.
12. Westra WH. Detection of human papillomavirus in clinical samples. Otolaryngol Clin North Am 2012;45:765–77.
13. El-Naggar AK, Westra WH. p16 Expression as a surrogate marker for HPV-related oropharyngeal carcinoma: a guide for interpretative relevance and consistency. Head Neck 2012;34(4):459–61.
14. AJCC cancer staging manual. 7th edition. Springer Science and Business Media; 2010. Available at: www.springer.com. Accessed September 16, 2012.
15. Kreppel M, Eich HT, Kubler A, et al. Prognostic value of the sixth edition of the UICC's TNM classification and stage grouping for oral cancer. J Surg Oncol 2010;102:443–9.
16. Huang SH, Hwang D, Lockwood G, et al. Predictive value of tumor thickness for cervical lymph node involvement in squamous cell carcinoma of the oral cavity: a meta-analysis of reported studies. Cancer 2009;115(7):1489–97.
17. Sparano A, Weinstein G, Chalian A, et al. Multivariate predictors of occult neck metastasis in early oral tongue cancer. Otolaryngol Head Neck Surg 2004;131:472–6.
18. Brandwein-Gensler M, Teixeira MS, Lewis CM, et al. Oral squamous cell carcinoma: histologic risk assessment, but not margin status, is strongly predictive of local disease-free and overall survival. Am J Surg Pathol 2005;29:167–78.
19. Binmadi NO, Basile JR. Perineural invasion in oral squamous cell carcinoma: a discussion of significance and review of the literature. Oral Oncol 2011;47:1005–10.
20. Woolgar JA. Histopathological prognosticators in oral and oropharyngeal squamous cell carcinoma. Oral Oncol 2006;42:229–39.
21. Woolgar JA, Scott J. Prediction of cervical lymph node metastasis in squamous cell carcinoma of the tongue/floor of mouth. Head Neck 1995;17:463–72.
22. Fan KH, Wang HM, Kang CJ, et al. Treatment results of postoperative radiotherapy on squamous cell carcinoma of the oral cavity: coexistence of multiple minor risk factors results in higher recurrence rates. Int J Radiat Oncol Biol Phys 2010;77(4):1024–9.
23. Johnson JT, Myers EN, Bedetti C, et al. Cervical lymph node metastasis. Arch Otolaryngol 1985;11:534–7.
24. Cherncok RD, Zhang Q, El-Mofty SK, et al. Human papillomavirus–related squamous cell carcinoma of the oropharynx: a comparative study in whites and African Americans. Arch Otolaryngol Head Neck Surg 2011;137(2):163–9.
25. Chaturvedi AK, Engels EA, Anderson WF, et al. Incidence trends for human papillomavirus-related and -unrelated oral squamous cell carcinomas in the United States. J Clin Oncol 2008;26:612–9.

26. Rischin D, Young RJ, Fisher R, et al. Prognostic significance of p16INK4A and human papillomavirus in patients with oropharyngeal cancer treated on TROG 02.02 phase III trial. J Clin Oncol 2010;28:4142–8.
27. Lassen P, Eriksen JG, Krogdahl A, et al. The influence of HPV-associated p16-expression on accelerated fractionated radiotherapy in head and neck cancer: evaluation of the randomised DAHANCA 6 and 7 trial. Radiother Oncol 2011; 100:49–55.
28. Posner MR, Lorch JH, Goloubeva O, et al. Survival and human papillomavirus in oropharynx cancer in tax 324: a subset analysis from an international phase III trial. Ann Oncol 2011;22:1071–7.
29. Gillison ML, D'Souza G, Westra W, et al. Distinct risk factor profiles for human papillomavirus type 16–positive and human papillomavirus type 16–negative head and neck cancers. J Natl Cancer Inst 2008;100:407–20.
30. D'Souza G, Zhang HH, D'Souza WD, et al. Moderate predictive value of demographic and behavioral characteristics for a diagnosis of HPV16-positive and HPV16-negative head and neck cancer. Oral Oncol 2010;46:100–4.
31. Hafkamp HC, Manni JJ, Haesevoets A, et al. Marked differences in survival rate between smokers and nonsmokers with HPV16-associated tonsillar carcinomas. Int J Cancer 2008;122:2656–64.
32. Kumar B, Cordell KG, Lee JS, et al. EGFR, p16, HPV Titer, Bcl-xL, and p53, sex, and smoking as indicators of response to therapy and survival in oropharyngeal cancer. J Clin Oncol 2008;26:3128–37.
33. Maxwell H, Kumar B, Feng FY, et al. Tobacco use in human papillomavirus-positive advanced oropharynx cancer patients related to increased risk of distant metastases and tumor recurrence. Clin Cancer Res 2010;16:1226–35.
34. Gillison ML, Zhang Q, Jordan R, et al. Tobacco smoking and increased risk of death and progression for patients with p16-positive and p16-negative oropharyngeal cancer. J Clin Oncol 2012;30(17):2102–11.
35. Haughey BH, Sinha P. Prognostic factors and survival unique to surgically treated p16+ oropharyngeal cancer. Laryngoscope 2012;122:S13–33.
36. Haughey BH, Hinni ML, Salassa JR, et al. Transoral laser microsurgery as primary treatment for advanced-stage oropharyngeal cancer: a United States multicenter study. Head Neck 2011;33:1683–94.
37. Straetmans JM, Olthof N, Mooren JJ, et al. Human papillomavirus reduces the prognostic value of nodal involvement in tonsillar squamous cell carcinomas. Laryngoscope 2009;119:1951–7.
38. Don DM, Anzai Y, Lufkin RB, et al. Evaluation of cervical lymph node metastases in squamous cell carcinoma of the head and neck. Laryngoscope 1995;105(7): 669–74.
39. Gourin CG, Conger BT, Porubsky ES, et al. The effect of occult nodal metastases on survival and regional control in patients with head and neck squamous cell carcinoma. Laryngoscope 2008;118(7):1191–4.
40. Tankere F, Camproux A, Barry B, et al. Prognostic value of lymph node involvement in oral cancers: a study of 137 cases. Laryngoscope 2000;110:2061–5.
41. van den Brekel MW, van der Waal I, Meijer CJ, et al. The incidence of micrometastases in neck dissection specimens obtained from elective neck dissections. Laryngoscope 1996;106:987–91.
42. Pitman KT, Johnson JT, Myers EN. Effectiveness of selective neck dissection for management of the clinically negative neck. Arch Otolaryngol Head Neck Surg 1997;123:917–22.

43. Byers RM, Wolf PF, Ballantyne AJ. Rationale for elective modified neck dissection. Head Neck Surg 1988;10:160–7.
44. Alkureishi LW, Burak Z, Alvarez JA, et al. Joint practice guidelines for radionuclide lymphoscintigraphy for sentinel node localization in oral/oropharyngeal squamous cell carcinoma. Ann Surg Oncol 2009;16:3190–210.
45. Stoeckli SJ, Broglie MA. Sentinel node biopsy for early oral carcinoma. Curr Opin Otolaryngol Head Neck Surg 2012;20(2):103–8.
46. Broglie MA, Haile SR, Stoeckli SJ. Long-term experience in sentinel node biopsy for early oral and oropharyngeal squamous cell carcinoma. Ann Surg Oncol 2011;18(10):2732–8.
47. Alkureishi LW, Ross GL, Shoaib T, et al. Sentinel node biopsy in head and neck squamous cell cancer: 5-year follow-up of a European multicenter trial. Ann Surg Oncol 2010;17:2459–64.
48. Civantos FJ, Zitsch RP, Schuller DE, et al. Sentinel lymph node biopsy accurately stages the regional lymph nodes for T1-T2 oral squamous cell carcinomas: results of a prospective multiinstitutional trial. J Clin Oncol 2010;28:1395–400.
49. Schiefke F, Akdemir M, Weber A, et al. Function, postoperative morbidity, and quality of life after cervical sentinel node biopsy and after selective neck dissection. Head Neck 2009;31:503–12.
50. Murer K, Huber GF, Haile SR, et al. Comparison of morbidity between sentinel node biopsy and elective neck dissection for treatment of the N0 neck in patients with oral squamous cell carcinoma. Head Neck 2011;33:1260–4.
51. Broglie MA, Haerle SK, Huber GF, et al. Occult metastases detected by sentinel node biopsy in patients with early oral and oropharyngeal squamous cell carcinomas: impact on survival. Head Neck 2012. http://dx.doi.org/10.1002/hed.23017.
52. Haerle SK, Stoeckli SJ. SPECT/CT for lymphatic mapping of sentinel nodes in early squamous cell carcinoma of the oral cavity and oropharynx. Int J Mol Imaging 2011;106068. Available at: http://www.hindawi.com/journals/ijmi/2011/106068.
53. Ferris RL, Xi L, Seethala RR, et al. Intraoperative qRT-PCR for detection of lymph node metastasis in head and neck cancer. Clin Cancer Res 2011;17:1858–66.
54. Vermeeren L, Valdés Olmos RA, Klop WM, et al. A portable gamma-camera for intraoperative detection of sentinel nodes in the head and neck region. J Nucl Med 2010;51(5):700–3.
55. Wendler T, Hartl A, Lasser T, et al. Towards intraoperative 3D nuclear imaging: reconstruction of 3D radioactive distributions using tracked gamma probes. Med Image Comput Comput Assist Interv 2007;10:909–17.
56. Aderson RS, Eifert B, Tartt S, et al. Radioimmunoguided surgery using indium-111 capromab pendetide (PROSTASCINT) to diagnose supraclavicular metastasis from prostate cancer. Urology 2000;56:669.
57. Available at: http://www.clinicaltrials.gov/ct2/show/NCT00911326?term=head+and+neck+cancer+sentinel+lymph+node&rank=5. Accessed September 3, 2012.
58. Cashman EC, MacMahon PJ, Shelly MJ, et al. Role of positron emission tomography–computed tomography in head and neck cancer. Ann Otol Rhinol Laryngol 2011;120(9):593–602.
59. Rudmik L, Lau HY, Matthews TW, et al. Clinical utility of PET/CT in the evaluation of head and neck squamous cell carcinoma with an unknown primary: a prospective clinical trial. Head Neck 2011;33:935–40.
60. Kim SY, Roh JL, Yeo NK, et al. Combined ^{18}F-fluorodeoxyglucose-positron emission tomography and computed tomography as a primary screening method for

detecting second primary cancers and distant metastases in patients with head and neck cancer. Ann Oncol 2007;18:1698–703.
61. Menda Y, Graham MM. Update on ^{18}F-fluorodeoxyglucose/positron emission tomography and positron emission tomography/computed tomography imaging of squamous head and neck cancers. Semin Nucl Med 2005;35:214–9.
62. Hyde NC, Prvulovich E, Newman L, et al. A new approach to pretreatment assessment of the N0 neck in oral squamous cell carcinoma: the role of sentinel node biopsy and positron emission tomography. Oral Oncol 2003;39:350–60.
63. Stoeckli SJ, Steinert H, Pfaltz M, et al. Is there a role for positron emission tomography with 18F-fluorodeoxyglucose in the initial staging of nodal negative oral and oropharyngeal squamous cell carcinoma. Head Neck 2002;24:345–9.
64. Civantos FJ, Gomez C, Duque C, et al. Sentinel node biopsy in oral cavity cancer: correlation with PET scan and immunohistochemistry. Head Neck 2003;25:1–9.
65. Xie P, Li M, Zhao H, et al. (18)F-FDG PET or PET-CT to evaluate prognosis for head and neck cancer: a meta-analysis. J Cancer Res Clin Oncol 2011;137:1085–93.

Surgical Innovations

Daniel R. Clayburgh, MD, PhD, Neil Gross, MD*

KEYWORDS

- Transoral robotic surgery (TORS) • Transoral laser microsurgery (TLM)
- Robotic surgery • Minimally invasive surgery • Head and neck surgery

KEY POINTS

- In preliminary studies, minimally invasive approaches to the oropharynx, including transoral laser microsurgery and transoral robotic surgery, show improved functional outcomes and similar oncologic outcomes to primary radiation.
- The application of sentinel lymph node biopsy techniques to oral cavity cancer may reduce the need for elective neck dissection and its associated morbidity.

INTRODUCTION

In 2012, an estimated 40,250 people in the United States were diagnosed with oral cavity or oropharyngeal squamous cell carcinoma (SCC), and 7850 people died of these diseases.[1] Although the overall incidence of oral cavity SCC has been decreasing by approximately 1% per year, the incidence of oropharyngeal SCC is rising, particularly in middle-aged patients, likely because of the increasing incidence of human papilloma virus (HPV)-associated oropharyngeal SCC.[2] Treatment of oral cavity and oropharyngeal SCC is particularly challenging, as these sites are involved in many crucial functions, including breathing, deglutition, and speech, and impairment of any of these functions may significantly affect quality of life. Thus, both functional and oncologic outcomes are important considerations in the treatment of oral cavity and oropharyngeal SCC.

Although surgical excision has always been a mainstay of treatment for oral cavity SCC, the treatment of oropharyngeal SCC in recent decades has been notable for the use of primary nonsurgical approaches, namely radiation or chemoradiation. Publication of the Veterans Affairs study in 1991[3] heralded an era of organ-preservation strategies that were extrapolated from the larynx to the oropharynx. Traditional surgical

Disclosures: Intuitive Surgical: Proctor (N. Gross).
Head and Neck Surgery and Oncology, Department of Otolaryngology-Head and Neck Surgery, Knight Cancer Institute, Oregon Health and Science University, 3181 Southwest Sam Jackson Park Road, PV01, Portland, OR 97239, USA
* Corresponding author.
E-mail address: grossn@ohsu.edu

Otolaryngol Clin N Am 46 (2013) 615–628
http://dx.doi.org/10.1016/j.otc.2013.04.003 oto.theclinics.com
0030-6665/13/$ – see front matter

Abbreviations: Surgical innovations	
HPV	Human papilloma virus
SCC	Squamous cell carcinoma
SLNB	Sentinel lymph node biopsy
TLM	Transoral laser microsurgery
TORS	Transoral robotic surgery

approaches to the oropharynx (eg, mandibulotomy) entailed significant morbidity, thus making nonsurgical approaches the more attractive treatment option. However, recent technological advances, including transoral laser microsurgery (TLM) and transoral robotic surgery (TORS), have afforded improved access to pathology and the opportunity for decreased treatment-related morbidity. The application of sentinel lymph node biopsy (SLNB) for oral cavity and oropharyngeal SCC may also allow for more minimally invasive management of the neck. Here, we review the evidence behind these surgical innovations to examine how they may be integrated into modern management strategies for oral cavity and oropharyngeal SCC.

TRADITIONAL SURGICAL APPROACHES

Surgical resection has long been a mainstay of treatment for head and neck cancer, including oral cavity and oropharyngeal SCC. Given the complex 3-dimensional anatomy and functional roles of the oral cavity and oropharynx, a variety of surgical approaches have been explored.

Direct Transoral Surgery

A direct transoral approach provides the quickest and most direct route to the oral cavity and oropharynx with the least potential for morbidity. As such, transoral surgery remains important for the treatment of oral cavity SCC and many oropharyngeal SCCs. The primary disadvantage of this approach can be related to exposure. Most oral cavity cancers, and some oropharyngeal cancers, can be adequately visualized via a direct transoral approach; however, larger cancers may be difficult or impossible to reach through the mouth without specialized techniques and/or instrumentation. Patient factors (trismus, kyphosis, dental obstruction) and tumor characteristics (tumor size, location) can limit direct line-of-site visualization of areas in the oral cavity and oropharynx, thereby preventing a traditional direct transoral approach from being used.

Mandibulotomy/Mandibulectomy Approach

The mandible can represent a barrier to exposure for resection of oral cavity and oropharyngeal SCC. Several techniques have been developed to improve access to the posterior oral cavity and oropharynx. Using either a visor flap or lip-splitting approach, the mandible may be divided and retracted laterally to allow broad access to the oral cavity and oropharynx. Internal fixation may be used to restore the mandibular arch at completion of the procedure. Alternatively, a section of involved mandible may be removed during extirpation and then reconstructed with or without restoration of the entire mandibular arch. Although these approaches greatly expand the scope of tumors that may be resected, they also entail significant additional morbidity. Complications from mandibulotomy or mandibulectomy range from 10% to 60%,[4] and include difficulty with speech and swallowing, malocclusion, temporomandibular joint pain, and cosmetic deformity.[5,6]

Pharyngotomy Approach

As an alternative to mandibulotomy or mandibulectomy, tumors of the tongue base, inferior tonsillar fossae, or pharyngeal wall may be approached via a pharyngotomy. Depending on the location of the tumor and the extent of exposure needed, a lateral pharyngotomy, transhyoid pharyngotomy, and/or suprahyoid pharyngotomy may be used. Acceptable oncologic outcomes have been reported using each of these approaches.[7–9] Although these approaches avoid many of the complications inherent in mandibulotomy and mandibulectomy, the access afforded is substantially more limited. In addition, patients undergoing pharyngotomy are at increased risk of pharyngocutaneous fistula formation and severe dysphagia, which have been reported to occur in 7% to 38% of patients.[7–9]

NECK DISSECTION AND SLNB FOR ORAL CAVITY SCC

Oral cavity SCC spreads via regional lymphatics. Metastasis to the cervical lymph nodes is an early event in the progression of oral cavity SCC, particularly of the oral tongue and oropharynx,[10] and has important prognostic implications.[11] This is reflected in the major contribution of cervical metastases in American Joint Committee on Cancer TNM Classification System for oral cavity SCC. Thus, management of cervical lymph nodes, and possible metastases, is critical to proper risk stratification and application of therapy. There is little controversy surrounding the need for neck dissection for advanced primary (T3 and T4) oral cavity SCC, and in patients who are clinically node positive (N+). Good evidence also exists to define the appropriate use of neck dissection for early primary (T1 and T2) clinically node-negative (N0) oral cavity SCC, particularly when located in the oral tongue or floor of mouth. Selective neck dissection is now widely accepted for elective management of the neck in early-stage oral cavity SCC. Recently, SLNB has been investigated as an even less invasive method of staging the clinically N0 neck in early-stage oral cavity SCC.

Neck Dissection in Early-Stage Oral Cavity SCC

Current imaging technologies, including positron emission tomography/computed tomography, cannot accurately identify metastatic disease smaller than 5 mm. Therefore, pathologic evaluation of cervical lymph nodes is necessary for the detection of microscopic disease. Tumor thickness can accurately predict the risk of nodal cervical metastases.[12] In particular, oral tongue SCC with thickness greater than 4 mm has been shown to have a significantly increased risk of occult metastasis, regional recurrence, worse disease-specific survival, and worse overall survival.[13–16] Furthermore, elective neck dissection at or near the time of resection of oral cavity SCC, rather than after a period of failed observation, improves locoregional control[14,17] and survival.[15] Finally, it has been shown that selective neck dissection of levels I to III is as effective as radical or modified radical neck dissection.[18,19] Based on these studies, elective selective neck dissection (levels I–III) is the current gold standard for management of the clinically N0 neck in early-stage oral cavity SCC with tumor thickness greater than 4 mm.[20]

Sentinel Node Biopsy for Oral Cavity SCC

The concept of the sentinel lymph node as the initial site of lymphatic tumor spread, and therefore a predictor of the metastases within the remainder of the nodal basin, was first introduced more than 50 years ago.[21,22] SLNB is most widely used in clinical practice for the treatment of cutaneous malignant melanoma.[23–25] SLNB has also been adopted into treatment algorithms for breast cancer,[26] colon cancer,[27] and vulvar cancer.[28]

Given the complex lymphatic drainage of the oral cavity and oropharynx, SLNB has the potential to detect micrometastatic disease in oral cavity SCC with less morbidity than elective neck dissection. Furthermore, finer specimen sectioning and immunohistochemistry routinely used with SLNB may improve the detection of micrometastasis. The first studies of SLNB in head and neck SCC compared the pathologic results of SLNB to the gold standard treatment: elective neck dissection. The SLN was identified in 90% to 100% of patients, and false-negative pathology results were 0% to 6%, suggesting that SLNB alone may be sufficient for accurate neck nodal classification.[29–32] These encouraging results have been replicated in a recent large-scale multi-institutional clinical trial.[33] Observational studies have also validated the efficacy of SLNB biopsy in oral cavity SCC.[34] For example, a long-term study found a negative predictive value of 90%, and a disease-free survival of 96% in patients with initial negative SLNB.[35] A multicenter European trial of 134 patients showed that 5-year overall survival was comparable between patients receiving SLNB alone versus SLNB and elective neck dissection.[36,37] Finally, SLNB has been shown to be less morbid than elective neck dissection,[38] validating the primary rationale for the approach.

Based on the available literature, guidelines for the use of SLNB in oral cavity SCC have been proposed by the European Association of Nuclear Medicine and the Sentinel European Node Trial Committee.[39] SLNB should be confined to patients with early-stage (T1-2N0) oral cavity SCC. Larger primary cancers are considered large enough to drain to multiple nodal basins, and therefore not recommended for SLNB. Floor-of-mouth SCC is also potentially problematic, as the sentinel nodes can be obscured by close proximity to the primary tumor site. Indications for use of SLNB include staging of the ipsilateral N0 neck for a unilateral primary oral cavity SCC, staging of the ipsilateral and contralateral N0 neck for primary oral cavity SCC involving the midline, or staging of the contralateral N0 neck for an oral cavity SCC near the midline with an ipsilateral N+ neck. It is important to note that randomized studies comparing oncologic outcomes of SLNB to elective neck dissection in oral cavity SCC have not yet been performed. Thus, SLNB for oral cavity SCC is currently not advised outside the setting of a clinical trial but may be incorporated into standard practice algorithms for oral cavity SCC in the near future.

SURGICAL INNOVATIONS IN OROPHARYNGEAL CANCER

Until recently, radiation or chemoradiation was the treatment of choice for the vast majority of oropharyngeal SCCs. However, recent technological advances have expanded transoral access to the oropharynx, reinvigorating the use of primary surgical treatment for selected oropharyngeal SCCs. Two primary innovations have been at the forefront in this shift: TLM and TORS.

TLM

TLM was first introduced in the 1970s for the treatment of laryngeal papillomas,[40,41] and is now accepted for the treatment of early-stage laryngeal SCC with good oncologic results.[42,43] More recently, TLM has been applied to oropharyngeal SCC. One early series of 48 patients treated with TLM for base-of-tongue SCC yielded an 85% 5-year local control rate.[44] A retrospective review of 166 patients treated for tonsillar SCC also found an 82% 5-year local control rate.[45,46] Excellent oncologic results have been replicated by groups performing TLM for oropharyngeal SCC treated with and without neck dissection and without adjuvant radiation therapy.[47,48] Despite these encouraging results, no randomized studies have been performed comparing TLM with or without adjuvant treatment to nonsurgical approaches. TLM requires the use of rigid laryngoscopes with a narrow field of view to provide line-of-sight access to the site of resection. This makes the technique technically challenging to perform in the complex anatomy of the oropharynx. Thus, TLM is largely restricted to a few high-volume centers with extensive experience and may not be easily adapted into widespread clinical use.

TORS

The use of robotic assistance in surgery was first pioneered in the 1980s in neurosurgical and urological surgery.[49,50] Over the past 2 decades, robotic surgery has proliferated, and several indications have been approved by the Food and Drug Administration (FDA), including applications in prostate surgery, gynecologic surgery, laparoscopic surgery, cardiac surgery, and head and neck surgery. The use of surgical robotic systems provides several advantages, including increased instrument degrees of freedom of movement, improved visualization (particularly outside of line-of-site), potential reduction of hand tremor, and a relatively short learning curve.[51–53] These advantages are partially offset by the lack of haptic feedback. Nevertheless, TORS has recently emerged as a viable technique for the initial treatment of oropharyngeal SCC.

Development of TORS

In 2003, the first potential head and neck applications for robotic surgery were reported, including neck dissection and salivary gland surgery in a porcine model.[54] However, TORS, as it is known today, originated with studies performed at the University of Pennsylvania, where Hockstein and colleagues[55] demonstrated in an airway mannequin that the da Vinci surgical system (Intuitive Surgical, Inc, Sunnyvale, CA.) could be safely manipulated to access the oropharynx and larynx. Furthermore, this group showed that multiple oropharyngeal and laryngeal procedures were technically feasible and refined the proper use of oral retractors and surgical instrumentation in both canine and cadaveric models, thereby paving the way for the use of this technique in humans.[56]

The first use of TORS for oropharyngeal SCC was reported by O'Malley and colleagues,[57] whereby they demonstrated the importance of oral retractor use and detailed the steps of tongue-base resection using this approach. In this initial series of 3 patients, 2 patients received planned tracheotomies and were successfully decannulated after surgery, and all patients tolerated a regular diet within 6 weeks of surgery. Shortly thereafter, robot-assisted supraglottic laryngectomy was reported with good postoperative functional results and no complications.[58,59]

The first larger series of the use of TORS in oropharynx SCC included 27 patients, all of whom received prophylactic gastrostomy tube placement, and showed an overall complication rate of 19%. Early oncologic results were promising at 6-month follow-up, with no patients having evidence of locoregional recurrence.[60] Three independent groups then reported initial case series ranging from 20 to 45 patients.[61–63] Oncologic results from these studies were similarly encouraging, with negative margins in all patients and high rates of locoregional disease control and no life-threatening perioperative complications reported. However, it must be pointed out that most patients in these TORS retrospective series received postoperative radiation as part of the treatment package. Functional results were also promising, with temporary tracheostomy needed in 10% to 31% of patients and temporary enteral feeding needed in 31% to 48%.[62,64] Those with prolonged feeding tube dependence and tracheostomy tube dependence tended to have advanced (T3-T4) disease. Based on these encouraging results at multiple institutions, TORS was approved by the FDA (December 2009) for resection of tumors of the oral cavity and oropharynx.

Functional Results

The primary rationale for the shift from a primary surgical approach to a primary nonsurgical approach for the treatment of oropharyngeal SCC over the past several decades was the significant functional morbidity entailed with most traditional surgical approaches to the oropharynx; however, the application of chemoradiation to the oropharynx is not without risk of significant functional impairment. The rate of severe late toxicity from chemoradiation for oropharyngeal cancer ranges from 35% to 43%.[65] A prospective study of 104 patients with head and neck cancer treated with chemoradiation found that 26% remained feeding tube dependent at 1 year, and 14% remained tracheostomy dependent.[66] In addition, there is a small but real risk of death in patients treated with chemoradiation.[67] However, in a recent prospective multi-institutional trial specifically for oropharyngeal cancer and using modern radiotherapy techniques, long-term toxicities were quite modest.[68] Proponents of TORS argue that functional outcomes may be significantly improved without compromising oncologic control.

Several studies have assessed the early functional outcomes following TORS (**Table 1**). In these studies, 0% to 31% of patients received temporary tracheostomy. Of the patients who required tracheostomy, most were decannulated within 14 days of TORS. Of a total of 204 patients treated with TORS, 1 (0.5%) patient remained tracheostomy dependent at 1 year after surgery. Importantly, 83% to 100% of patients returned to an oral diet within 2 weeks after TORS. The rate of temporary feeding tube use varies significantly across studies, depending on surgeon preference and possible need for postoperative radiation. However, only 0% to 17% of patients required a feeding tube at 1 year, and many of these patients already had impaired swallowing before TORS.[61–64,69–71] A case-control study comparing quality of life between patients receiving TORS and patients receiving primary chemoradiation found that patients receiving TORS scored significantly higher in swallowing, eating, and diet domains 2 weeks after treatment, although these differences disappeared at 3 to 6 months after treatment.[72] At 1 year, patients who received TORS had returned to baseline scores on subjective measures of swallowing and oral intake, whereas patients who received chemoradiation continued to score below pretreatment levels.[72] These early functional results compare favorably with previously reported functional outcomes of primary chemoradiation; however, further prospective, large-scale and long-term data comparing a primary TORS approach with a primary chemoradiation approach are necessary to better define potential differences in functional outcomes.

Oncologic Results

Although the application of TORS for the initial treatment of oropharyngeal SCC offers the potential for decreased overall toxicity and improved long-term functional outcomes, oncologic control remains the most important outcome. Long-term survival outcomes are not yet available for patients treated with TORS; however, several recent studies have reported 1-year to 3-year oncologic outcome data (**Table 2**). Across these studies, regional recurrence rates ranged from 2% to 8%, and distant metastases developed in 1% to 9% of patients.[70–74] Two of these studies stratified their results based on HPV status. Cohen and colleagues[73] found patients who were HPV positive (HPV+) experienced 81% 2-year overall survival and 90% 2-year disease-specific survival. Patients who were HPV negative (HPV–) experienced 80% 2-year overall survival and 100% 2-year disease-specific survival. There were no significant differences in

Table 1
Functional outcomes of TORS

Study	No. Patients	Site(s)	Tracheostomy, %	Tracheostomy Dependence >1 y, %	Exclusively Oral Diet ≤6 wk, %	G-Tube, %	Permanent G-Tube, %	Preoperative MDADI	1-mo Postoperative MDADI
Boudreaux et al,[61] 2009	36	OC+OP +larynx	3	0	79	25	17	77	61
Gendon et al,[63] 2009	18	OP +larynx	0	0	100	0	0	nr	nr
Iseli et al,[64] 2009	54	OC+OP +larynx	9	0	83	17	17	75	65
Moore et al,[62] 2009	45	OP	31	0	89	18	0	nr	nr
Weinstein et al,[71] 2010	47	OP	11	nr	nr	nr	2	nr	nr
White et al,[74] 2010	89	OP +larynx	nr	nr	nr	nr	0	nr	nr
Gendon et al,[72] 2011	30	OP +larynx	13	0	nr	nr	nr	nr	nr
Hurtuk et al,[69] 2011	64	OP +larynx	n/a	n/a	100	19	2	nr	nr
Moore et al,[70] 2012	66	OP	26	2	97	27	5	nr	nr

Abbreviations: G-tube, gastrostomy tube; MDADI, MD Anderson Dysphagia Inventory; n/a, not applicable, nr, not reported; OC, oral cavity; OP, oropharynx.

Table 2
TORS oncologic outcomes

Study	No. Patients	HPV+, n (%)	Post-TORS Adjuvant XRT, %	Overall Survival			Disease-Specific Survival			Recurrence-Free Survival		
				1 y, %	2 y, %	3 y, %	1 y, %	2 y, %	3 y, %	1 y, %	2 y, %	3 y, %
Weinstein et al,[71] 2010	47	nr	85	96	82	nr	98	90	nr	96	79	nr
White et al,[74] 2010	89	nr	63	nr	nr	nr	nr	nr	nr	89	86	nr
Cohen et al,[73] 2011	50	37 (74)	78	96	81	nr	98	93	nr	nr	nr	nr
Gendon et al,[72] 2011	30	nr	83	nr	90[a]	nr	nr	nr	nr	nr	78[a]	nr
Moore et al,[70] 2012	66	44 (67)	83%	nr	nr	96	nr	nr	95	nr	nr	92

Abbreviations: nr, not reported; TORS, transoral robotic surgery; XRT, radiation therapy.

[a] 1.5-year survival rates.

overall survival, disease-specific survival, or disease-free survival between the HPV+ and HPV– groups in this study. Moore and colleagues[70] reported 3-year disease-specific survival to be 98% in patients who were HPV+ and 89% in patients who were HPV–. Although these studies are limited by relatively small patient numbers, they compare favorably with previously reported oncologic outcomes achieved with primary chemoradiation; however, it must be noted that most patients (63%–85%; see **Table 2**) received adjuvant radiotherapy after TORS.[71–74]

Incorporating TORS into the Management of Oropharyngeal SCC

Appropriate integration of TORS into treatment algorithms for oropharyngeal SCC has yet to be established. National Comprehensive Cancer Network consensus guidelines allow for either surgery, including the use of TORS, or radiation as definitive treatment for T1-2N0-1 oropharyngeal SCC.[75–82] Patients with more extensive nodal disease (N2-3) are recommended multimodality therapy, either primary surgery and adjuvant radiation/chemoradiation or primary concurrent chemoradiation.[83] For patients with N+ disease treated with TORS, there are clear indications for the use of adjuvant chemotherapy with postoperative radiation therapy, such as lymph node extracapsular spread and positive surgical margins.[84] However, there can be considerable differences in the delivery of adjuvant therapies after TORS for advanced-stage oropharyngeal SCC (eg, dose and extent of radiation, choice and dosing of chemotherapy). This heterogeneity, often compounded by considerations of HPV status, complicates decision making in the treatment of oropharyngeal SCC. Proponents of TORS argue that surgical resection, including selective neck dissection, provides the most accurate staging information that more accurately risk-stratifies patients and may allow for de-intensification of adjuvant therapy.[85] In particular, a reduction in postoperative radiation dose to 54 to 60 Gy, rather than a definitive treatment dose of 66 to 70 Gy, is believed to reduce the potential for long-term toxicities. Although long-term outcomes data are lacking, there is evidence demonstrating a direct correlation between radiation dose and apical peridontitis.[85] In a post hoc analysis of patients from several Radiation Therapy Oncology Group studies, radiation dose was shown to be a predictor of late toxicities in univariate analysis, but was not significant on multivariate analysis.[65] Therefore, further research is needed to fully define the role of TORS in the treatment of patients with oropharyngeal SCC.

SUMMARY

The management of oral cavity and oropharyngeal SCC remains challenging. Minimizing treatment morbidity is a significant consideration in addition to oncologic success when assessing any treatment modality aimed at the oral cavity and oropharynx. Surgical innovations, including TLM and TORS, offer the potential for improved preservation of speech and swallowing without compromising survival. Similarly, the application of SLNB to oral cavity SCC shows great promise in potentially avoiding treatment sequelae associated with elective neck dissection while maintaining oncologic outcomes. Rigorous studies are still required to validate these innovative approaches and to define their optimal utility in patients with oral cavity and oropharyngeal SCC.

REFERENCES

1. Howlader NA, Krapcho M, Neyman N, et al, editors. SEER Cancer Statistics Review, 1975-2009 (Vintage 2009 Populations). 2012. Available at: http://seer.cancer.gov/csr/1975_2009_pops09/. Accessed 13th August 2012.

2. Brown LM, Check DP, Devesa SS. Oral cavity and pharynx cancer incidence trends by subsite in the United States: changing gender patterns. J Oncol 2012;2012:649498.
3. Induction chemotherapy plus radiation compared with surgery plus radiation in patients with advanced laryngeal cancer. The Department of Veterans Affairs Laryngeal Cancer Study Group. N Engl J Med 1991;324(24):1685–90.
4. Dziegielewski PT, Mlynarek AM, Dimitry J, et al. The mandibulotomy: friend or foe? Safety outcomes and literature review. Laryngoscope 2009;119(12): 2369–75.
5. Babin R, Calcaterra TC. The lip-splitting approach to resection of oropharyngeal cancer. J Surg Oncol 1976;8(5):433–6.
6. Sessions DG. Surgical resection and reconstruction for cancer of the base of the tongue. Otolaryngol Clin North Am 1983;16(2):309–29.
7. Nasri S, Oh Y, Calcaterra TC. Transpharyngeal approach to base of tongue tumors: a comparative study. Laryngoscope 1996;106(8):945–50.
8. Moore DM, Calcaterra TC. Cancer of the tongue base treated by a transpharyngeal approach. Ann Otol Rhinol Laryngol 1990;99(4 Pt 1):300–3.
9. Zeitels SM, Vaughan CW, Ruh S. Suprahyoid pharyngotomy for oropharynx cancer including the tongue base. Arch Otolaryngol Head Neck Surg 1991;117(7): 757–60.
10. Haddadin KJ, Soutar DS, Webster MH, et al. Natural history and patterns of recurrence of tongue tumours. Br J Plast Surg 2000;53(4):279–85.
11. Shah JP. Cervical lymph node metastases—diagnostic, therapeutic, and prognostic implications. Oncology (Williston Park) 1990;4(10):61–9 [discussion: 72, 76].
12. Pentenero M, Gandolfo S, Carrozzo M. Importance of tumor thickness and depth of invasion in nodal involvement and prognosis of oral squamous cell carcinoma: a review of the literature. Head Neck 2005;27(12):1080–91.
13. Asakage T, Yokose T, Mukai K, et al. Tumor thickness predicts cervical metastasis in patients with stage I/II carcinoma of the tongue. Cancer 1998;82(8): 1443–8.
14. Fakih AR, Rao RS, Borges AM, et al. Elective versus therapeutic neck dissection in early carcinoma of the oral tongue. Am J Surg 1989;158(4):309–13.
15. Kligerman J, Lima RA, Soares JR, et al. Supraomohyoid neck dissection in the treatment of T1/T2 squamous cell carcinoma of oral cavity. Am J Surg 1994; 168(5):391–4.
16. Kurokawa H, Yamashita Y, Takeda S, et al. Risk factors for late cervical lymph node metastases in patients with stage I or II carcinoma of the tongue. Head Neck 2002;24(8):731–6.
17. Vandenbrouck C, Sancho-Garnier H, Chassagne D, et al. Elective versus therapeutic radical neck dissection in epidermoid carcinoma of the oral cavity: results of a randomized clinical trial. Cancer 1980;46(2):386–90.
18. Results of a prospective trial on elective modified radical classical versus supraomohyoid neck dissection in the management of oral squamous carcinoma. Brazilian Head and Neck Cancer Study Group. Am J Surg 1998;176(5):422–7.
19. Bier J, Schlums D, Metelmann H, et al. A comparison of radical and conservative neck dissection. Int J Oral Maxillofac Surg 1993;22(2):102–7.
20. Bessell A, Glenny AM, Furness S, et al. Interventions for the treatment of oral and oropharyngeal cancers: surgical treatment. Cochrane Database Syst Rev 2011;(9):CD006205.
21. Seaman WB, Powers WE. Studies on the distribution of radioactive colloidal gold in regional lymph nodes containing cancer. Cancer 1955;8(5):1044–6.

22. Gould EA, Winship T, Philbin PH, et al. Observations on a "sentinel node" in cancer of the parotid. Cancer 1960;13:77–8.
23. Morton DL, Wen DR, Wong JH, et al. Technical details of intraoperative lymphatic mapping for early stage melanoma. Arch Surg 1992;127(4):392–9.
24. Morton DL, Thompson JF, Essner R, et al. Validation of the accuracy of intraoperative lymphatic mapping and sentinel lymphadenectomy for early-stage melanoma: a multicenter trial. Multicenter Selective Lymphadenectomy Trial Group. Ann Surg 1999;230(4):453–63 [discussion: 463–5].
25. Pijpers R, Collet GJ, Meijer S, et al. The impact of dynamic lymphoscintigraphy and gamma probe guidance on sentinel node biopsy in melanoma. Eur J Nucl Med 1995;22(11):1238–41.
26. Giuliano AE, Dale PS, Turner RR, et al. Improved axillary staging of breast cancer with sentinel lymphadenectomy. Ann Surg 1995;222(3):394–9 [discussion: 399–401].
27. Hamy A, Curtet C, Paineau J, et al. Feasibility of radioimmunoguided surgery of colorectal carcinoma using indium 111 CEA specific antibody and simulation with a phantom using 2 steps targetting with bispecific antibody. Tumori 1995; 81(Suppl 3):103–6.
28. Levenback C, Burke TW, Morris M, et al. Potential applications of intraoperative lymphatic mapping in vulvar cancer. Gynecol Oncol 1995;59(2):216–20.
29. Taylor RJ, Wahl RL, Sharma PK, et al. Sentinel node localization in oral cavity and oropharynx squamous cell cancer. Arch Otolaryngol Head Neck Surg 2001;127(8):970–4.
30. Stoeckli SJ, Steinert H, Pfaltz M, et al. Sentinel lymph node evaluation in squamous cell carcinoma of the head and neck. Otolaryngol Head Neck Surg 2001; 125(3):221–6.
31. Zitsch RP 3rd, Todd DW, Renner GJ, et al. Intraoperative radiolymphoscintigraphy for detection of occult nodal metastasis in patients with head and neck squamous cell carcinoma. Otolaryngol Head Neck Surg 2000;122(5):662–6.
32. Mozzillo N, Chiesa F, Botti G, et al. Sentinel node biopsy in head and neck cancer. Ann Surg Oncol 2001;8(Suppl 9):103S–5S.
33. Civantos FJ, Zitsch RP, Schuller DE, et al. Sentinel lymph node biopsy accurately stages the regional lymph nodes for T1-T2 oral squamous cell carcinomas: results of a prospective multi-institutional trial. J Clin Oncol 2010;28(8):1395–400.
34. Stoeckli SJ. Sentinel node biopsy for oral and oropharyngeal squamous cell carcinoma of the head and neck. Laryngoscope 2007;117(9):1539–51.
35. Broglie MA, Haile SR, Stoeckli SJ. Long-term experience in sentinel node biopsy for early oral and oropharyngeal squamous cell carcinoma. Ann Surg Oncol 2011;18(10):2732–8.
36. Ross GL, Soutar DS, MacDonald DG, et al. Improved staging of cervical metastases in clinically node-negative patients with head and neck squamous cell carcinoma. Ann Surg Oncol 2004;11(2):213–8.
37. Alkureishi LW, Ross GL, Shoaib T, et al. Sentinel node biopsy in head and neck squamous cell cancer: 5-year follow-up of a European multicenter trial. Ann Surg Oncol 2010;17(9):2459–64.
38. Murer K, Huber GF, Haile SR, et al. Comparison of morbidity between sentinel node biopsy and elective neck dissection for treatment of the N0 neck in patients with oral squamous cell carcinoma. Head Neck 2011;33(9):1260–4.
39. Alkureishi LW, Burak Z, Alvarez JA, et al. Joint practice guidelines for radionuclide lymphoscintigraphy for sentinel node localization in oral/oropharyngeal squamous cell carcinoma. Ann Surg Oncol 2009;16(11):3190–210.

40. Holinger PH, Andrews AH Jr. The carbon dioxide laser in management of papilloma of the larynx. JFORL J Fr Otorhinolaryngol Audiophonol Chir Maxillofac 1974;23(2):177–8.
41. Strong MS, Vaughan CW, Cooperband SR, et al. Recurrent respiratory papillomatosis: management with the CO2 laser. Ann Otol Rhinol Laryngol 1976; 85(4 Pt 1):508–16.
42. Grant DG, Salassa JR, Hinni ML, et al. Transoral laser microsurgery for untreated glottic carcinoma. Otolaryngol Head Neck Surg 2007;137(3):482–6.
43. Grant DG, Salassa JR, Hinni ML, et al. Transoral laser microsurgery for carcinoma of the supraglottic larynx. Otolaryngol Head Neck Surg 2007;136(6): 900–6.
44. Steiner W, Fierek O, Ambrosch P, et al. Transoral laser microsurgery for squamous cell carcinoma of the base of the tongue. Arch Otolaryngol Head Neck Surg 2003;129(1):36–43.
45. Holsinger FC, McWhorter AJ, Menard M, et al. Transoral lateral oropharyngectomy for squamous cell carcinoma of the tonsillar region: I. Technique, complications, and functional results. Arch Otolaryngol Head Neck Surg 2005;131(7): 583–91.
46. Laccourreye O, Hans S, Menard M, et al. Transoral lateral oropharyngectomy for squamous cell carcinoma of the tonsillar region: II. An analysis of the incidence, related variables, and consequences of local recurrence. Arch Otolaryngol Head Neck Surg 2005;131(7):592–9.
47. Grant DG, Hinni ML, Salassa JR, et al. Oropharyngeal cancer: a case for single modality treatment with transoral laser microsurgery. Arch Otolaryngol Head Neck Surg 2009;135(12):1225–30.
48. Rich JT, Milov S, Lewis JS Jr, et al. Transoral laser microsurgery (TLM) +/– adjuvant therapy for advanced stage oropharyngeal cancer: outcomes and prognostic factors. Laryngoscope 2009;119(9):1709–19.
49. Kwoh YS, Hou J, Jonckheere EA, et al. A robot with improved absolute positioning accuracy for CT guided stereotactic brain surgery. IEEE Trans Biomed Eng 1988;35(2):153–60.
50. Davies B. A review of robotics in surgery. Proc Inst Mech Eng H 2000;214(1): 129–40.
51. Hagen ME, Meehan JJ, Inan I, et al. Visual clues act as a substitute for haptic feedback in robotic surgery. Surg Endosc 2008;22(6):1505–8.
52. Maan ZN, Gibbins N, Al-Jabri T, et al. The use of robotics in otolaryngology-head and neck surgery: a systematic review. Am J Otol 2012;33(1):137–46.
53. Chandra V, Nehra D, Parent R, et al. A comparison of laparoscopic and robotic assisted suturing performance by experts and novices. Surgery 2010;147(6): 830–9.
54. Haus BM, Kambham N, Le D, et al. Surgical robotic applications in otolaryngology. Laryngoscope 2003;113(7):1139–44.
55. Hockstein NG, Nolan JP, O'Malley BW Jr, et al. Robotic microlaryngeal surgery: a technical feasibility study using the daVinci surgical robot and an airway mannequin. Laryngoscope 2005;115(5):780–5.
56. Weinstein GS, O'Malley BW Jr, Hockstein NG. Transoral robotic surgery: supraglottic laryngectomy in a canine model. Laryngoscope 2005;115(7):1315–9.
57. O'Malley BW Jr, Weinstein GS, Snyder W, et al. Transoral robotic surgery (TORS) for base of tongue neoplasms. Laryngoscope 2006;116(8):1465–72.
58. Weinstein GS, O'Malley BW Jr, Snyder W, et al. Transoral robotic surgery: supraglottic partial laryngectomy. Ann Otol Rhinol Laryngol 2007;116(1):19–23.

59. Solares CA, Strome M. Transoral robot-assisted CO2 laser supraglottic laryngectomy: experimental and clinical data. Laryngoscope 2007;117(5):817–20.
60. Weinstein GS, O'Malley BW Jr, Snyder W, et al. Transoral robotic surgery: radical tonsillectomy. Arch Otolaryngol Head Neck Surg 2007;133(12):1220–6.
61. Boudreaux BA, Rosenthal EL, Magnuson JS, et al. Robot-assisted surgery for upper aerodigestive tract neoplasms. Arch Otolaryngol Head Neck Surg 2009; 135(4):397–401.
62. Moore EJ, Olsen KD, Kasperbauer JL. Transoral robotic surgery for oropharyngeal squamous cell carcinoma: a prospective study of feasibility and functional outcomes. Laryngoscope 2009;119(11):2156–64.
63. Genden EM, Desai S, Sung CK. Transoral robotic surgery for the management of head and neck cancer: a preliminary experience. Head Neck 2009;31(3): 283–9.
64. Iseli TA, Kulbersh BD, Iseli CE, et al. Functional outcomes after transoral robotic surgery for head and neck cancer. Otolaryngol Head Neck Surg 2009;141(2): 166–71.
65. Machtay M, Moughan J, Trotti A, et al. Factors associated with severe late toxicity after concurrent chemoradiation for locally advanced head and neck cancer: an RTOG analysis. J Clin Oncol 2008;26(21):3582–9.
66. Givens DJ, Karnell LH, Gupta AK, et al. Adverse events associated with concurrent chemoradiation therapy in patients with head and neck cancer. Arch Otolaryngol Head Neck Surg 2009;135(12):1209–17.
67. Calais G, Alfonsi M, Bardet E, et al. Randomized trial of radiation therapy versus concomitant chemotherapy and radiation therapy for advanced-stage oropharynx carcinoma. J Natl Cancer Inst 1999;91(24):2081–6.
68. Eisbruch A, Harris J, Garden A, et al. Multi-institutional trial of accelerated hypofractionated intensity-modulated radiation therapy for early-stage oropharyngeal cancer. Int J Radiat Oncol Biol Phys 2009;76(5):1333–8.
69. Hurtuk A, Agrawal A, Old M, et al. Outcomes of transoral robotic surgery: a preliminary clinical experience. Otolaryngol Head Neck Surg 2011;145(2): 248–53.
70. Moore EJ, Olsen SM, Laborde RR, et al. Long-term functional and oncologic results of transoral robotic surgery for oropharyngeal squamous cell carcinoma. Mayo Clin Proc 2012;87(3):219–25.
71. Weinstein GS, O'Malley BW Jr, Cohen MA, et al. Transoral robotic surgery for advanced oropharyngeal carcinoma. Arch Otolaryngol Head Neck Surg 2010; 136(11):1079–85.
72. Genden EM, Kotz T, Tong CC, et al. Transoral robotic resection and reconstruction for head and neck cancer. Laryngoscope 2011;121(8):1668–74.
73. Cohen MA, Weinstein GS, O'Malley BW Jr, et al. Transoral robotic surgery and human papillomavirus status: oncologic results. Head Neck 2011;33(4): 573–80.
74. White HN, Moore EJ, Rosenthal EL, et al. Transoral robotic-assisted surgery for head and neck squamous cell carcinoma: one- and 2-year survival analysis. Arch Otolaryngol Head Neck Surg 2010;136(12):1248–52.
75. Chao KS, Ozyigit G, Blanco AI, et al. Intensity-modulated radiation therapy for oropharyngeal carcinoma: impact of tumor volume. Int J Radiat Oncol Biol Phys 2004;59(1):43–50.
76. de Arruda FF, Puri DR, Zhung J, et al. Intensity-modulated radiation therapy for the treatment of oropharyngeal carcinoma: the Memorial Sloan-Kettering Cancer Center experience. Int J Radiat Oncol Biol Phys 2006;64(2):363–73.

77. Eisbruch A, Harris J, Garden AS, et al. Multi-institutional trial of accelerated hypofractionated intensity-modulated radiation therapy for early-stage oropharyngeal cancer (RTOG 00-22). Int J Radiat Oncol Biol Phys 2010;76(5):1333–8.
78. Garden AS, Morrison WH, Wong PF, et al. Disease-control rates following intensity-modulated radiation therapy for small primary oropharyngeal carcinoma. Int J Radiat Oncol Biol Phys 2007;67(2):438–44.
79. Yao M, Nguyen T, Buatti JM, et al. Changing failure patterns in oropharyngeal squamous cell carcinoma treated with intensity modulated radiotherapy and implications for future research. Am J Clin Oncol 2006;29(6):606–12.
80. Sanguineti G, Gunn GB, Endres EJ, et al. Patterns of locoregional failure after exclusive IMRT for oropharyngeal carcinoma. Int J Radiat Oncol Biol Phys 2008;72(3):737–46.
81. Chepeha DB, Hoff PT, Taylor RJ, et al. Selective neck dissection for the treatment of neck metastasis from squamous cell carcinoma of the head and neck. Laryngoscope 2002;112(3):434–8.
82. National Comprehensive Cancer Network. NCCN Clinical Practice Guidelines in Oncology: Head and Neck Cancers. 2012. Available at: http://www.nccn.org/professionals/physician_gls/pdf/head-and-neck.pdf. Accessed June 23, 2012.
83. Ferlito A, Rinaldo A, Silver CE, et al. Elective and therapeutic selective neck dissection. Oral Oncol 2006;42(1):14–25.
84. Bernier J, Cooper JS, Pajak TF, et al. Defining risk levels in locally advanced head and neck cancers: a comparative analysis of concurrent postoperative radiation plus chemotherapy trials of the EORTC (#22931) and RTOG (# 9501). Head Neck 2005;27(10):843–50.
85. Weinstein GS, Quon H, O'Malley BW Jr, et al. Selective neck dissection and deintensified postoperative radiation and chemotherapy for oropharyngeal cancer: a subset analysis of the University of Pennsylvania transoral robotic surgery trial. Laryngoscope 2010;120(9):1749–55.

Advances in Radiation Oncology for the Management of Oropharyngeal Tumors

G. Brandon Gunn, MD[a], Steven J. Frank, MD[b,*]

KEYWORDS

• Radiation therapy • Oropharyngeal tumors • Head and neck cancer
• Intensity-modulated proton therapy • Intensity-modulated radiation therapy

KEY POINTS

- Altered-fractionation radiation therapy improves locoregional control and survival over that obtained with conventionally fractionated radiation therapy when either is used as single-modality treatment.
- Radiation therapy alone can achieve excellent locoregional control of early T-category oropharyngeal carcinoma.
- Advances in radiation therapy techniques such as intensity-modulated radiation therapy (IMRT) have improved patient functional and quality of life outcomes through parotid sparing with resultant reduction in xerostomia.
- Protons have unique physical properties compared with x-rays or photons owing to the Bragg peak.
- Intensity-modulated proton therapy may offer additional advantages over IMRT by reducing the toxicity associated with multiple beams passing through critical structures and by improving quality of life during and after treatment.

Radiation therapy (RT) has long been a standard approach for the definitive treatment of oropharyngeal carcinoma (OPC), with the dual treatment goals of cure and functional organ preservation.[1] Current RT standards for patients with head and neck cancer (HNC) were defined through the sequential execution of several large randomized phase III clinical trials conducted over the past 2 to 3 decades, which led to improved disease control rates[2,3] and improved survival.[4–6] These important trials, along with

Disclosure: The authors report no financial conflicts of interest.
[a] Department of Radiation Oncology, The University of Texas MD Anderson Cancer Center, Unit 97, 1515 Holcombe Boulevard, Houston, TX 77030, USA; [b] Department of Radiation Oncology, The University of Texas MD Anderson Cancer Center, Unit 1202, 1220 Holcombe Boulevard, Houston, TX 77030, USA
* Corresponding author.
E-mail address: sjfrank@mdanderson.org

Otolaryngol Clin N Am 46 (2013) 629–643
http://dx.doi.org/10.1016/j.otc.2013.04.004 oto.theclinics.com
0030-6665/13/$ – see front matter

Abbreviations: Radiation Oncology for Oropharyngeal Tumors	
EGFR	Epidermal growth factor receptor
GORTEC	Groupe d'Oncologie Radiothérapie Tête et Cou
HNC	Head and neck cancer
HPV	Human papillomavirus
IMPT	Intensity-modulated proton therapy
IMRT	Intensity-modulated radiation therapy
LRC	Locoregional control
OPC	Oropharyngeal carcinoma
OS	Overall survival
RFS	Recurrence-free survival
RT	Radiation therapy

data from meta-analyses,[7,8] helped established the optimal radiation fractionation schedules[2,3] and the benefit of concurrent radiosensitizing systemic therapy (chemoradiation).[4–6]

Over the past decade, advances in RT planning and delivery techniques (eg, intensity-modulated RT [IMRT]) led to improved dose distributions compared with previous methods. These dosimetric gains, most notably the reduction of unnecessary irradiation of the parotid glands, translated into improved functional outcomes and quality of life for patients.[9] More recently, advances in proton therapy planning and delivery are providing new opportunities to investigate whether proton therapy can further improve outcomes over those obtained with modern-day IMRT, specifically with regard to reducing treatment-related toxicity and symptoms and improving quality of life.

The goals of this article are to (1) highlight some key trials that established the current standards of care; (2) discuss some major studies that helped to guide current practice; (3) review some of the specific advantages and limitations of IMRT, the current standard of care for OPC, and (4) briefly describe features of proton therapy and its potential to further improve patient outcomes.

RT FRACTIONATION

Two aspects of the RT schedule generally regarded as important for tumor control and acute normal tissue reactions are the total radiation dose and overall treatment time; late normal tissue reactions depend more on other variables, such as radiation fraction size. Attempts to modify or alter fractionation schedules have been made in an effort to improve locoregional control rates over those that can be achieved with conventionally fractionated RT, through either decreasing the overall treatment time, increasing the total dose, or often both. Altered fractionation schedules typically involve the delivery of multiple smaller daily fractions as a component of the treatment schedule.[10]

Landmark Fractionation Studies

Several institutions have developed and refined various altered fractionation schedules for locally advanced HNC during the past few decades. One landmark cooperative group trial, the Radiation Therapy Oncology Group (RTOG) trial 9003, compared 3 altered fractionation schedules against conventionally fractionated RT (70 Gy in 35 fractions over 7 weeks) for HNC. Most of the 1000 patients in this randomized trial had OPC. Fu and colleagues[2] reported an absolute improvement in locoregional tumor control at 2 years of approximately 8% from continuous altered fractionation schedules compared with conventional fractionation, with a trend toward improved disease-specific survival. Acute reactions were noted to be worse in the groups given altered fractionation, but without an increase in long-term late radiation effects.[2] These results led the RTOG to adopt altered fractionation as their standard schedule for RT in subsequent trials.

Likewise, Overgaard and colleagues,[3] in the Danish Head and Neck Cancer Study Group trials, showed a similar magnitude of benefit in locoregional control for accelerated RT compared with conventionally fractionated RT. Importantly, a recent meta-analysis[11] of 15 trials that included the aforementioned fractionation studies demonstrated that altered fractionation produced an overall survival advantage in HNC. For example, hyperfractionated RT conveyed an absolute overall survival advantage of 8% at 5 years compared with conventional fractionation, further establishing the advantage of altered fractionation schedules over conventionally fractionated RT when RT is given as monotherapy.

CHEMORADIATION

Historically, the predominant pattern of disease relapse after RT for locally advanced HNC has been locoregional recurrence, which has been attributed to the "radioresistance" of tumor-cell clonogens that persist after therapy. One approach taken to improve locoregional control was to add concurrent chemotherapy to RT with the intent of sensitizing malignant cells to the damaging effects of ionizing radiation. Although recent studies have refined induction chemotherapy regimens,[12] this discussion of chemotherapy and RT will focus on concurrent chemoradiation, the current standard of care that is supported by the largest body of evidence.

Landmark Chemoradiation Studies

Calais and colleagues[4] in the Groupe d'Oncologie Radiothérapie Tête et Cou (GORTEC) conducted an important trial in the late 1990s comparing chemoradiation with concurrent 5-flourouracil and carboplatin versus RT alone for locally advanced OPC. Increased rates of acute reactions were seen in the combined-modality arm; for example, high-grade mucositis was experienced by 71% of patients in the chemoradiation group versus 39% in the RT-only group.[4] The rate of late reactions was substantial, occurring in 56% of patients receiving chemoradiation, and in a similar proportion of the RT-only group. Long-term follow-up revealed a benefit from chemoradiation in terms of both locoregional control rates at 5 years (48% vs 25%; $P = .002$) and long-term survival (22% vs 16%; $P = .05$).[13]

Pignon and colleagues[8] reported updated results from their meta-analysis of more than 16,000 patients participating in trials that incorporated chemotherapy and locoregional treatment. Overall, the addition of chemotherapy improved survival (5% absolute benefit at 5 years), with the greatest benefit seen among patients receiving concurrent chemotherapy (6.5% absolute benefit at 5 years).[8] Another recent analysis from this same group showed that patients with primary OPC obtained the greatest magnitude of survival benefit from the addition of concurrent chemotherapy relative to those with HNC at other primary sites.[14]

EPIDERMAL GROWTH FACTOR RECEPTOR INHIBITION AND RT

On the basis of important preclinical work and retrospective validation with pathology tumor specimens demonstrating the importance of tumor-cell expression of epidermal growth factor receptor (EGFR) in HNC,[15] Bonner and colleagues[5,6] performed a phase III randomized clinical trial comparing RT alone and RT plus concurrent cetuximab, a monoclonal antibody inhibitor of EGFR, in patients with locally advanced HNC. Assessments of toxicity revealed that those patients who received cetuximab experienced a greater number of high-grade acute reactions, such as infusion reaction and acneiform-like rash. However, the addition of cetuximab did not increase the reported rates of high-grade mucosal reactions or dysphagia[5,6] and did not negatively affect patient quality of life compared with RT alone.[16] Overall, the addition of cetuximab to RT improved locoregional control and overall survival rates (the latter being 45.6% vs 36.4% for RT only at 5 years; $P = .018$), and extended the median overall survival time from 29 to 49 months.[5,6] This trial established RT and concurrent cetuximab as a standard treatment option for patients with locally advanced HNC.

RT AS MONOTHERAPY FOR EARLY T-CATEGORY OROPHARYNGEAL CANCER

Most of the patients who participated in the randomized trials that established the survival advantage for chemoradiation had higher T-category tumors; patients with T1 primary tumors were often excluded from these trials. For example, more than 80% of the patients in the GORTEC study had T3 or T4 disease. Although RT with concurrent systemic therapy remains the standard of care for patients with locally advanced disease, excellent locoregional control rates can be achieved with RT used as a single modality (ie, without systemic therapy), and this strategy may minimize the severity of treatment-related reactions.

For example, as part of a large single-institution series, Garden and colleagues[17] reported excellent locoregional control rates for patients with T1 or T2 primary OPC tumors but with stage III through IVA disease (ie, patients who had smaller primary tumors but higher stage grouping because of nodal disease) treated with RT alone, and no benefit to the addition of concurrent chemotherapy for this early T-category group was seen (**Fig. 1**). The authors' current approach is to consider both the local and regional extent of disease when considering therapeutic strategies for individual patients; in terms of local therapy, they typically select concurrent chemoradiation as a component of treatment for advanced T-category tumors, but often treat early T-category OPC with RT alone.

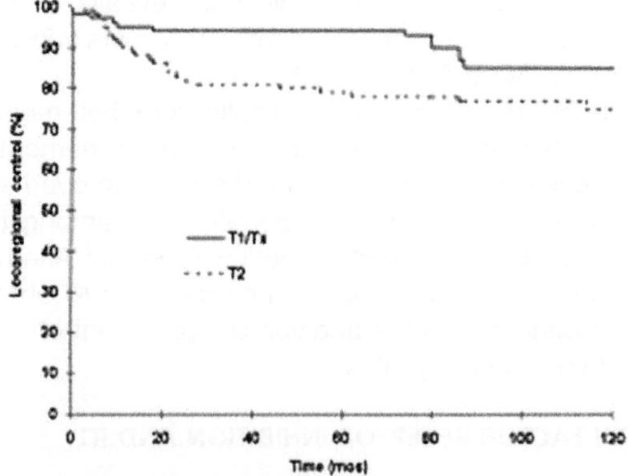

Fig. 1. Locoregional control rates stratified by T-category for oropharyngeal cancer treated with definitive RT. (*From* Garden AS, Kies MS, Morrison WH, et al. Outcomes and patterns of care of patients with locally advanced oropharyngeal carcinoma treated in the early 21st century. Radiat Oncol 2013;8:21.)

Unilateral RT for Tonsillar Carcinoma

In carefully selected cases of lateralized tonsillar carcinoma, the RT treatment volume can often be restricted to treatment of the primary site and ipsilateral cervical and retropharyngeal lymph nodes; this treatment can result in excellent locoregional control, low contralateral cervical lymph node failure rates, and less toxicity than that expected from bilateral neck treatment.[18,19] Compared with bilateral neck irradiation, this approach substantially reduces the dose to contralateral major salivary glands, nontarget upper aerodigestive tract mucosa, and important swallowing structures.

Chronowski and colleagues[20] recently reported findings from 102 patients treated with this unilateral approach at The University of Texas MD Anderson Cancer Center. The ideal patients for this approach had T2 or lower primary site disease, no more than minimal soft palate invasion, and no base of tongue invasion. Only 5 of the patients in this series received systemic therapy as a component of treatment, and most received IMRT. Locoregional control rates for both the primary site and ipsilateral neck were 100% at 5 years. At a median follow-up interval of 39 months, only 2 patients had developed a contralateral recurrence. With regard to toxicity, only 9 patients required placement of a feeding tube during therapy, and no patient experienced long-term dependence on a feeding tube. A representative case of this unilateral approach is shown in **Fig. 2**.

RT FOR UNKNOWN PRIMARY METASTATIC TO CERVICAL LYMPH NODES

For patients with squamous carcinoma metastatic to cervical lymph nodes, without an identifiable primary site after adequate clinical evaluation, and for whom a head and neck mucosal source is suspected, the authors' preferred approach is primary RT that targets both the neck and at-risk mucosal sites. Frank and colleagues[21] recently reported outcomes for patients treated with IMRT at MD Anderson Cancer Center according to this general treatment philosophy, which yielded 5-year mucosal and regional control rates of 98% and 94%, respectively. Rates of disease-free and overall survival at 5 years were 88% and 81%, respectively. As for late toxicity, only 2 patients had high-grade swallowing toxicity, with 1 requiring a long-term feeding tube and the other requiring esophageal dilatation.[21]

The authors' current practice and their IMRT target volumes are guided by the anatomic location of the involved nodes, the patient's smoking history, and the tumor's human papillomavirus (HPV) status. For example, for patients without an identifiable primary site when examined under anesthesia and laryngoscopy and no evidence of disease on directed biopsies or tonsillectomies, the authors target the involved lymph nodes with curative intent, electively irradiate the uninvolved bilateral neck and retropharyngeal lymph nodes at risk, and electively irradiate the pharyngeal axis mucosal sites to doses designed to eradicate subclinical microscopic disease. For patients who have never smoked and for those with viral-associated carcinomas, the authors typically shield the larynx and hypopharynx from radiation to minimize swallowing dysfunction after RT, because the occult primary site is unlikely to reside in the larynx or hypopharynx in these cases.

IMRT FOR OROPHARYNGEAL CARCINOMA

Because HNCs are adjacent to several normal tissues that are critical to a variety of important functions, the ideal means of delivering RT would conform the dose distributions tightly to the target areas and spare these nearby nontarget organs. Traditional RT approaches typically were restricted to lateral x-ray beams aimed across

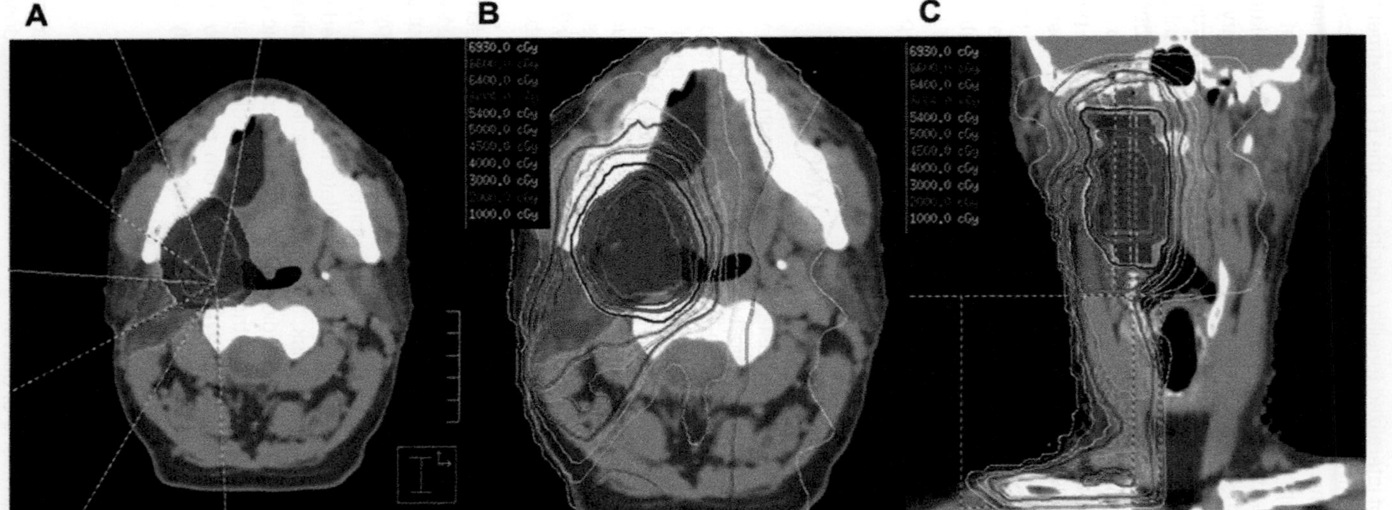

Fig. 2. Computed tomography (CT)–based treatment plans for a patient with a squamous cell carcinoma of the right tonsil (cTXN0M0 after diagnostic tonsillectomy) to be treated with unilateral IMRT. (*A*) Axial CT scan illustrates clinical target volumes to be treated with a 7-field IMRT beam arrangement to 66 Gy (*red*), 60 Gy (*blue*), and 54 Gy (*yellow*). (*B*) Axial CT scan of the same patient shows representative isodose distributions for IMRT to be delivered in 30 daily fractions. A custom fabricated tongue-deviating stent was used to displace the anterior tongue to the left, away from the intermediate dose distribution. (*C*) Coronal CT scan of the same patient demonstrates the split-field IMRT technique used to facilitate maximal sparing of the larynx, esophageal inlet, and esophagus. The ipsilateral lateral retropharyngeal lymph node region was included in the volume to be treated to 54 Gy. Mean doses to the contralateral parotid were kept lower than 6.4 Gy, and doses to the submandibular gland were kept lower than 10.0 Gy.

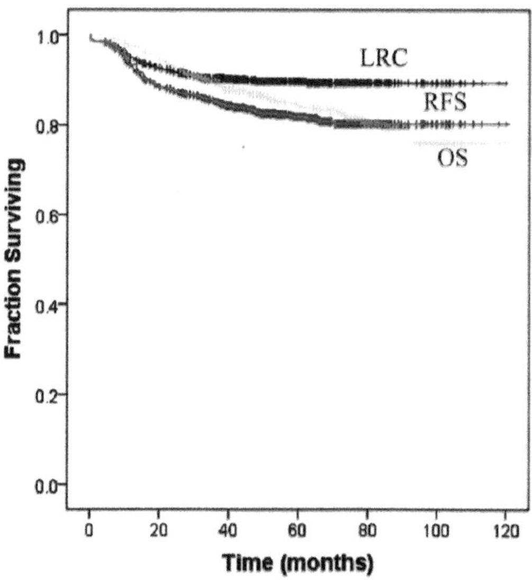

Fig. 3. Rates of locoregional control (LRC), recurrence-free survival (RFS), and overall survival (OS) among patients treated with IMRT for oropharyngeal carcinoma. (*From* Garden AS, Dong L, Morrison WH, et al. Patterns of disease recurrence following treatment of oropharyngeal cancer with intensity modulated radiation therapy. Int J Radiat Oncol Biol Phys 2013;85:941–7; with permission.)

the patient, with little ability to account for 3-dimensional relationships between targets and organs to be avoided. Advances in computer-based treatment-planning systems coupled with modern-day linear accelerator technology provided the ability to apply several treatment fields of nonuniform beam intensities to generate more conformal dose distributions, an approach known as IMRT.

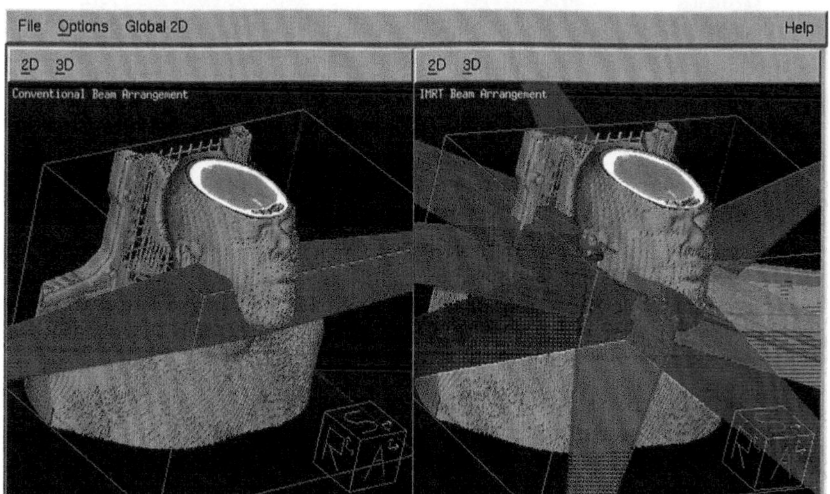

Fig. 4. Comparison of nontarget beam paths in IMRT (*right*) versus conventional 3-dimensional technique (*left*). (*From* Rosenthal DI, Chambers MS, Fuller CD, et al. Beam path toxicities to non-target structures during intensity-modulated radiation therapy for head and neck cancer. Int J Radiat Oncol Biol Phys 2008;72:747–55; with permission.)

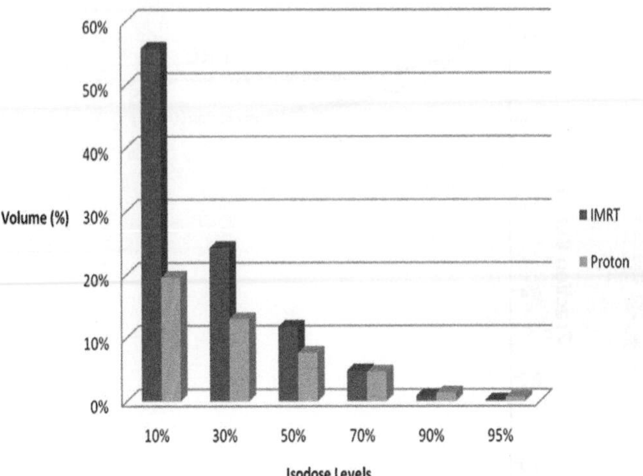

Fig. 5. The mean volumes of tissues irradiated at different isodose levels for IMRT (*blue bars*) versus for IMPT. IMRT delivers significantly more radiation to normal tissues in what is commonly referred to as the "dose bath," which can result in beam-path toxicities, such as nausea and vomiting, anterior oral mucositis, xerostomia, dysgeusia, odynophagia, hoarseness, and dysphagia.

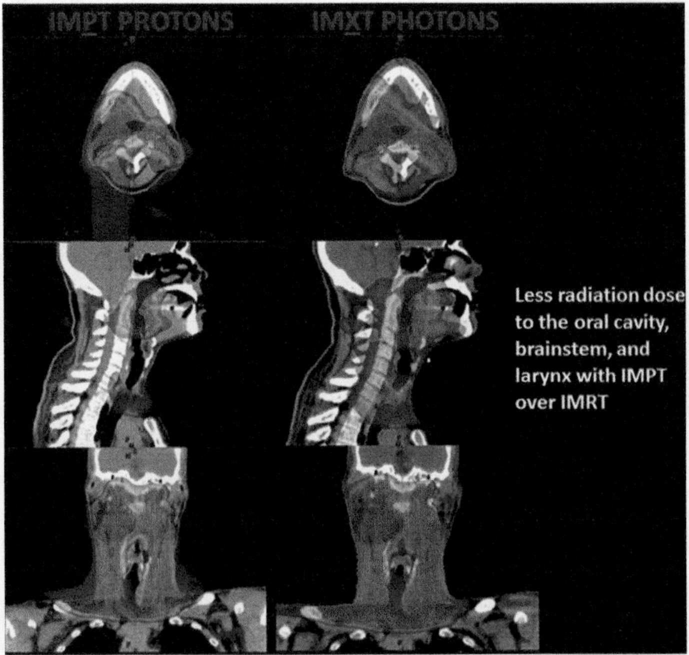

Fig. 6. A radiation dose comparison of treatment plans for IMPT versus IMX[R]T (photon) for a T2N2b squamous cell carcinoma of the right tonsil. The IMPT plan would result in less radiation dose being delivered to the oral cavity, brainstem, and larynx compared with the IMRT plan.

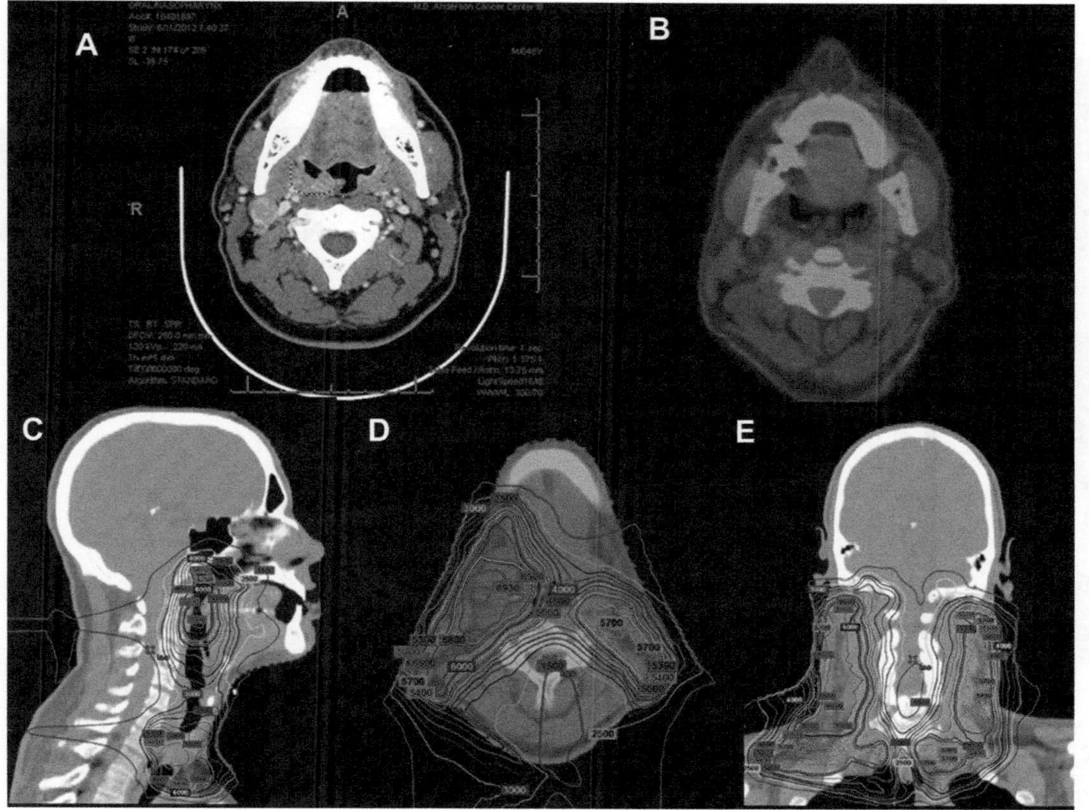

Fig. 7. Images used for disease staging and treatment planning for a 48-year-old man with T2N2b (stage IVa), HPV/p16–positive squamous cell carcinoma of the right tonsil. Computed tomography (*A*) and positron emission tomography (*B*) scans demonstrate a primary tumor in the right tonsil with right neck adenopathy. The treatment plan called for IMPT to 66 GyE in 30 fractions with cetuximab. The IMPT dose distributions in the sagittal (*C*) axial (*D*), and coronal (*E*) planes illustrate the minimal exposure of the oral cavity, brainstem, and larynx from IMPT.

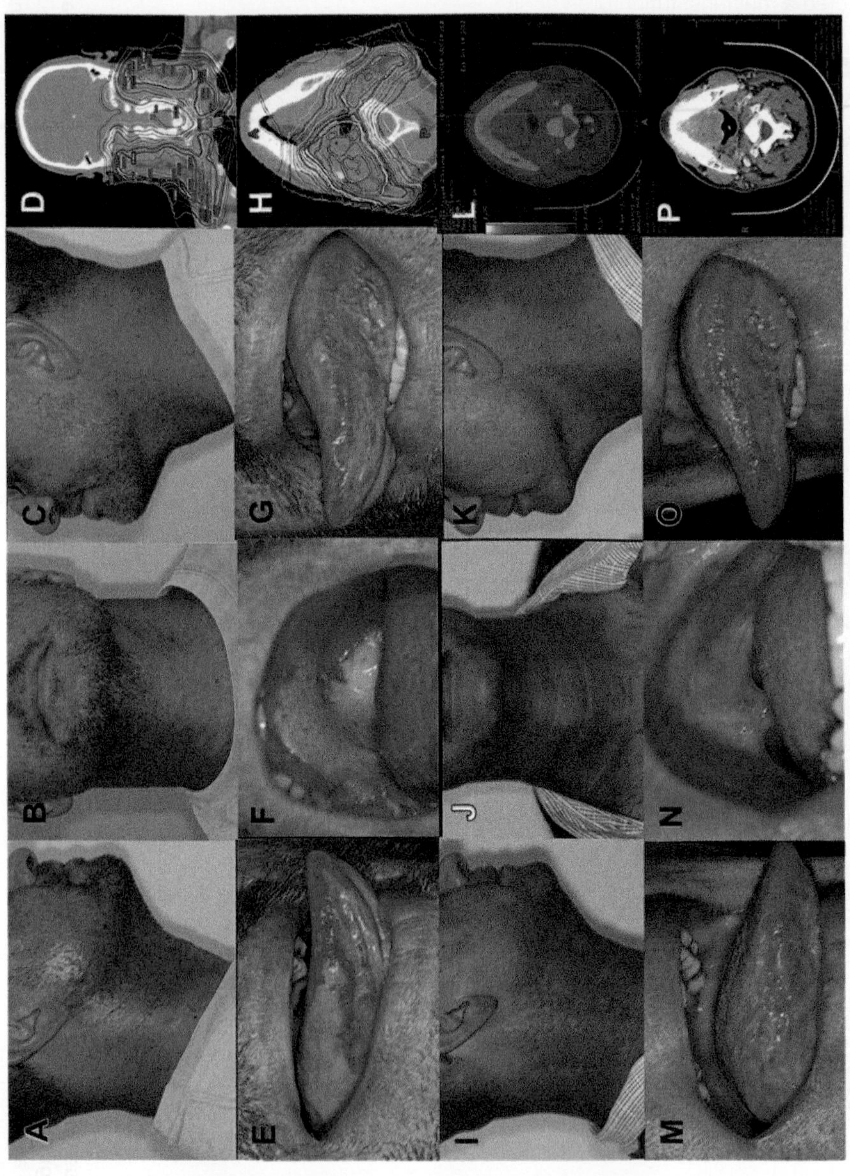

One of the main benefits of IMRT compared with traditional methods of treating HNC is the ability to conform the dose distributions around tumors, which allows relative sparing of the parotid glands. The ability to spare the parotids with IMRT has translated into reduced xerostomia and improved functional and quality-of-life outcomes, as has been borne out in several prospective studies. For example, the RTOG conducted a multi-institution prospective study of IMRT alone for early OPC. Overall, parotid dose constraints could be met for most patients, and the xerostomia rate was encouragingly low at only 16% at 2 years.[22] More recently, Nutting and colleagues[23] reported results from the PARSPORT trial, a landmark multi-institutional, randomized phase III trial comparing IMRT versus conventional RT for pharyngeal cancers, which confirmed the ability of IMRT to reduce xerostomia and improve patient quality of life.

Garden and colleagues[24] at MD Anderson recently reported excellent long-term clinical outcomes and described the patterns of failure after IMRT for OPC. In this study of more than 700 patients, with a median follow-up interval of 54 months, rates of locoregional control, relapse-free survival, and overall survival were 90%, 82%, and 84% at 5 years (**Fig. 3**). Most patients also received systemic therapy. As for toxicity, 47% of patients had a feeding tube placed during therapy, but only 18 patients had a feeding tube in place at the last follow-up. No patient experienced disease recurrence in or immediately adjacent to a spared parotid gland, further justifying the use of a parotid-sparing IMRT approach for most patients with OPC.[24]

Although the benefit of IMRT in terms of reduction in xerostomia has been clearly demonstrated, some tradeoffs have been made to achieve these results. For example, Rosenthal and colleagues[25] reported the potential for negative clinical effects from the use of IMRT, wherein multiple beams surround the patient, compared with the classic lateral beam arrangement (**Fig. 4**). The use of multiple oblique IMRT beams increases the volume of irradiation, and the beams traverse several tissues that were essentially unirradiated during the previous classical-beam eras. In this retrospective comparison study, the dose to far-posterior structures such as the occipital scalp and brainstem from IMRT correlated with occipital alopecia and nausea and vomiting, respectively. Similarly, the dose to the far-anterior mandible correlated with anterior oral cavity mucositis.[25] Others have also pointed out the potential negative effects of IMRT in terms of increased doses to skin, larynx, and esophagus. These studies highlight the importance of selecting the appropriate IMRT technique and careful treatment planning, with attention to the intermediate-dose regions because of the potential for toxicity associated with exposure of these regions.[9]

Fig. 8. Treatment plans and side effects and treatment response after IMPT to 66 GyE in 30 fractions given with concurrent cetuximab for the 48-year-old man in **Fig. 7** with T2N2b (stage IVa) HPV/p16–positive squamous cell carcinoma of the right tonsil. (*A–C*) Photographs illustrate grade 2 radiation dermatitis in the right neck and grade 1 radiation dermatitis in the left neck. (*D*) Treatment plan in the coronal plane shows the radiation dose distribution from the base of skull to the clavicles. (*E–G*) Mucositis is evident within the treatment field on the right lateral tongue, tonsillar fossa, and soft palate but not on the left lateral or anterior tongue. (*H*) Treatment plan in the axial plane shows the radiation dose distribution, with a left tongue–deviating stent used to minimize dose to the left lateral and anterior oral tongue. (*I–K*) Photographs taken at 5 months after treatment show good healing of the bilateral neck with mild radiation-induced changes remaining. (*L*) Positron emission tomography and (*P*) computed tomography scans in the axial plane show a complete response. (*M–O*) Photographs taken at 5 months show good healing of the tongue, soft palate, and right tonsillar fossa, with moist mucous membranes.

INTENSITY-MODULATED PROTON THERAPY FOR OROPHARYNGEAL CARCINOMA

Protons have unique physical properties that confer advantages to proton therapy over more traditional forms of photon-based RT. IMRT involves the use of photons (X rays), which deposit the greatest radiation dose near the surface of the skin, with the dose slowly diminishing in intensity with increasing depth. In contrast, intensity-modulated proton therapy (IMPT) involves the use of protons, which deposit minimal dose near the surface of the skin and on the way to the tumor, depositing most of the radiation dose at a finite depth because of the so-called Bragg peak phenomenon.[26] Proton therapy can be delivered by several methods; IMPT requires the use of an active scanning proton beam.[27] IMPT also incorporates magnets to deflect the narrow proton beam (called a *pencil beam*) to conform the radiation dose to the target, in a layer-by-layer fashion, by using protons or "spots" of different energies. Thus protons delivered via IMPT can in theory deliver lower total radiation doses to nontarget normal tissues than can photons delivered via IMRT, because photons by their nature deposit most of their dose to the entry and exit portions of the beam path. As a result, IMPT has the potential to further improve the therapeutic ratio over that of IMRT for the treatment of HNCs by reducing the so-called beam-path toxicities resulting from inadvertent multi-beam irradiation of the oral cavity, brainstem, and larynx and by potentially allowing higher radiation doses to be delivered to the tumor, thereby enhancing tumor control.

Several treatment-planning studies (studies that compare the dosimetric characteristics of treatment plans generated for different types of therapy) have showed the dosimetric superiority of IMPT over IMRT[28,29] (**Figs. 5** and **6**). Investigators at MD Anderson recently overcame significant technological challenges associated with quality assurance in proton therapy to permit the safe delivery of IMPT for OPC, and their initial clinical experience with using IMPT to treat HNC validates the feasibility of this novel technique.[30] This early experience involved treating 15 patients with IMPT for tumors of the oropharynx (8), nasopharynx (4), paranasal sinus (2), or an unknown primary (1). Patients who were to receive concurrent chemotherapy were treated to a total dose of 70 GyE (Gray-equivalents) in 33 fractions, whereas those to be treated with proton therapy alone received a total dose of 66 GyE in 30 fractions. A simultaneous integrated boost technique was used to deliver lower doses to elective anatomic sites in all patients. Plans for a representative case are shown in **Fig. 7**. Dosimetric comparisons of IMPT versus IMRT performed before treatment showed no significant differences in target volume coverage but significant reductions of dose from IMPT to the whole brain ($P = .01$), brainstem ($P = .03$), anterior oral cavity ($P = .01$), and larynx ($P = .04$).[31] All patients were able to complete the proton therapy as prescribed, without the need for treatment breaks or hospitalization. Specifically noted were low radiation doses to the brainstem, with resultant low rates of nausea and vomiting, and low radiation doses to the oral cavity, with resultant lack of anterior oral cavity mucositis. All 8 of the patients with OPC had a complete response, demonstrating that IMPT is clinically feasible, can potentially reduce the incidence and severity of acute side effects, and can generate clinical responses that are consistent with treatment plans (**Fig. 8**).[30]

Since 2011, the MD Anderson group has treated 26 patients with oropharyngeal squamous cell carcinoma using IMPT, with a median follow-up time of 10 months (range, 0–22 months). The median age of these patients at presentation was 61.5 years; most (92%) were men, 85% were white, and 50% had never smoked; 100% had HPV/p16+ tumors; 69% had tonsillar disease and 31% had base-of-tongue disease; and 77% had stage IV disease. Systemic therapy was a component of treatment for 20 patients (77%), and the prescribed radiation dose was 70 Gy in 33 fractions. During treatment, 5 patients (19%) developed grade 3 dysphagia requiring a gastrostomy tube, a rate that is less than half of that in a recently published experience with IMRT.[32] No patient given IMPT had aspiration or stricture, and all patients were disease-free at last follow-up. On the basis of these encouraging preliminary findings of reduced grade 3 toxicity and consistent disease response with IMPT, investigators at MD Anderson are initiating a phase II/III randomized trial of IMPT versus IMRT for advanced-stage OPC with the goal of confirming the predicted reduction in the beam-path toxicities associated with IMRT.

OTHER AREAS OF ACTIVE INVESTIGATION

Because most patients with OPC diagnosed in the modern era have HPV-related cancers and are expected to have a good chance of long-term survival after RT-based therapy,[33] recent investigational treatment strategies undertaken by clinical trial cooperative groups have focused on the potential for treatment "deintensification" for selected patients, with the goals of maintaining high cure rates and reducing treatment-related toxicity. Along these same lines, clinicians have sought to improve patient outcomes, not only through the development and investigation of advanced RT modalities but also through detailed prospective study of symptoms as reported by patients with HNC,[34] and to that end the authors are currently conducting prospective randomized clinical trials with pharmaceutical agents targeting key symptom development and symptom-expression pathways.

REFERENCES

1. Parsons JT, Mendenhall WM, Stringer SP, et al. Squamous cell carcinoma of the oropharynx: surgery, radiation therapy, or both. Cancer 2002;94:2967–80.
2. Fu KK, Pajak TF, Trotti A, et al. A Radiation Therapy Oncology Group (RTOG) phase III randomized study to compare hyperfractionation and two variants of accelerated fractionation to standard fractionation radiotherapy for head and neck squamous cell carcinomas: first report of RTOG 9003. Int J Radiat Oncol Biol Phys 2000;48:7–16.
3. Overgaard J, Hansen HS, Specht L, et al. Five compared with six fractions per week of conventional radiotherapy of squamous-cell carcinoma of head and neck: DAHANCA 6 and 7 randomised controlled trial. Lancet 2003;362:933–40.
4. Calais G, Alfonsi M, Bardet E, et al. Randomized trial of radiation therapy versus concomitant chemotherapy and radiation therapy for advanced-stage oropharynx carcinoma. J Natl Cancer Inst 1999;91:2081–6.
5. Bonner JA, Harari PM, Giralt J, et al. Radiotherapy plus cetuximab for squamous-cell carcinoma of the head and neck. N Engl J Med 2006;354:567–78.
6. Bonner JA, Harari PM, Giralt J, et al. Radiotherapy plus cetuximab for locoregionally advanced head and neck cancer: 5-year survival data from a phase 3 randomised trial, and relation between cetuximab-induced rash and survival. Lancet Oncol 2010;11:21–8.
7. Bourhis J, Overgaard J, Audry H, et al. Hyperfractionated or accelerated radiotherapy in head and neck cancer: a meta-analysis. Lancet 2006;368:843–54.
8. Pignon JP, Le Maître A, Maillard E, et al. Meta-analysis of chemotherapy in head and neck cancer (MACH-NC): an update on 93 randomised trials and 17,346 patients. Radiother Oncol 2009;92:4–14.
9. Gunn GB, Garden A. Intensity-modulated radiation therapy for head and neck cancer: a decade of experience demonstrates improved patient outcomes.

In: Heron D, Tishler R, Thomas CR Jr, editors. Radiation medicine rounds: head and neck cancer, vol. 2, Issue 2. New York: Demos Medical; 2011. p. 173–81.
10. Ang KK. Altered fractionation in the management of head and neck cancer. Int J Radiat Biol 1998;73:395–9.
11. Baujat B, Bourhis J, Blanchard P, et al. Hyperfractionated or accelerated radiotherapy for head and neck cancer. Cochrane Database Syst Rev 2010;(12):CD002026.
12. Posner MR, Hershock DM, Blajman CR, et al. Cisplatin and fluorouracil alone or with docetaxel in head and neck cancer. N Engl J Med 2007;357:1705–15.
13. Denis F, Garaud P, Bardet E, et al. Final results of the 94-01 French Head and Neck Oncology and Radiotherapy Group randomized trial comparing radiotherapy alone with concomitant radiochemotherapy in advanced-stage oropharynx carcinoma. J Clin Oncol 2004;22:69–76.
14. Blanchard P, Baujat B, Holostenco V, et al. Meta-analysis of chemotherapy in head and neck cancer (MACH-NC): a comprehensive analysis by tumour site. Radiother Oncol 2011;100:33–40.
15. Ang KK, Berkey BA, Tu X, et al. Impact of epidermal growth factor receptor expression on survival and pattern of relapse in patients with advanced head and neck carcinoma. Cancer Res 2002;62:7350–6.
16. Curran D, Giralt J, Harari PM, et al. Quality of life in head and neck cancer patients after treatment with high-dose radiotherapy alone or in combination with cetuximab. J Clin Oncol 2007;25:2191–7.
17. Garden AS, Kies MS, Morrison WH, et al. Outcomes and patterns of care of patients with locally advanced oropharyngeal carcinoma treated in the early 21st century. Radiat Oncol 2013;8:21.
18. O'Sullivan B, Warde P, Grice B, et al. The benefits and pitfalls of ipsilateral radiotherapy in carcinoma of the tonsillar region. Int J Radiat Oncol Biol Phys 2001;51:332–43.
19. Rusthoven KE, Raben D, Schneider C, et al. Freedom from local and regional failure of contralateral neck with ipsilateral neck radiotherapy for node-positive tonsil cancer: results of a prospective management approach. Int J Radiat Oncol Biol Phys 2009;74:1365–70.
20. Chronowski GM, Garden AS, Morrison WH, et al. Unilateral radiotherapy for the treatment of tonsil cancer. Int J Radiat Oncol Biol Phys 2012;83:204–9.
21. Frank SJ, Rosenthal DI, Petsuksiri J, et al. Intensity-modulated radiotherapy for cervical node squamous cell carcinoma metastases from unknown head-and-neck primary site: MD Anderson Cancer Center outcomes and patterns of failure. Int J Radiat Oncol Biol Phys 2010;78:1005–10.
22. Eisbruch A, Harris J, Garden AS, et al. Multi-institutional trial of accelerated hypofractionated intensity-modulated radiation therapy for early-stage oropharyngeal cancer (RTOG 00-22). Int J Radiat Oncol Biol Phys 2010;76:1333–8.
23. Nutting CM, Morden JP, Harrington KJ, et al. Parotid-sparing intensity modulated versus conventional radiotherapy in head and neck cancer (PARSPORT): a phase 3 multicentre randomised controlled trial. Lancet Oncol 2011;12:127–36.
24. Garden AS, Dong L, Morrison WH, et al. Patterns of disease recurrence following treatment of oropharyngeal cancer with intensity modulated radiation therapy. Int J Radiat Oncol Biol Phys 2012;85(4):941–7.
25. Rosenthal DI, Chambers MS, Fuller CD, et al. Beam path toxicities to non-target structures during intensity-modulated radiation therapy for head and neck cancer. Int J Radiat Oncol Biol Phys 2008;72:747–55.

26. Gerweck L, Paganetti H. Radiobiology of charged particles. In: DeLaney TF, Kooy HM, editors. Proton and charged particle radiotherapy. Philadelphia: Lippincott Williams & Wilkins; 2008. p. 8–18.
27. Gottschalk B, Pedroni E. Treatment delivery systems. In: DeLaney TF, Kooy HM, editors. Proton and charged particle radiotherapy. Philadelphia: Lippincott Williams & Wilkins; 2008. p. 33–49.
28. van de Water TA, Bijl HP, Schilstra C, et al. The potential benefit of radiotherapy with protons in head and neck cancer with respect to normal tissue sparing: a systematic review of literature. Oncologist 2011;16:366–77.
29. Kandula S, Zhu XR, Garden AS. Spot scanning beam proton therapy versus intensity-modulated radiation therapy for ipsilateral head and neck malignancies: a treatment planning comparison. Med Dosim 2013 (in press).
30. Frank S, Cox J, Gillin M, et al. Intensity-modulated proton therapy for head and neck cancer: the first clinical experience [abstract]. Int J Radiat Oncol Biol Phys 2012;84:S474.
31. Yeh B, Zhu XR, Palmer MB, et al. Intensity-modulated proton therapy is dosimetrically superior to intensity-modulated radiation therapy for head and neck cancers [abstract]. Int J Radiat Oncol Biol Phys 2012;84:S840.
32. Bhayani MK, Hutcheson KA, Barringer DA, et al. Gastrostomy tube placement in patients with oropharyngeal carcinoma treated with radiotherapy or chemoradiotherapy: factors affecting placement and dependence. Head Neck 2013. http://dx.doi.org/10.1002/hed.23200.
33. Ang KK, Harris J, Wheeler R, et al. Human papillomavirus and survival of patients with oropharyngeal cancer. N Engl J Med 2010;363:24–35.
34. Gunn GB, Mendoza TR, Fuller CD, et al. High symptom burden prior to radiation therapy for head and neck cancer: a patient-reported outcomes study. Head Neck 2012. http://dx.doi.org/10.1002/hed.23181.

The Role of Systemic Treatment Before, During, and After Definitive Treatment

Kathryn A. Gold, MD, Michele Neskey, PA,
William N. William Jr, MD*

KEYWORDS

• Systemic treatment • Squamous cell carcinoma
• Oropharyngeal squamous cell carcinomas • Chemotherapy • Targeted therapy

KEY POINTS

- Patients with squamous cell carcinoma of the head and neck frequently present with locally advanced disease. In this setting, outcomes can be improved by the incorporation of multimodality treatment, often with chemotherapy.
- In locally advanced oropharyngeal squamous cell carcinomas, concurrent chemoradiation with cisplatin is the standard of care and improves outcomes compared with radiation alone.
- In patients with oropharyngeal squamous cell carcinomas, radiation with concurrent cetuximab improves disease-free and overall survival compared with radiation alone and is another treatment option for patients with locally advanced disease.
- The use of induction chemotherapy before definitive radiation has been extensively studied and may improve outcomes in certain groups. Its use, however, remains controversial.
- Following surgical resection, adjuvant concurrent chemoradiation with cisplatin improves outcomes for patients with nodal extracapsular extension or positive margins.

INTRODUCTION

In locoregionally advanced head and neck squamous cell carcinomas, outcomes using single-modality therapy are usually poor. Head and neck cancers are chemosensitive malignancies, with response rates as high as 90% described with chemotherapy in treatment-naïve patients.[1] Although chemotherapy alone is not considered a curative therapy, the addition of chemotherapy to other modalities can lead to improved

Funding Source: This work was supported by the National Institutes of Health grants P30 CA016672-36 and P50 CA097007-09.
Department of Thoracic/Head and Neck Medical Oncology, The University of Texas MD Anderson Cancer Center, 1515 Holcombe Boulevard, Houston, TX 77030, USA
* Corresponding author. Department of Thoracic/Head and Neck Medical Oncology, The University of Texas MD Anderson Cancer Center, 1515 Holcombe Boulevard, Unit 432, Houston, TX 77030.
E-mail address: wnwillia@mdanderson.org

Otolaryngol Clin N Am 46 (2013) 645–656
http://dx.doi.org/10.1016/j.otc.2013.04.005 oto.theclinics.com

outcomes. Discussed here is the use of chemotherapy for oropharyngeal and/or oral cavity squamous cell carcinomas in 3 settings:

1. In combination with radiation as definitive therapy
2. As induction treatment before definitive therapy
3. In combination with radiation therapy as adjuvant treatment following surgical resection

The authors also discuss the role of the targeted agent cetuximab in combination with radiation therapy for locally advanced disease.

CONCURRENT CHEMORADIATION THERAPY

Definitive radiation treatment of patients with unresectable or locoregionally advanced head and neck cancer has been associated with high rates of both locoregional failure and distant recurrence. The addition of chemotherapy to radiation therapy has been studied in an attempt to improve cure rates and functional outcomes as well as survival rates.

Locally Advanced Oropharyngeal Cancer

For patients with locally advanced oropharyngeal cancer, a pivotal randomized phase III trial by the French Groupe Oncologie Radiotherapie Tete et Cou (GORTEC) group was designed to compare radiotherapy alone to radiotherapy and concomitant chemotherapy.[2]

- Both groups received identical radiation therapy with conventional fractionation of 70 Gy in 35 fractions.
- Patients in the chemotherapy arm received a 4-day chemotherapy regimen consisting of carboplatin (70 mg/m^2/d) and 5-flourouracil (600 mg/m^2/d) by continuous infusion for the duration of radiotherapy.

Results yielded the following:

- An improvement in both progression-free survival and overall survival at three years for patients receiving combined modality therapy (42% and 51%) versus radiation therapy alone (20% and 31%)
- Improvement in locoregional control rates in the chemoradiation arm (66%) versus radiation therapy alone (42%)
- Similar rates of distant metastases in both arms (11%)
- Higher hematologic toxicities and incidence of grade 3 and 4 mucositis in the chemotherapy arm, leading to a need for a temporary feeding tube more frequently when compared with the radiation therapy alone arm

These results suggest that the addition of chemotherapy concurrently to radiation therapy improves locoregional control, which translates into both an overall and progression-free survival benefit for these patients, at the expense of more acute toxicities. Long-term follow-up of this study confirms the results in favor of the concurrent chemoradiation therapy arm, with an improvement in overall survival primarily secondary to a reduced incidence of locoregional failure.[3]

Resectable or Unresectable Head and Neck Cancer

To better assess the impact of chemotherapy on the treatment of head and neck cancer and overall survival, an updated meta-analysis of 87 randomized trials between 1965 and 2000 was performed.

The Meta-Analysis of Chemotherapy in Head and Neck Cancer (MACH-NC) pooled data from clinical trials in which patients with resectable or unresectable disease were randomized to receive definitive local therapy (surgery or radiation) or definitive local therapy plus chemotherapy.[4,5] Trials included patients who had received chemotherapy in the induction, concurrent, or adjuvant setting and had a diagnosis of oral cavity, oropharynx, hypopharynx, or larynx cancer.

Results yielded the following:

- The addition of chemotherapy in any setting had a statistically significant overall absolute survival benefit of 4.5% at 5 years and an even greater benefit of 6.5% at 5 years in the concurrent chemoradiation trials.
- As in the GORTEC trial, the improvement in survival was primarily caused by an impact of concurrent chemotherapy on locoregional control, with an absolute reduction of the cumulative rate of locoregional recurrence of 9.3% in the concurrent group at 5 years.
- Concurrent chemotherapy also reduced the cumulative rate of distant metastases but to a lesser extent (absolute reduction of 2.5% at 5 years).[5] This analysis did not define an optimal concurrent chemotherapy regimen but found a greater benefit of platinum-based chemotherapy. Multidrug regimens including 5-flourouracil had similar benefit when compared with single-agent cisplatin; however, monotherapy with a drug other than cisplatin yielded inferior results.

High-Dose Cisplatin Concurrent with Radiation Therapy

High-dose cisplatin administered at 100 mg/m^2 on days 1, 22, and 43 concurrent with radiation therapy has been associated with an improvement in overall survival and has been considered the preferred regimen for definitive treatment.[6,7] Because of both acute and late toxicities, it is reserved for patients with a good performance status and limited comorbidities. Alternative schedules and dosing of cisplatin including daily and weekly treatment have demonstrated improvements in both locoregional control and survival but have not been directly compared with high-dose cisplatin.[8,9] Because of a more tolerable side-effect profile, specifically less nephrotoxicity, ototoxicity, and neurotoxicity, carboplatin has also been investigated as an alternative option, although it has not been directly compared as a single agent against cisplatin. However, when carboplatin is used in combination with another agent, such as 5-flourouracil, there is a survival benefit when compared with radiation therapy alone.[2] Definitive radiation therapy with carboplatin monotherapy is occasionally used for patients with a poor performance status, multiple comorbidities, or a contraindication to cisplatin therapy.

Accelerated Radiation Therapy and Hyperfractionation

The impact of altered radiation schedules with concurrent chemotherapy on overall survival and locoregional control has also been studied. Accelerated radiation, which delivers the same dose as conventional therapy over a shorter period of time, and hyperfractionation, which gives higher doses of radiation therapy via multiple small fractions, were developed to help improve locoregional control rates. For patients receiving radiation therapy alone, studies have shown hyperfractionation to have an 8% absolute benefit in the 5-year overall survival.[10] When combined with chemotherapy, the value of these techniques remains unclear. In a comparison of conventional radiation with 3 cycles of standard high-dose cisplatin to accelerated boost radiation with 2 cycles of high-dose cisplatin, there was no statistically significant difference in overall survival, locoregional failure, progression-free survival, or development of distant metastases between the 2 chemoradiation schedules.[11]

RADIATION WITH CONCURRENT CETUXIMAB

The use of targeted therapies for the treatment of head and neck cancer has been of high interest because of, potentially, a more favorable side-effect profile than platinum-based therapies. Cetuximab is a monoclonal antibody against the epidermal growth factor receptor (EGFR) and is the only targeted agent currently approved for the management of locally advanced and/or recurrent and metastatic head and neck squamous cell carcinomas.[12–14] Preclinically, EGFR-targeted agents have been demonstrated to reduce cancer cell proliferation, increase apoptosis, inhibit invasiveness and metastatic potential, and augment sensitivity to chemotherapy and radiation therapy.[15]

In a multinational study, weekly cetuximab in combination with radiation therapy was compared with radiation therapy alone.

- Eligibility criteria included previously untreated stage III or IV nonmetastatic cancer of the oropharynx, larynx, or hypopharynx and a Karnofsky performance score of at least 60.
- Three radiotherapy schedules were allowed and chosen by the investigators before patient registration (70.0 Gy in once-daily fractions, 72.0–76.8 Gy in twice-daily fractions, or 72.0 Gy in once-daily fractions with a concomitant twice-daily boost in the last 2.4 weeks of treatment).
- In the experimental arm, cetuximab was added to the elected radiotherapy treatment, given at a loading dose of 400 mg/m^2 (starting 1 week before radiation) followed by a weekly 250 mg/m^2 maintenance dose for the duration of radiotherapy.
- Patients were stratified according to performance status, nodal involvement, tumor stage, and radiation-fractionation regimen.

Results yielded the following:

- The 3-year rates of locoregional control (the study's primary endpoint) were significantly higher for the cetuximab-radiotherapy arm as compared with the radiotherapy alone arm (47% vs 34%, respectively, $P<.01$).
- Median progression-free survival was 17.1 months versus 12.4 months for the experimental and control arms, respectively ($P = .006$).
- The 3-year overall survival was 55% among patients treated with the combined modality versus 45% among those given radiation only ($P = .03$).
- Response rates were significantly higher for the experimental group as compared with control patients (74% vs 64%, respectively, $P = .02$).
- The cumulative rates of distant metastases were similar between the two groups. Grade 3 to 5 mucositis and dermatitis occurred in 56% and 23% of the experimental group versus 52% and 18% of the control group.
- Other toxicities were similar between the arms, except for acneiform rash (17% in the cetuximab arm vs 1% in the radiation alone arm, $P<.001$) and infusion-related side effects (3% for cetuximab).

Taken together, this study demonstrates that cetuximab increases survival and locoregional control rates without significant additional toxicity.[14]

Long-Term Follow-up

On long-term follow-up, the survival benefits of cetuximab added to radiation therapy remained (overall survival of 46% and 36% at 5 years for the experimental and control arms, respectively). Subgroup analysis demonstrated more pronounced improvement in survival by the addition of cetuximab in the following cohorts: patients with oropharyngeal cancers (compared with larynx or hypopharynx), T1 to T3 primary tumor (vs T4), N1 to N3 nodal status (vs N0), treatment in the United States, use of concomitant boost radiotherapy, Karnofsky performance status of 90 to 100, male gender, and younger age (<65 years). These results should be interpreted with caution, given the low number of patients in each group and the exploratory nature of the analysis.[16]

Although this study showed a benefit of concurrent cetuximab versus radiation alone, there has been no head-to-head comparison with concurrent cisplatin with radiation therapy, the standard of care, and it is unknown which patients would derive greater benefits from one approach versus the other.

In a follow-up to the trial of Bonner and colleagues described above, The Radiation Therapy Oncology Group (RTOG) study 0522 randomized patients to cisplatin chemoradiation therapy with or without cetuximab.[17] The combination with cetuximab did not improve progression-free or overall survival and increased adverse events when compared with cisplatin and radiation, and this strategy should not be used.

Unfortunately, despite extensive efforts, no predictive biomarkers of the efficacy of cetuximab have been identified to date. The demographics of the patients who had improved survival in the study by Bonner and colleagues[18] suggest that patients with human papillomavirus (HPV)-positive oropharyngeal tumors could be appropriate candidates for this therapy because they typically present at a younger age, with a low T primary tumor and more advanced nodal stage. Nonetheless, exploratory analysis of a recent trial in the recurrent/metastatic setting evaluating chemotherapy ± panitumumab (another anti-EGFR antibody) demonstrated a survival benefit of the targeted agent in the HPV-negative group only. It is unknown whether these results hold true in the setting of locally advanced disease, using cetuximab combined with radiation therapy. Currently, the RTOG1016 study is evaluating cetuximab and radiation therapy versus cisplatin and radiation therapy in locally advanced, HPV-positive oropharyngeal squamous cell carcinomas using a noninferiority phase III trial design (NCT01302834).

INDUCTION CHEMOTHERAPY

Induction chemotherapy in locally advanced head and neck cancer offers several theoretical benefits[19,20]:

- It allows for administration of more intensified chemotherapy than with concurrent therapy, with a potential for reducing the risk of distant metastases by treatment of micrometastatic disease.
- It can be used to reduce tumor bulk before a definitive approach to therapy and has been used to select patients for organ preservation.

Despite these advantages, clinical trial data have not definitively shown a survival benefit of induction chemotherapy, and its use remains controversial.

Early Induction Chemotherapy Studies

In the 1970s, several groups studied cisplatin-based combinations with methotrexate, bleomycin, or vinca alkaloids in the induction setting, before either surgery or radiation therapy.[21–23] They found that these regimens were feasible and active. A group at Wayne State University first studied the combination of cisplatin and fluorouracil (PF) in a phase II pilot trial.[1] Cisplatin (100 mg/m^2 intravenously [IV] on day 1) followed by a 5-day infusion of fluorouracil (1000 mg/m^2/d) resulted in a response rate of 93% and a complete response rate of 54%. All patients went on to receive surgery and/or radiation, and median survival was not reached after 18 months of follow-up. With these promising efficacy data, this regimen became the basis for many other trials.

Paccagnella and colleagues[24] randomized patients with locally advanced squamous cell carcinoma of the oropharynx, oral cavity, hypopharynx, and paranasal sinus to either induction chemotherapy followed by locoregional treatment or locoregional treatment alone. A significant reduction in the rate of distant metastases was seen with induction chemotherapy (15% vs 36% at 2 years). For patients deemed inoperable, induction chemotherapy led to improved local control and overall survival. This survival benefit persisted with longer follow-up.[25] Another trial with a similar design enrolled only patients with oropharyngeal cancer.[26] This trial demonstrated an improvement in overall survival with induction chemotherapy (median overall survival 5.1 years vs 3.3 years, P = .03).

The MACH-NC also summarized the experience with induction chemotherapy added to locoregional therapy.[4,5] The hazard ratio for death with induction chemotherapy was 0.96 (95% confidence interval 0.90–1.02), translating into an absolute improvement in survival at 5 years of 2.4%. This figure compares unfavorably with the benefits in survival seen with concurrent chemoradiation therapy (absolute improvement in survival of 6.5% at 5 years). As a result, induction chemotherapy failed to be considered the standard regimen for the management of locally advanced head and neck cancers. Nonetheless, a more detailed analysis of the data presented by the MACH-NC collaborative group demonstrated that when only trials using platinum/fluorouracil induction regimens were considered, the hazard ration for death was 0.90 (95% confidence interval 0.82–0.99) in favor of induction treatment.[5] Furthermore, induction chemotherapy led to an absolute reduction in the cumulative rate of distant metastases of 4.3%, whereas the absolute reduction in the rate of locoregional failure was only 1.0% at 5 years. Taken together, these results demonstrate that there might be a role for induction chemotherapy, especially when treatment goals are to reduce the risk of distant metastases. However, the benefits in locoregional failure and overall survival are marginal and less striking than what is observed with concurrent chemoradiation therapy regimens.

Induction Chemotherapy with Taxane-Containing Regimens

In hopes of improving outcomes with induction chemotherapy, several groups studied the addition of docetaxel to cisplatin and fluorouracil. Docetaxel was known to be an active agent in squamous cell carcinoma of the head and neck, with single-agent activity in recurrent or metastatic disease.[27] Two initial phase III trials used docetaxel, cisplatin, and fluorouracil (TPF) as induction chemotherapy.

In the TAX 324 study, 501 patients with locally advanced head and neck cancer were randomized to receive 3 cycles of induction chemotherapy with either TPF (docetaxel 75 mg/m^2, cisplatin 100 mg/m^2, and infusional fluorouracil 1000 mg/m^2/d for 4 days every 3 weeks) or PF (cisplatin 100 mg/m^2 and fluorouracil 1000 mg/m^2/d for 5 days), followed by concurrent chemoradiation with weekly carboplatin (area under the curve 1.5).

Results of the TAX 324 study yielded the following:

- Median overall survival was significantly prolonged in the group receiving TPF (71 vs 40 months, P = .0006).

- Rates of locoregional recurrence were decreased with TPF, but the rate of distant metastatic disease was not significantly different between the groups.[28]
- Results remained similar on long-term follow-up, demonstrating a 5-year overall survival rate of 52% for TPF compared with 42% for PF (P = .014).[29]

The TAX 323 study had a similar design, with patients randomized to induction chemotherapy with either TPF or PF followed by radiation therapy alone. The TPF regimen used (docetaxel 75 mg/m^2, cisplatin 75 mg/m^2, and infusional fluorouracil 750 mg/m^2/d for 5 days every 3 weeks) was slightly different than that used in the TAX 324 study.

Results of the TAX 323 study yielded the following:

- The median overall survival was significantly improved with TPF (18.8 vs 14.5 months, P = .02).[30] Patient selection criteria for these trials were different, perhaps accounting for the differences in overall survival seen between the two studies, although the use of concurrent carboplatin in the TAX 324 study compared with radiation alone in TAX 323 might also contribute to the differences.

Although these studies were able to show conclusively that TPF is superior to PF as an induction chemotherapy regimen, they did not address what the optimal concurrent treatment following induction chemotherapy is or whether concurrent chemoradiation with cisplatin up front is superior to an induction approach. Several recent studies have attempted to address these questions.

A phase II, single-arm Southwest Oncology Group study, S0216, treated patients with 2 cycles of induction TPF, followed by concurrent chemoradiation, with cisplatin 100 mg/m^2 on days 1 and 22.[31] There were 74 patients enrolled for this study; 61 patients were able to complete induction and begin concurrent chemoradiation. Four deaths occurred during treatment, and 50 patients were able to complete all planned treatment. A total 85% and 91% of patients had at least grade 3 toxicity during induction chemotherapy and concurrent chemoradiation, respectively.

Results of the Southwest Oncology Group study

- Suggest that high-dose cisplatin following induction TPF leads to excessive toxicity and should be reserved for carefully selected patients
- Demonstrates that sequential therapy, with induction chemotherapy followed by concurrent chemoradiation, may compromise administration of concurrent therapy

Two recently reported studies compared a sequential approach (with induction chemotherapy followed by concurrent chemoradiation) with concurrent chemoradiation alone.

In the PARADIGM trial, patients with locally advanced head and neck cancer were randomized to concurrent chemoradiation with cisplatin or induction chemotherapy with three cycles of TPF followed by chemoradiation with either weekly carboplatin (for patients with a complete response to induction treatment) or weekly docetaxel (for patients with less than a complete response to induction treatment).[32] Planned accrual was 300 patients, but because of slow enrollment, only 145 patients were treated on study. There were no clear survival differences between the arms, with a 3-year survival of 73% with induction chemotherapy and 78% with concurrent therapy.

In the Docetaxel Based Chemoradiotherapy Plus or Minus Induction Chemotherapy to Decrease Events in Head and Neck Cancer (DeCIDE) trial, patients were randomized to receive either concurrent chemoradiation with docetaxel, fluorouracil, and hydroxyurea with or without induction chemotherapy with 2 cycles of TPF.[33] The 3-year overall survival was similar between the arms (75% with induction therapy vs 73% with concurrent therapy only, P = .70), although the induction arm had a lower risk of distant failure (10% vs 19%, P = .025).

Induction Chemotherapy Versus Concurrent Chemoradiation Trial Results

DeCIDE and PARADIGM were limited by the small sample size and a reduced power to detect survival differences between the arms because the outcomes in both studies (three-year overall survival greater than 70% in all arms) outperformed original estimations. Although these studies cannot definitely exclude a benefit from TPF induction chemotherapy before chemoradiation therapy, they illustrate that the magnitude of improvement in survival in an unselected patient population is marginal, at best, especially in an era when a significant proportion of patients are alive and disease-free following nonsurgical treatment of head and neck cancers. Almost certainly, the increased incidence of HPV-positive oropharyngeal cancers is contributing to the improvement in prognosis seen in recent studies. Patients with HPV-positive cancers have high survival rates when treated with induction chemotherapy,[34,35] but it is yet to be determined if HPV status serves as a predictive marker of benefit from induction treatment.

In summary, to date, no trials have shown a clear survival benefit for induction chemotherapy over concurrent chemoradiation, and concurrent chemoradiation with cisplatin is still considered the standard of care for most patients with locally advanced squamous cell carcinoma of the head and neck. As locoregional treatment improves, distant metastatic failure is becoming a more frequent cause of treatment failure. Induction chemotherapy may reduce this risk; however, we do not yet know which patients may derive a benefit. Induction chemotherapy should be used only following multidisciplinary discussion between medical oncologists, radiation oncologists, and head and neck surgeons. Preferably, induction chemotherapy should be used in the setting of a clinical trial.

Newer approaches to induction chemotherapy include regimens containing targeted agents like cetuximab,[36] selection of patients for organ preservation approaches following only one cycle of induction therapy,[37] and the use of chemotherapy alone as the definitive treatment in carefully selected, closely monitored patients.[38]

ADJUVANT CONCURRENT CHEMORADIATION THERAPY

The risk of recurrence for locally advanced squamous cell carcinomas of the head and neck following surgical resection is high. For patients with adverse features like perineural invasion, multiple positive lymph nodes, and T3 or T4 tumors, postoperative radiation therapy has long been known to provide a benefit.[39] Even with radiotherapy, however, tumors frequently recur. Because chemotherapy can act as a radiation sensitizer, combined chemoradiation has been studied as adjuvant treatment of surgically treated tumors.

In the European Organisation for Research and Treatment of Cancer (EORTC) study 22931, patients with surgically resected head and neck cancer were randomized to postoperative irradiation alone or with concurrent chemotherapy (cisplatin 100 mg/m^2 on days 1, 22, and 43).[40] Eligible patients had tumor stage T3 or T4 or nodal stage N2 or N3. Patients with earlier stage tumors but unfavorable pathologic conditions (extracapsular extension, positive margins, perineural involvement, or vascular emboli) were also eligible.

Results yielded the following:

- Progression-free survival was significantly greater in the group that received chemotherapy (55 months with chemoradiation vs 23 months with radiation alone, $P = .04$)
- Overall survival was significantly greater in the chemotherapy group (72 months vs 32 months, $P = .02$), although at the cost of increased grade 3 or higher adverse effects (41% vs 21%, $P = .001$).

RTOG 9501 had a very similar design, although with slightly different inclusion criteria.[41] Patients with extracapsular extension, positive margins, and 2 or more involved lymph nodes were eligible. Both studies used an identical chemotherapy schedule: cisplatin 100 mg/m^2 IV on days 1, 22, and 43 of radiation.

Results yielded the following:

- There was significantly improved locoregional control (hazard ratio 0.61 with chemoradiation, $P = .01$) and disease-free survival with concurrent chemoradiation (hazard ratio 0.78, $P = .04$).
- In contrast to the EORTC trial, there was no significant increase in overall survival (hazard ratio for death 0.84, $P = .19$).

Because there are significant side effects of concurrent chemoradiation, efforts have been made to identify which patients might derive the greatest benefit from this approach. The data from the 2 studies described, EORTC 22931 and RTOG 9501, were included in a collaborative comparative analysis.[42] The criteria that predicted an improved outcome with the addition of chemotherapy to radiation therapy were positive surgical margins and extracapsular extension. The other criteria used in these studies to identify patients at high risk for recurrence (vascular emboli, perineural invasion, stage III or IV disease, and 2 or more involved lymph nodes) were not associated with a significant benefit from chemotherapy.

SUMMARY

For many patients with locally advanced head and neck cancer, chemotherapy represents a key component of optimal multimodality therapy. Cisplatin administered concurrently with radiation has been shown to improve outcomes when compared with radiation alone and is considered the standard of care for many patients with squamous cell carcinomas of the oropharynx, hypopharynx, or larynx. Radiation therapy with cetuximab is also superior to radiation therapy alone and is a viable treatment option, although cisplatin remains the standard of care for most patients that are candidates for concurrent cytotoxic therapy.

Induction chemotherapy has the potential to improve outcomes by reducing the disease burden before definitive treatment and by reducing the risk of distant metastatic disease but at the cost of increased adverse events and a reduction in the intensity of subsequent therapy. However, its use is controversial, and it is not yet known which patients may derive benefit from this approach. Before the use of induction chemotherapy, patients should be evaluated and discussed by a multidisciplinary group. This treatment approach is best used at a tertiary care center, and clinical trials should always be considered.

Following surgical resection, adjuvant concurrent chemoradiation improves disease-free and overall survival in selected patients. The greatest benefit is in those with positive surgical margins or extracapsular extension. High-dose cisplatin is the most widely studied regimen in this setting.

REFERENCES

1. Rooney M, Kish J, Jacobs J, et al. Improved complete response rate and survival in advanced head and neck cancer after three-course induction therapy with 120-hour 5-FU infusion and cisplatin. Cancer 1985;55:1123–8.
2. Calais G, Alfonsi M, Bardet E, et al. Randomized trial of radiation therapy versus concomitant chemotherapy and radiation therapy for advanced-stage oropharynx carcinoma. J Natl Cancer Inst 1999;91:2081–6.
3. Denis F, Garaud P, Bardet E, et al. Final results of the 94-01 French Head and Neck Oncology and Radiotherapy Group randomized trial comparing radiotherapy alone with concomitant radiochemotherapy in advanced-stage oropharynx carcinoma. J Clin Oncol 2004;22:69–76.
4. Pignon JP, Bourhis J, Domenge C, et al. Chemotherapy added to locoregional treatment for head and neck squamous-cell carcinoma: three meta-analyses of updated individual data. MACH-NC Collaborative Group. Meta-analysis of chemotherapy on head and neck cancer. Lancet 2000;355:949–55.
5. Pignon JP, le Maitre A, Maillard E, et al. Meta-analysis of chemotherapy in head and neck cancer (MACH-NC): an update on 93 randomised trials and 17,346 patients. Radiother Oncol 2009;92:4–14.
6. Adelstein DJ, Li Y, Adams GL, et al. An intergroup phase III comparison of standard radiation therapy and two schedules of concurrent chemoradiotherapy in patients with unresectable squamous cell head and neck cancer. J Clin Oncol 2003;21:92–8.
7. Forastiere AA, Goepfert H, Maor M, et al. Concurrent chemotherapy and radiotherapy for organ preservation in advanced laryngeal cancer. N Engl J Med 2003;349:2091–8.
8. Sharma A, Mohanti BK, Thakar A, et al. Concomitant chemoradiation versus radical radiotherapy in advanced squamous cell carcinoma of oropharynx and nasopharynx using weekly cisplatin: a phase II randomized trial. Ann Oncol 2010;21:2272–7.
9. Jeremic B, Shibamoto Y, Stanisavljevic B, et al. Radiation therapy alone or with concurrent low-dose daily either cisplatin or carboplatin in locally advanced unresectable squamous cell carcinoma of the head and neck: a prospective randomized trial. Radiother Oncol 1997;43:29–37.
10. Budach W, Hehr T, Budach V, et al. A meta-analysis of hyperfractionated and accelerated radiotherapy and combined chemotherapy and radiotherapy regimens in unresected locally advanced squamous cell carcinoma of the head and neck. BMC Cancer 2006;6:28.
11. Ang KK, Zhang Q, Wheeler RH, et al. A phase III trial (RTOG 0129) of two radiation-cisplatin regimens for head and neck carcinomas: impact of radiation and cisplatin intensity on outcome. 2010 ASCO Annual Meeting Proceedings. J Clin Oncol 2010;28:5507.
12. Vermorken JB, Mesia R, Rivera F, et al. Platinum-based chemotherapy plus cetuximab in head and neck cancer. N Engl J Med 2008;359:1116–27.
13. Vermorken JB, Trigo J, Hitt R, et al. Open-label, uncontrolled, multicenter phase II study to evaluate the efficacy and toxicity of cetuximab as a single agent in patients with recurrent and/or metastatic squamous cell carcinoma of the head and neck who failed to respond to platinum-based therapy. J Clin Oncol 2007;25:2171–7.
14. Bonner JA, Harari PM, Giralt J, et al. Radiotherapy plus cetuximab for squamous-cell carcinoma of the head and neck. N Engl J Med 2006;354:567–78.

15. Ciardiello F, Tortora G. EGFR antagonists in cancer treatment. N Engl J Med 2008; 358:1160–74.
16. Bonner JA, Harari PM, Giralt J, et al. Radiotherapy plus cetuximab for locoregionally advanced head and neck cancer: 5-year survival data from a phase 3 randomised trial, and relation between cetuximab-induced rash and survival. Lancet Oncol 2010;11:21–8.
17. Ang KK, Zhang QE, Rosenthal DI, et al. A randomized phase III trial (RTOG 0522) of concurrent accelerated radiation plus cisplatin with or without cetuximab for stage III-IV head and neck squamous cell carcinomas. 2011 ASCO Annual Meeting Proceedings. J Clin Oncol 2011;29:5500.
18. Stoehlmacher-Williams J, Villaneuva C, Foa P, et al. Safety and efficacy of panitumumab in HPV-positive and HPV-negative recurrent/metastatic squamous cell carcinoma of the head and neck: analysis of the global phase III SPECTRUM trial. 2012 ASCO Annual Meeting Proceedings. J Clin Oncol 2012;30:5504.
19. The Department of Veterans Affairs Laryngeal Cancer Study Group. Induction chemotherapy plus radiation compared with surgery plus radiation in patients with advanced laryngeal cancer. The Department of Veterans Affairs Laryngeal Cancer Study Group. N Engl J Med 1991;324:1685–90.
20. Lefebvre JL, Chevalier D, Luboinski B, et al. Larynx preservation in pyriform sinus cancer: preliminary results of a European Organization for Research and Treatment of Cancer phase III trial. EORTC Head and Neck Cancer Cooperative Group. J Natl Cancer Inst 1996;88:890–9.
21. Al-Sarraf M, Amer MH, Vaishampayan G, et al. A multidisciplinary therapeutic approach for advanced previously untreated epidermoid cancer of the head and neck: preliminary report. Int J Radiat Oncol Biol Phys 1979;5:1421–3.
22. Elias EG, Chretien PB, Monnard E, et al. Chemotherapy prior to local therapy in advanced squamous cell carcinoma of the head and neck: preliminary assessment of an intensive drug regimen. Cancer 1979;43:1025–31.
23. Hong WK, Shapshay SM, Bhutani R, et al. Induction chemotherapy in advanced squamous head and neck carcinoma with high-dose cis-platinum and bleomycin infusion. Cancer 1979;44:19–25.
24. Paccagnella A, Orlando A, Marchiori C, et al. Phase III trial of initial chemotherapy in stage III or IV head and neck cancers: a study by the Gruppo di Studio sui Tumori della Testa e del Collo. J Natl Cancer Inst 1994;86:265–72.
25. Zorat PL, Paccagnella A, Cavaniglia G, et al. Randomized phase III trial of neoadjuvant chemotherapy in head and neck cancer: 10-year follow-up. J Natl Cancer Inst 2004;96:1714–7.
26. Domenge C, Hill C, Lefebvre JL, et al. Randomized trial of neoadjuvant chemotherapy in oropharyngeal carcinoma. French Groupe d'Etude des Tumeurs de la Tete et du Cou (GETTEC). Br J Cancer 2000;83:1594–8.
27. Dreyfuss AI, Clark JR, Norris CM, et al. Docetaxel: an active drug for squamous cell carcinoma of the head and neck. J Clin Oncol 1996;14:1672–8.
28. Posner MR, Hershock DM, Blajman CR, et al. Cisplatin and fluorouracil alone or with docetaxel in head and neck cancer. N Engl J Med 2007;357:1705–15.
29. Lorch JH, Goloubeva O, Haddad RI, et al. Induction chemotherapy with cisplatin and fluorouracil alone or in combination with docetaxel in locally advanced squamous-cell cancer of the head and neck: long-term results of the TAX 324 randomised phase 3 trial. Lancet Oncol 2011;12:153–9.
30. Vermorken JB, Remenar E, van Herpen C, et al. Cisplatin, fluorouracil, and docetaxel in unresectable head and neck cancer. N Engl J Med 2007;357: 1695–704.

31. Adelstein DJ, Moon J, Hanna E, et al. Docetaxel, cisplatin, and fluorouracil induction chemotherapy followed by accelerated fractionation/concomitant boost radiation and concurrent cisplatin in patients with advanced squamous cell head and neck cancer: A Southwest Oncology Group phase II trial (S0216). Head Neck 2010;32:221–8.
32. Haddad RI, Rabinowits G, Tishler RB, et al. The PARADIGM trial: a phase II study comparing sequential therapy to concurrent chemoradiotherapy in locally advanced head and neck cancer. 2012 ASCO Annual Meeting Proceedings. J Clin Oncol 2012;30:5501.
33. Cohen EE, Karrison T, Kocherginsky M, et al. DeCIDE: a phase III randomized trial of docetaxel, cisplatin, 5-fluorouracil induction chemotherapy in patients with N2/N3 locally advanced squamous cell carcinoma of the head and neck. 2012 ASCO Annual Meeting Proceedings. J Clin Oncol 2012;30:5500.
34. Posner MR, Lorch JH, Goloubeva O, et al. Survival and human papillomavirus in oropharynx cancer in TAX 324: a subset analysis from an international phase III trial. Ann Oncol 2011;22:1071–7.
35. Fakhry C, Westra WH, Li S, et al. Improved survival of patients with human papillomavirus-positive head and neck squamous cell carcinoma in a prospective clinical trial. J Natl Cancer Inst 2008;100:261–9.
36. Kies MS, Holsinger FC, Lee JJ, et al. Induction chemotherapy and cetuximab for locally advanced squamous cell carcinoma of the head and neck: results from a phase II prospective trial. J Clin Oncol 2010;28:8–14.
37. Urba S, Wolf G, Eisbruch A, et al. Single-cycle induction chemotherapy selects patients with advanced laryngeal cancer for combined chemoradiation: a new treatment paradigm. J Clin Oncol 2006;24:593–8.
38. Holsinger FC, Kies MS, Diaz EM Jr, et al. Durable long-term remission with chemotherapy alone for stage II to IV laryngeal cancer. J Clin Oncol 2009;27:1976–82.
39. Fletcher GH, Evers WT. Radiotherapeutic management of surgical recurrences and postoperative residuals in tumors of the head and neck. Radiology 1970;95:185–8.
40. Bernier J, Domenge C, Ozsahin M, et al. Postoperative irradiation with or without concomitant chemotherapy for locally advanced head and neck cancer. N Engl J Med 2004;350:1945–52.
41. Cooper JS, Pajak TF, Forastiere AA, et al. Postoperative concurrent radiotherapy and chemotherapy for high-risk squamous-cell carcinoma of the head and neck. N Engl J Med 2004;350:1937–44.
42. Bernier J, Cooper JS, Pajak TF, et al. Defining risk levels in locally advanced head and neck cancers: a comparative analysis of concurrent postoperative radiation plus chemotherapy trials of the EORTC (#22931) and RTOG (# 9501). Head Neck 2005;27:843–50.

Quality of Life and Quality of Care

Functional Assessment and Rehabilitation

How to Maximize Outcomes

Katherine A. Hutcheson, PhD*, Jan S. Lewin, PhD

KEYWORDS

• Swallowing • Speech • Rehabilitation • Survivorship

KEY POINTS

- The number of long-term oral cavity and oropharyngeal cancer survivors is increasing. Speech and swallowing outcomes are critical survivorship end points.
- Pretreatment functional assessment is essential to plan rehabilitation and supportive care, to predict functional outcomes, and to select the modality of therapy most likely to maximize functional outcomes.
- Refinements in surgical reconstruction, conformal radiotherapy techniques, and preventive therapy can be used to reduce functional problems after treatment.
- Posttreatment rehabilitation requires individualized planning on the basis of standardized, instrumental assessments.

INTRODUCTION

The number of oral cavity and oropharyngeal cancer survivors is rising owing to the increased incidence of oropharyngeal cancer and improved survival rates. By 2030, oropharyngeal cancers are projected to account for almost half of all head and neck cancers.[1] The oral cavity and oropharynx are essential to normal speech, swallowing,

Funding Sources: Dr Hutcheson acknowledges funding from the UT Health Innovation for Cancer Prevention Research Fellowship, The University of Texas School of Public Health – Cancer Prevention and Research Institute of Texas (CPRIT) grant #RP101503. Disclaimer: The content is solely the responsibility of the authors and does not necessarily represent the official views of the CPRIT (K.A. Hutcheson). None (J.S. Lewin).
The University of Texas MD Anderson Cancer Center is supported in part by a Cancer Center Support Grant (CA016672) from the National Institutes of Health.
Conflicts of Interest: None.
Department of Head and Neck Surgery, Section of Speech Pathology & Audiology, The University of Texas MD Anderson Cancer Center, 1515 Holcombe Boulevard, Unit 1445, Houston, TX 77030, USA
* Corresponding author.
E-mail address: karnold@mdanderson.org

Otolaryngol Clin N Am 46 (2013) 657–670
http://dx.doi.org/10.1016/j.otc.2013.04.006 **oto.theclinics.com**
0030-6665/13/$ – see front matter

Abbreviations: Maximizing Outcomes of Rehabilitation	
IMRT	Intensity-modulated radiotherapy
TLM	Transoral laser microsurgery
TORS	Transoral robotic surgery
UADT	Upper aerodigestive tract

and respiration. This review summarizes the clinically distinct functional outcomes of patients with oral cavity and oropharyngeal cancers, methods of pretreatment functional assessments, strategies to reduce or prevent functional complications, and posttreatment rehabilitation considerations.

OVERVIEW OF FUNCTIONAL OUTCOMES

Oral Cavity Cancer

Surgical resection remains the primary treatment for many cancers of the oral cavity.[2,3] Surgery disrupts the complex anatomy and functions of the upper aerodigestive tract (UADT) and may lead to lifelong disability, despite advances in minimally invasive approaches and microsurgical reconstruction. Radiotherapy or chemoradiation, often delivered as an adjuvant therapy, exacerbates postsurgical effects by way of added fibrosis and neuromuscular insult.

Speech production is dependent on 4 processes: respiration, phonation, resonation, and articulation.[4] Each process involves precise biomechanical coordination of multiple structures in the oral cavity and UADT. Consequently, the type and degree of speech impairment varies depending on the location and extent of tumor within the oral cavity. In general, speech production is most adversely affected when oral cavity resections involve the mobile tongue or extend to include the soft palate.

Oral cavity cancers involving the tongue most commonly impair articulation. A recent systematic review suggested that speech remains largely intelligible (92%–98% intelligible at the sentence level [blinded ratings of unfamiliar listeners]) for most surgically treated patients with advanced-stage oral cancer (tumor category $\geq$T2), including those with tumors involving the tongue. Deviant speech characteristics were common findings across published studies, despite intelligible speech ratings.[5] That is, data suggest that speech is largely understandable but not normal after surgical resection of advanced stage oral cancers. In addition, the extent of tongue resection greatly affects the accuracy of articulation and intelligibility. Most patients will ultimately acquire good intelligibility after partial or hemiglossectomy procedures that preserve half or more of the native tongue, but outcomes are more variable after subtotal and total glossectomy.[5]

Treatment of oral cavity cancers can also disrupt speech resonance. Resections of cancers involving the maxilla cause significant rhinolalia until the oronasal defect is adequately sealed. Acceptable speech quality is achieved in most patients after successful prosthetic obturation or surgical reconstruction of the oronasal defect,[6,7] but surveys find that self-reported speech function is still significantly lower in patients with cancer with maxillary defects relative to normal controls.[8] In addition, obturation is typically less successful when the defect extends to involve the soft palate because of the soft palate's dynamic involvement in the process of velopharyngeal closure.[9]

Speech and swallowing function are closely related because they rely on common UADT structures. Swallowing occurs in 4 phases: oral preparatory, oral, pharyngeal, and esophageal. Treatment of oral cavity cancers most commonly affects the first 3 phases of swallowing. Oropharyngeal swallowing function can be impaired by the direct effects of oral cavity resection on oral preparatory functions (ie, mastication, collecting a bolus in the mouth) and oral transit (ie, posterior propulsion from the mouth to the pharynx). Oral cavity resection can also indirectly affect pharyngeal bolus transit by way of premature spillage that accompanies the loss of oral control, decreased lingual driving pressure on a bolus through the pharynx, or disrupted stabilization of the hyolaryngeal complex required for airway closure and upper esophageal opening. In addition, adverse effects of adjuvant radiotherapy or chemoradiation on pharyngeal swallowing function are well established. Data from a systematic review suggest that swallowing efficiency is commonly impaired after surgical management of advanced-stage oral cavity cancers (ie, prolonged bolus transit times and incomplete bolus clearance), but chronic aspiration is a less common consequence of surgical management (12%–25% prevalence). Therefore, it is not surprising that patients surgically treated for oral cavity cancer perceive the greatest degree of trouble swallowing dry or hard foods when polled about specific dysphagia symptoms.[10]

Oropharyngeal Cancer

Survival after oropharyngeal cancer has dramatically improved in the past 20 years owing to intensified organ preservation strategies and the rising proportion of human papillomavirus-attributable cancer. Options for organ preservation include nonsurgical therapy (ie, radiotherapy and chemoradiation) and minimally invasive surgery (ie, transoral robotic surgery [TORS] or transoral laser microsurgery [TLM]).

Organ preservation strategies seek to achieve locoregional control and optimize functional outcomes. The oropharyngeal region is the crossroads where nasal, oral, laryngeal, and pharyngeal cavities meet. Swallowing function relies heavily on the coordinated response of these structures to propel a bolus safely from the mouth through the pharynx. Thus, pharyngeal dysphagia is the principal functional toxicity of treatment for oropharyngeal cancer, and is recognized as a key end point measure in the contemporary management of this disease. As Weinstein and colleagues[11] noted, "...if it is found that the oncologic outcomes are equivalent...then the most important factor for triaging patients to TORS or chemoradiation will be swallowing outcomes."

Swallowing is a complex biomechanical process involving 5 cranial nerves and more than 25 muscles in the UADT. Swallowing impairments can occur as the result of surgery alone, radiotherapy alone, or chemoradiation. Data specific to patients with oropharyngeal primary tumors demonstrate a high burden of dysphagia. In a population-based Surveillance, Epidemiology, and End Results–Medicare analysis of more than 8000 patients with head and neck cancer, patients with cancers of the oropharynx had the second-highest prevalence of dysphagia.[12] In a pooled analysis of 3 Radiation Therapy Oncology Group chemoradiation trials, 35% of 101 patients with oropharyngeal cancer with adequate baseline function experienced late grade 3 or 4 laryngeal or pharyngeal toxicity, often including dysphagia.[13]

Even in the era of conformal radiotherapy (ie, intensity-modulated radiotherapy [IMRT]) for oropharyngeal cancer, as many as 85% of patients require feeding tubes during therapy, and investigators report 6% to 31% rates of aspiration 1 year or more after treatment and 4% to 8% rates of chronic feeding tube dependence.[14–16] In a trial evaluating treatment for oropharyngeal cancer with chemoIMRT that was designed to protect dysphagia-organs-at-risk using swallowing-specific dose constraints, 31% of patients had higher occurrences of aspiration 1 year or more after treatment relative to baseline, and 22% developed pneumonia.[16] Aspiration was significantly predictive of pneumonia in this trial ($P = .017$, sensitivity = 80%, specificity = 60%), and silent aspiration was evident on modified barium swallow (MBS) studies in 63% of patients who developed pneumonia. In addition, pharyngeal residue on MBS studies was significantly associated with the development of pneumonia after chemoIMRT ($P<.01$).[17]

Particularly concerning is the risk of severe, late radiation-associated dysphagia (late-RAD) that presents up to decades after radiotherapy in long-term survivors of oropharyngeal cancer. Although the prevalence of severe late-RAD is likely rare data suggest that the level of impairment is profound, often accompanied by a constellation of neuromuscular pathologies, including lower cranial neuropathies. In addition, late-RAD is largely refractory to standard, nonsurgical dysphagia therapies and leads to recurrent pneumonias requiring lifelong gastrostomy or elective functional laryngectomy.[18]

TORS is emerging as a minimally invasive surgical alternative to nonsurgical organ preservation for oropharyngeal cancer, proposed to offer several functional advantages relative to open surgery or definitive chemoradiation. TORS allows access for resection without pharyngotomy or mandibulotomy, maintaining the critical muscular framework of the laryngopharynx. Tracheostomy, typically required for airway management after open resection, is also not needed for most patients who undergo TORS (70%–100%). Furthermore, published series suggest that 9% to 27% of patients treated with frontline TORS avoid postoperative radiotherapy and 34% to 45% avoid chemoradiation. Crude end points of functional recovery after TORS suggest promising early outcomes relative to radiation-based organ preservation regimens. Rates of percutaneous endoscopic gastrostomy tube placement (18%–23%) and chronic dependence (0%–7%) after TORS are lower than those reported for patients receiving definitive chemoradiation.[19–23] However, patient-reported swallowing outcomes after TORS, according to the MD Anderson Dysphagia Inventory, are fairly similar to those of chemoradiation cohorts,[19] and findings of gold-standard instrumental swallowing assessments are rarely reported after TORS. In addition, functional outcomes have been studied almost exclusively in the first year after TORS. Thus, further comparisons of long-term outcomes and swallowing outcomes based on instrumental examinations are needed to better understand the functional differences in surgical and nonsurgical organ preservation strategies for oropharyngeal cancer.

PRETREATMENT FUNCTIONAL ASSESSMENT

Pretreatment functional assessment is a critical component of comprehensive care. Baseline functional status has been shown to predict posttreatment functional outcomes. Finding of baseline functional assessments also, contribute to clinical decisions about supportive care to optimize treatment tolerance, such as the need for feeding tube placement prior to treatment or dietary changes necessary to prevent aspiration. Pretreatment functional status is also important to consider when selecting the modality of cancer therapy most likely to maximize functional outcomes, particularly when various modalities offer a similar likelihood of cure. Pretreatment examination by a speech pathologist should include, at a minimum, an *oral motor/cranial nerve examination*, *motor speech evaluation* (articulation, resonance, voice quality, speech intelligibility), and a *clinical swallow evaluation*. An instrumental swallowing examination is indicated in many cases, particularly in patients who present with advanced-stage primary tumors who have an increased risk of baseline aspiration.[24] For patients with cancers of the oral cavity and oropharynx, the radiographic *MBS* study is the instrumental examination of choice because it allows evaluation of both oral and pharyngeal phases of swallowing.[25] *Laryngeal videostroboscopy* is also useful in assessing laryngopharyngeal function, particularly in patients with advanced-stage oropharyngeal cancer that extends to involve the larynx.

Instrumental examinations are considered the gold-standard methods of assessment because they objectively assess oropharyngeal swallowing physiology and bolus transit, and predict adverse health outcomes (eg, pneumonia and malnutrition). Functional outcomes can also be assessed by patient-reported outcome (PRO) measures. PRO measures provide complementary data to instrumental or clinician-rated examinations, mainly regarding the impact of functional impairments on daily activities and quality of life. However, there is often a lack of agreement about the severity of impairment between subjective PRO measures and clinician-rated examinations, and PRO measures do not fully reflect true swallowing competency. Thus, the consensus is that both metrics (instrumental, clinician-rated examinations and PROs) should be combined for comprehensive evaluation of functional outcomes.

Standardized functional assessments offer critical data, but functional assessments lack uniformity in clinical practice and research. Minimum standards for functional assessment have been suggested on the basis of a recent systematic review to include the following measures, longitudinally assessed at least 3 to 4 times during the treatment trajectory of patients with oral cavity or oropharyngeal cancer: (1) instrumental/objective swallowing assessment (eg, MBS study) with supplemental clinical data, (2) assessment of speech intelligibility, (3) supplemental speech assessment of specific impairments relevant to oral cavity and oropharyngeal cancer (eg, articulation, resonance), and (4) PRO measures related to speech and swallowing.[25] **Table 1** describes various methods of pretreatment functional assessment.

Table 1
Pretreatment functional assessment methods

Pretreatment Functional Assessment	Domains Assessed
Clinical examinations	
Cranial nerve/oral motor examination	Symmetry/range of motion oral musculature Oral opening
Motor speech examination	Articulation Resonance Voice quality Subjective intelligibility rating
Clinical swallowing evaluation	Oral preparatory functions: mastication, oral containment, bolus consolidation Oral phase functions: oral control, oral clearance Pharyngeal phase functions (inferred): airway protection, pharyngeal transit
Instrumental examinations	
Modified barium swallow	Oral, pharyngeal, and laryngeal physiology Airway protection: laryngeal penetration, aspiration Pharyngeal transit: residue
Fiberoptic endoscopic evaluation of swallowing	Laryngeal and pharyngeal physiology Airway protection: laryngeal penetration, aspiration Pharyngeal transit: residue No direct observation of oral phase
Laryngeal videostroboscopy	Vocal fold mobility Symmetry, amplitude, periodicity Mucosal wave Laryngeal pathology

PREVENTING OR REDUCING FUNCTIONAL PROBLEMS

The severity of functional impairment can be influenced by a number of clinical factors. Current literature indicates that the percentage of oral tongue resection, type of reconstruction, contour of the free flap, and primary tumor stage affect postsurgical speech and swallowing outcomes.[5,10,26] Functional outcomes also vary depending on the schedule of radiation, radiotherapy dose distribution, and the use of concurrent chemotherapy. Finally, swallowing outcomes can be influenced by supportive care practices, including the timing and type of feeding tube placement and the provision of targeted preventive exercise in patients receiving radiotherapy or chemoradiation. Disease characteristics (ie, subsite and tumor volume) that influence functional outcomes are unchangeable; thus, this section is focused on factors that can potentially be modified to prevent or reduce functional problems after treatment. These include surgical reconstructive factors, radiotherapy techniques, and supportive care/preventive therapy.

Surgical and Reconstructive Factors

Microvascular reconstruction is typically considered to benefit functional outcomes. Some studies, however, report significantly worse swallowing outcomes in patients who have reconstruction after oral cavity and oropharyngeal resections,[26] largely due to the confounding effects of greater tumor burden and greater surgical defects in patients who require reconstruction rather than primary closure. Reconstructive factors that drive functional outcomes include sensory repair and the contour and volume of the flap.

Intraoral sensation has been shown to be correlated with UADT function, including pharyngeal swallowing competency,[27,28] and sensory reinnervation can be performed during microvascular reconstruction.

Published studies report conflicting results regarding the functional outcomes of sensory reinnervation in oral cavity reconstructions. For instance, objective swallowing ratings according to MBS studies did not differ between patients with reinnervated flaps and those with noninnervated flaps in a prospective functional analysis of 44 patients.[29] In contrast, Yu[30] found significantly higher diet levels in patients with reinnervated anterolateral thigh flaps compared with those with noninnervated flaps after near-total or total glossectomy. Nonetheless, investigators have advocated that a relatively simple reinnervation procedure improves intraoral sensation and should be attempted when possible.[31]

In addition, the shape and volume of the reconstructed tongue has been shown to affect postoperative speech and swallowing outcomes. Reconstructed flaps that are protuberant or semiprotuberant and those with greater volume are associated with significantly better speech intelligibility and dietary outcomes.[32,33] On the basis of these findings, investigators have suggested overcorrection of the defect to account for volume loss that occurs with atrophy and postoperative radiotherapy.[32,33] Finally, the utility of laryngeal suspension in patients requiring total or subtotal glossectomy has been demonstrated both to help protect the airway from aspiration and prevent prolapse of the flap.[32,34]

Radiotherapy Techniques

Radiotherapy techniques can vary greatly, particularly the conformal methods used to spare normal tissue. Normal tissue constraints using IMRT have historically limited the dose to the salivary glands to reduce xerostomia. Swallowing-specific dose-constraints using IMRT have only recently been explored[16] after a number of studies (most commonly in oropharyngeal cancer) elucidated the core swallowing-related organs at risk.[35] The anterior oral cavity, superior pharyngeal musculature, and inferior larynx/esophageal inlet have been identified as swallowing-specific organs at risk, for which dose-volume coverage is correlated with short-term and long-term swallowing outcomes after IMRT. Data suggest that integrating swallowing-specific organ dose constraints into IMRT plans may reduce gastrostomy dependence, improve oropharyngeal swallowing efficiency, minimize aspiration, and optimize swallowing-related quality of life.[14,16,36–39]

Pharyngeal and oral cavity constraints can be integrated into IMRT plans, whereas laryngeal dose-sparing can be achieved by integrating laryngeal dose constraints into full-field IMRT plans or a larynx block can be accomplished using a split-field technique. A split-field laryngeal block technique matches IMRT fields at the level of the arytenoid cartilages with a conventional supraclavicular laryngeal block (3 × 3 cm) using anteroposterior bilateral low neck fields. In patients with oropharyngeal cancer, the split-field technique has been shown to achieve a lower laryngeal and esophageal inlet dose compared with full IMRT fields.[14,37] Current evidence supports the potential for laryngeal shielding and dysphagia-specific dose constraints to reduce the risk of dysphagia after conformal radiotherapy.

Preventive Therapy

Preventive swallowing therapy encourages ongoing use of the swallowing musculature during radiotherapy under the “Use it or lose it” paradigm. In preventive swallowing therapy, speech pathologists train patients to perform targeted swallowing exercises before and during the course of radiotherapy (although not during actual radiotherapy treatment sessions), and prescribe compensatory swallowing techniques or dietary modifications to discourage even brief NPO (nothing per oral) periods. Three randomized clinical trials have shown a benefit of early initiation of swallowing exercises during chemoradiation.[40–42] One trial reported a 36% absolute risk reduction for loss of functional swallowing ability among patients randomized to receive swallowing exercises during chemoradiation.[41] Favorable outcomes reported with preventive swallowing exercises include superior swallowing-related quality of life scores[43,44]; better base of tongue retraction and epiglottic inversion[45]; larger postradiotherapy muscle mass and magnetic resonance imaging T2 signal intensity of the genioglossus, mylohyoid, and hyoglossus muscles[41]; more normal oral diet levels after chemoradiation[40]; and shorter duration of gastrostomy dependence.[46,47]

In addition, maintenance of *any* oral intake during radiotherapy (ie, avoidance of NPO intervals) has been found to independently predict long-term swallowing-related quality of life outcomes according to the MD Anderson Dysphagia Inventory and significantly predicts diet levels up to 1 year after radiotherapy.[48,49] Multidisciplinary management of acute radiation toxicities, including odynophagia, dysgeusia, weight loss, and dysphagia, is necessary to help patients safely maintain oral intake during therapy. The evidence in favor of proactive swallowing therapy in patients with head and neck cancer who are treated with radiotherapy is summarized in **Table 2**.

POSTTREATMENT REHABILITATION

Functional rehabilitation after cancer therapy is individualized to meet the needs of each patient. In general, patients with oral cavity cancers who have had surgery (and often postoperative radiotherapy or chemoradiation) require both speech and swallowing therapy, whereas patients who receive radiotherapy or chemoradiation for oropharyngeal cancers are most likely to require dysphagia therapy. In either

Table 2
Evidence for preventive "use it or lose it" swallowing therapy in patients with head and neck cancer treated with radiotherapy

Institution	Study Design	Comparison	Outcomes
"Use it or lose it" principle: early swallowing exercises			
University of Alabama–Birmingham	Retrospective[a]	Pretreatment exercise vs standard care[b]	Superior MDADI scores,[43] Better base of tongue and epiglottic movement[45]
The University of Texas MD Anderson Cancer Center	Retrospective[a]	Adherent to pretreatment exercise vs not adherent	Shorter duration of percutaneous endoscopic gastrostomy[46,47] Superior MDADI scores[44]
University of Florida	Randomized controlled trial	Pretreatment exercise vs pretreatment sham exercise vs standard care[b]	Significant preservation of muscle mass according to magnetic resonance imaging[41]
Netherlands Cancer Institute	Randomized clinical trial	Pretreatment exercise vs pretreatment exercise + Therabite[c]	Improved mouth opening[50]
Mount Sinai	Randomized controlled trial	Pretreatment exercise vs standard care[b]	Superior diet levels (3–6 mo after conformal radiotherapy)[40]
"Use it or lose it" principle: avoid NPO			
Medical University of South Carolina	Retrospective with cross-sectional survey[a]	Prolonged NPO (>2 wk) vs no prolonged NPO interval	Significantly lower MDADI scores with prolonged NPO[48]
Boston University	Retrospective[a]	Partial or fully PO at end of radiotherapy vs 100% NPO	Partial or fully PO led to significantly better diet levels (through 12 mo) after radiotherapy[49]

Abbreviations: MDADI, MD Anderson Dysphagia Inventory; NPO, no enteral nutrition.
[a] Observational between-group comparisons; not randomized.
[b] Standard care = no pretreatment exercise, posttreatment exercise provided as indicated.
[c] Atos Medical, Horby, Sweden.

case, rehabilitation should be planned to target physiologic and functional impairments identified on standardized, instrumental assessments. That is, effective rehabilitation begins with comprehensive and standardized functional assessment. Functional assessment includes, for all cases, oral motor/cranial nerve examination and motor speech assessment. Standardized articulation and intelligibility batteries are available to identify goals for speech intervention, and swallowing therapy goals should be determined on the basis of instrumental examinations (eg, the MBS study or fiberoptic endoscopic evaluation of swallowing).

Patients with postoperative dysarthria can be taught compensatory mechanisms of articulation that rely on exaggeration of the remaining labial, mandibular, pharyngeal, and laryngeal structures. Glossectomy-specific compensatory phonetic strategies pioneered by the work of Skelly and colleagues[51,52] in the 1970s remain useful in contemporary practice. Articulation targets are selected on the basis of standardized batteries, such as the Fisher-Logemann Test of Articulation. Speech pathologists also use findings of articulation testing to collaborate with maxillofacial prosthodontists in the process of designing palatal augmentation prostheses. Palatal augmentation prostheses improve the accuracy of consonant production and can normalize vowel production by reshaping the contour of the hard palate for better contact by the surgically altered tongue.[53] A systematic review that evaluated studies over more than 35 years found that palatal prostheses improve objective ratings of both speech and swallowing function in roughly 85% of patients. Published data also suggested an inverse relationship between the efficacy of a palatal prosthesis and mobility of the residual tongue. That is, the prognosis for improving speech with a palatal prosthesis is less favorable as the mobility of the residual tongue increases.[54]

Evidence-based compensatory swallowing techniques have been shown to improve airway protection and bolus clearance in patients with oropharyngeal dysphagia after cancer therapy.[55] Compensatory techniques may include postures, such as a chin tuck or head rotation, strategies, such as the supraglottic swallow, and/or dietary modifications, such as thickening liquids or blending foods. Instrumental examination is critical to match appropriate compensations with the specific swallowing impairment and to test the efficacy of compensations in individual patients. In some cases, compensations are used for a short interval to ensure safe oral intake during acute periods of recovery, whereas patients with chronic dysphagia may adopt swallowing compensations as a lifelong tool to prevent aspiration compromise.

Evidence-based swallowing exercises are also selected on the basis of the pathophysiology of dysphagia identified during instrumental examinations.[56–63] Exercise therapy is maximized by attending to defined principles of strength training and neuroplasticity. Exercises must challenge the system beyond its normal capacity in a systematic fashion, and skills-training encourages relearning and neuroplasticity through direct swallowing activities. Adjunctive biofeedback measures, such as surface electromyography or endoscopic monitoring, coupled with swallowing therapy, can help the patient examine, modify, and challenge the therapeutic task.[64,65] In addition, investigations are ongoing to determine the efficacy of transcutaneous neuromuscular electrical stimulation (NMES) as a treatment for dysphagia after cancer therapy. Current evidence suggests that NMES often lowers the hyolaryngeal complex because the superficial infrahyoid strap muscles receive more intense levels of stimulation than the deeper laryngeal elevators.[66] This finding suggests that transcutaneous NMES may benefit only patients who are able to sufficiently elevate the larynx during swallowing against the resistance (ie, downward pull) induced by the stimulation. This premise requires further investigation; if confirmed, it indicates that the physiologic effect of NMES on hyolaryngeal movement must be examined under videofluoroscopy in each patient before applying this therapy to avoid potential harm or unintended physiologic effects. Finally, the intensity of swallowing therapy matters. Dose-response data are lacking for most swallowing therapies, but intensive “boot-camp” paradigms show promise to improve swallowing outcomes in patients with chronic or severe dysphagia.[57]

SUMMARY

In summary, the number of long-term oral cavity and oropharyngeal cancer survivors is rising, and speech and swallowing outcomes are principal determinants of quality of life during cancer survivorship. Thus, maximizing long-term functional outcomes is a priority of contemporary multidisciplinary head and neck cancer care. Optimizing functional outcomes begins with a standardized, comprehensive baseline assessment. Pretreatment functional assessment should combine complementary instrumental, clinician-rated examinations with PRO measures. Functional analysis before treatment is critical to plan rehabilitation and supportive care, predict outcomes, and select the optimal cancer therapy. A number of strategies can be targeted to prevent or reduce the burden of functional problems. Therapeutic techniques that can maximize function include attention to flap volume and contour and consideration of sensory reinnervation in surgical cases requiring reconstruction. Current evidence also supports the potential for laryngeal shielding and dysphagia-specific IMRT dose constraints to diminish pharyngeal dysphagia after radiotherapy. Finally, preventive swallowing therapy that couples targeted swallowing exercises with avoidance of NPO intervals has been shown to positively affect a number of important functional endpoints. Functional rehabilitation after treatment requires individualized planning and should be guided by physiologic findings of instrumental examinations. Functional success is best achieved with a multidisciplinary team that includes speech pathologists specialized in assessment and management of head and neck cancer.

REFERENCES

1. Chaturvedi AK, Engels EA, Pfeiffer RM, et al. Human papillomavirus and rising oropharyngeal cancer incidence in the United States. J Clin Oncol 2011;29: 4294–301.
2. Cooper JS, Porter K, Mallin K, et al. National Cancer Database report on cancer of the head and neck: 10-year update. Head Neck 2009;31:748–58.
3. Funk GF, Karnell LH, Robinson RA, et al. Presentation, treatment, and outcome of oral cavity cancer: a National Cancer Data Base report. Head Neck 2002;24: 165–80.
4. Seikel JA, King DW, Drumright DG, editors. Anatomy & physiology for speech, language, and hearing. 4th edition. Clifton Park (NY): Cengage Learning; 2009.
5. Kreeft AM, van der Molen L, Hilgers FJ, et al. Speech and swallowing after surgical treatment of advanced oral and oropharyngeal carcinoma: a systematic review of the literature. Eur Arch Otorhinolaryngol 2009;266:1687–98.
6. Andrades P, Rosenthal EL, Carroll WR, et al. Zygomatic-maxillary buttress reconstruction of midface defects with the osteocutaneous radial forearm free flap. Head Neck 2008;30:1295–302.
7. Futran ND, Wadsworth JT, Villaret D, et al. Midface reconstruction with the fibula free flap. Arch Otolaryngol Head Neck Surg 2002;128:161–6.
8. Hertrampf K, Wenz HJ, Lehmann KM, et al. Quality of life of patients with maxillofacial defects after treatment for malignancy. Int J Prosthodont 2004;17: 657–65.
9. McCombe D, Lyons B, Winkler R, et al. Speech and swallowing following radial forearm flap reconstruction of major soft palate defects. Br J Plast Surg 2005;58: 306–11.
10. Dwivedi RC, St Rose S, Chisholm EJ, et al. Evaluation of swallowing by Sydney Swallow Questionnaire (SSQ) in oral and oropharyngeal cancer patients treated with primary surgery [published online ahead of print February 21, 2012]. Dysphagia 2012. Available at: http://www.springerlink.com/content/l87t8788u5871g11/?MUD=MP. Accessed July 1, 2012.
11. Weinstein GS, O'Malley BW Jr, Desai SC, et al. Transoral robotic surgery: does the ends justify the means? Curr Opin Otolaryngol Head Neck Surg 2009;17: 126–31.

12. Francis DO, Weymuller EA Jr, Parvathaneni U, et al. Dysphagia, stricture, and pneumonia in head and neck cancer patients: does treatment modality matter? Ann Otol Rhinol Laryngol 2010;119:391–7.
13. Machtay M, Moughan J, Trotti A, et al. Factors associated with severe late toxicity after concurrent chemoradiation for locally advanced head and neck cancer: an RTOG analysis. J Clin Oncol 2008;26:3582–9.
14. Schwartz DL, Hutcheson KA, Barringer DA, et al. Candidate dosimetric predictors of long-term swallowing dysfunction after oropharyngeal intensity-modulated radiotherapy. Int J Radiat Oncol Biol Phys 2010;78:1356–65.
15. Caudell JJ, Schaner PE, Meredith RF, et al. Factors associated with long-term dysphagia after definitive radiotherapy for locally advanced head-and-neck cancer. Int J Radiat Oncol Biol Phys 2009;73:410–5.
16. Eisbruch A, Kim HM, Feng FY, et al. Chemo-IMRT of oropharyngeal cancer aiming to reduce dysphagia: swallowing organs late complication probabilities and dosimetric correlates. Int J Radiat Oncol Biol Phys 2011;81:e93–9.
17. Hunter KU, Feng FY, Schipper M, et al. What is the clinical relevance of objective studies in head and neck cancer patients receiving chemoirradiation? Analysis of aspiration in swallow studies vs. risk of aspiration pneumonia. Paper presented at: American Society for Radiation Oncology (ASTRO) Annual Meeting. Miami, October 2–6, 2011.
18. Hutcheson KA, Lewin JS, Barringer DA, et al. Late dysphagia after radiotherapy-based treatment of head and neck cancer. Cancer 2012;118(23):5793–9.
19. Sinclair CF, McColloch NL, Carroll WR, et al. Patient-perceived and objective functional outcomes following transoral robotic surgery for early oropharyngeal carcinoma. Arch Otolaryngol Head Neck Surg 2011;137:1112–6.
20. Hurtuk A, Agrawal A, Old M, et al. Outcomes of transoral robotic surgery: a preliminary clinical experience. Otolaryngol Head Neck Surg 2011;145:248–53.
21. Genden EM, Park R, Smith C, et al. The role of reconstruction for transoral robotic pharyngectomy and concomitant neck dissection. Arch Otolaryngol Head Neck Surg 2011;137:151–6.
22. Weinstein GS, O'Malley BW Jr, Cohen MA, et al. Transoral robotic surgery for advanced oropharyngeal carcinoma. Arch Otolaryngol Head Neck Surg 2010; 136:1079–85.
23. Moore EJ, Olsen KD, Kasperbauer JL. Transoral robotic surgery for oropharyngeal squamous cell carcinoma: a prospective study of feasibility and functional outcomes. Laryngoscope 2009;119:2156–64.
24. Starmer H, Gourin C, Lua LL, et al. Pretreatment swallowing assessment in head and neck cancer patients. Laryngoscope 2011;121:1208–11.
25. Mylnarek AM, Rieger JM, Harris JR, et al. Methods of functional outcomes assessment following treatment of oral and oropharyngeal cancer: review of the literature. J Otolaryngol Head Neck Surg 2008;37:2–10.
26. Dwivedi RC, Chisholm EJ, Khan AS, et al. An exploratory study of the influence of clinico-demographic variables on swallowing and swallowing-related quality of life in a cohort of oral and oropharyngeal cancer patients treated with primary surgery. Eur Arch Otorhinolaryngol 2012;269:1233–9.
27. Jaghagen EL, Bodin I, Isberg A. Pharyngeal swallowing dysfunction following treatment for oral and pharyngeal cancer—association with diminished intraoral sensation and discrimination ability. Head Neck 2008;30:1344–51.
28. O'Connell DA, Reiger J, Dziegielewski PT, et al. Effect of lingual and hypoglossal nerve reconstruction on swallowing function in head and neck surgery: prospective functional outcomes study. J Otolaryngol Head Neck Surg 2009;38:246–54.

29. Markkanen-Leppanen M, Isotalo E, Makitie AA, et al. Swallowing after free-flap reconstruction in patients with oral and pharyngeal cancer. Oral Oncol 2006;42: 501–9.
30. Yu P. Reinnervated anterolateral thigh flap for tongue reconstruction. Head Neck 2004;26:1038–44.
31. Kimata Y, Uchiyama K, Ebihara S, et al. Comparison of innervated and noninnervated free flaps in oral reconstruction. Plast Reconstr Surg 1999;104:1307–13.
32. Kimata Y, Sakuraba M, Hishinuma S, et al. Analysis of the relations between the shape of the reconstructed tongue and postoperative functions after subtotal or total glossectomy. Laryngoscope 2003;113:905–9.
33. Yun IS, Lee DW, Lee WJ, et al. Correlation of neotongue volume changes with functional outcomes after long-term follow-up of total glossectomy. J Craniofac Surg 2010;21:111–6.
34. Weber RS, Ohlms L, Bowman J, et al. Functional results after total or near total glossectomy with laryngeal preservation. Arch Otolaryngol Head Neck Surg 1991;117:512–5.
35. Roe JW, Carding PN, Dwivedi RC, et al. Swallowing outcomes following intensity modulated radiation therapy (IMRT) for head & neck cancer—a systematic review. Oral Oncol 2010;46:727–33.
36. Eisbruch A, Schwartz M, Rasch C, et al. Dysphagia and aspiration after chemoradiotherapy for head-and-neck cancer: which anatomic structures are affected and can they be spared by IMRT? Int J Radiat Oncol Biol Phys 2004;60:1425–39.
37. Feng FY, Kim HM, Lyden TH, et al. Intensity-modulated radiotherapy of head and neck cancer aiming to reduce dysphagia: early dose-effect relationships for the swallowing structures. Int J Radiat Oncol Biol Phys 2007;68:1289–98.
38. Caglar HB, Tishler RB, Othus M, et al. Dose to larynx predicts for swallowing complications after intensity-modulated radiotherapy. Int J Radiat Oncol Biol Phys 2008;72:1110–8.
39. Levendag PC, Teguh DN, Voet P, et al. Dysphagia disorders in patients with cancer of the oropharynx are significantly affected by the radiation therapy dose to the superior and middle constrictor muscle: a dose-effect relationship. Radiother Oncol 2007;85:64–73.
40. Kotz T, Federman AD, Kao J, et al. Prophylactic swallowing exercises in patients with head and neck cancer undergoing chemoradiation: a randomized trial. Arch Otolaryngol Head Neck Surg 2012;138:376–82.
41. Carnaby-Mann G, Crary MA, Schmalfuss I, et al. "Pharyngocise": randomized controlled trial of preventative exercises to maintain muscle structure and swallowing function during head-and-neck chemoradiotherapy. Int J Radiat Oncol Biol Phys 2012;83:210–9.
42. Carnaby-Mann GD, Lagorio L, Crary MA, et al. Dysphagia prevention exercises in head and neck cancer: pharyngocise dose response study. Paper presented at: 20th Annual Dysphagia Research Society Meeting. Toronto (Canada), March 7–10, 2012.
43. Kulbersh BD, Rosenthal EL, McGrew BM, et al. Pretreatment, preoperative swallowing exercises may improve dysphagia quality of life. Laryngoscope 2006; 116:883–6.
44. Shinn EH, Basen-Engquist KM, Guam G, et al. Observation of adherence patterns to preventative swallowing exercises in oropharynx cancer survivors. Head Neck, in press.
45. Carroll WR, Locher JL, Canon CL, et al. Pretreatment swallowing exercises improve swallow function after chemoradiation. Laryngoscope 2008;118:39–43.

46. Bhayani M, Hutcheson KA, Barringer DA, et al. Gastrostomy tube placement in patients with hypopharyngeal cancer treated with chemoradiotherapy: factors affecting placement and dependence. Head Neck, Available at: http://www.ncbi.nlm.nih.gov/pubmed/23322545.
47. Bhayani M, Hutcheson KA, Barringer DA, et al. Gastrostomy tube placement in patients with oropharyngeal cancer treated with chemoradiotherapy: factors affecting placement and dependence. Head Neck, Available at: http://www.ncbi.nlm.nih.gov/pubmed/23322563.
48. Gillespie MB, Brodsky MB, Day TA, et al. Swallowing-related quality of life after head and neck cancer treatment. Laryngoscope 2004;114:1362–7.
49. Langmore S, Krisciunas GP, Miloro KV, et al. Does PEG use cause dysphagia in head and neck cancer patients? Dysphagia 2012;27:251–9.
50. van der Molen L, van Rossum MA, Burkhead LM, et al. A randomized preventive rehabilitation trial in advanced head and neck cancer patients treated with chemoradiotherapy: feasibility, compliance, and short-term effects. Dysphagia 2011;26:155–70.
51. Skelly M, Donaldson RC, Fust RS, et al. Changes in phonatory aspects of glossectomee intelligibility through vocal parameter manipulation. J Speech Hear Disord 1972;37:379–89.
52. Skelly M, Spector DJ, Donaldson RC, et al. Compensatory physiologic phonetics for the glossectomee. J Speech Hear Disord 1971;36:101–14.
53. de Carvalho-Teles V, Sennes LU, Gielow I. Speech evaluation after palatal augmentation in patients undergoing glossectomy. Arch Otolaryngol Head Neck Surg 2008;134:1066–70.
54. Marunick M, Tselios N. The efficacy of palatal augmentation prostheses for speech and swallowing in patients undergoing glossectomy: a review of the literature. J Prosthet Dent 2004;91:67–74.
55. McCabe D, Ashford J, Wheeler-Hegland K, et al. Evidence-based systematic review: oropharyngeal dysphagia behavioral treatments. Part IV—impact of dysphagia treatment on individuals' postcancer treatments. J Rehabil Res Dev 2009;46:205–14.
56. Antunes EB, Lunet N. Effects of the head lift exercise on the swallow function: a systematic review [published online ahead of print May 21, 2012]. Gerodontology 2012. Available at: http://onlinelibrary.wiley.com/doi/10.1111/j.1741-2358.2012.00638.x/full. Accessed July 1, 2012.
57. Crary MA, Carnaby-Mann GD, Lagorio LA, et al. Functional and physiological outcomes from an exercise-based dysphagia therapy: a pilot investigation of the McNeill Dysphagia Therapy program. Arch Phys Med Rehabil 2012;93:1173–8.
58. Shaker R, Easterling C, Kern M, et al. Rehabilitation of swallowing by exercise in tube-fed patients with pharyngeal dysphagia secondary to abnormal UES opening. Gastroenterology 2002;122:1314–21.
59. Kahrilas PJ, Logemann JA, Krugler C, et al. Volitional augmentation of upper esophageal sphincter opening during swallowing. Am J Physiol 1991;260:G450–6.
60. Fujiu M, Logemann JA. Effect of a tongue holding maneuver on posterior pharyngeal wall movement during deglutition. Am J Speech Lang Pathol 1996;5:23–30.
61. Fujiu M, Logemann JA, Pauloski BR. Increased post-operative posterior pharyngeal wall movement in anterior oral cancer patients: preliminary findings and possible implications for treatment. Am J Speech Lang Pathol 1995;4:24–30.

62. Lazarus C, Logemann JA, Song CW, et al. Effects of voluntary maneuvers on tongue base function for swallowing. Folia Phoniatr Logop 2002;54:171–6.
63. Huckabee ML, Steele CM. An analysis of lingual contribution to submental surface electromyographic measures and pharyngeal pressure during effortful swallow. Arch Phys Med Rehabil 2006;87:1067–72.
64. Burkhead LM, Sapienza CM, Rosenbek JC. Strength-training exercise in dysphagia rehabilitation: principles, procedures, and directions for future research. Dysphagia 2007;22:251–65.
65. Robbins J, Butler SG, Daniels SK, et al. Swallowing and dysphagia rehabilitation: translating principles of neural plasticity into clinically oriented evidence. J Speech Lang Hear Res 2008;51:S276–300.
66. Humbert IA, Poletto CJ, Saxon KG, et al. The effect of surface electrical stimulation on hyolaryngeal movement in normal individuals at rest and during swallowing. J Appl Physiol 2006;101:1657–63.

Standardizing Treatment

A Crisis in Cancer Care

Carol M. Lewis, MD, MPH*, Randal S. Weber, MD

KEYWORDS

• Standardizing treatment • Treatment outcomes • Head and neck cancer
• Cancer treatment • Practice guidelines • Quality assessment

KEY POINTS

- Clinical practice guidelines are recommendations for patient care that are formulated by expert multidisciplinary panels and based on the best available evidence. They have an important role in daily practice, as well as implications for quality improvement and health policy.
- The goals of head and neck cancer care are to maximize function and clinical outcomes. Treatment should be based on the best evidence available and ad hoc management plans should be avoided.
- Multidisciplinary treatment planning represents quality improvement in determining an optimized and individualized management plan.
- There have been trends toward regionalization of head and neck cancer care; however, efforts to encourage and incentivize regionalization should be adopted to maximize the quality of care delivered to patients with head and neck cancers.

INTRODUCTION

Recent reports from the Institute of Medicine (IOM) emphasizing the need for quality improvement in health care coupled with unsustainable increases in health care spending have brought health care to a crossroads.[1,2] Solutions highlighted in the IOM's 2001 report *Crossing the Quality Chasm: A New Health System for the 21st Century* include avoiding the overuse of practices without proven benefit and underuse of those practices known to be effective[2]; reducing waste, increasing efficiency, and providing timely access to care optimizes quality and contains costs.

Specific to oncology, the IOM has outlined recommendations for ensuring the quality of cancer care that include formulating clinical practice guidelines (CPGs),

---

Disclosures: The authors have no conflicts to disclose.
Department of Head and Neck Surgery, University of Texas MD Anderson Cancer Center, 1515 Holcombe Boulevard, Unit 1445, Houston, TX 77030, USA
* Corresponding author.
E-mail address: cmlewis@mdanderson.org

Otolaryngol Clin N Am 46 (2013) 671–679
http://dx.doi.org/10.1016/j.otc.2013.04.007 oto.theclinics.com
0030-6665/13/$ – see front matter

emphasizing multidisciplinary evaluation, and the regionalization of care.[1] This review focuses on these elements, which are critical to improving the quality of head and neck cancer care.

CLINICAL PRACTICE GUIDELINES

Definition and Considerations

CPGs are formulated by expert multidisciplinary panels that review existing literature and make consensus recommendations based on the strongest available evidence. The IOM defines CPGs as "statements that include recommendations intended to optimize patient care that are informed by a systematic review of evidence and an assessment of the benefits and harms of alternative care options."[3] Stated another way, CPGs are consensus-based recommendations for patient care that are based on the best available evidence; their purpose is to empower individual physicians to deliver optimal evidence-based care to their patients.

CPGs are limited by the quality of available evidence; the literature can be classified into 5 levels of evidence from strongest (level 1) to weakest (level 5) (**Table 1**). The National Comprehensive Cancer Network (NCCN) has addressed this by categorizing their recommendations based on the strength of available evidence and the degree of consensus among panel members (**Table 2**); because the availability of level 1 data from randomized prospective clinical trials is limited, most guidelines for head and neck cancer care are based on a lower level of evidence with uniform NCCN consensus.[4] In the United Kingdom, the Scottish Intercollegiate Guidelines Network (SIGN) assigns each recommendation both a numeric score denoting the level of evidence and a letter grade indicating the strength of the recommendation.[5] Although most recommendations for head and neck cancer are based on a lower level of evidence, level 1 studies have significantly changed NCCN guidelines for head and neck cancer.[6–8]

Because CPGs are created by an expert multidisciplinary panel, there is the potential for conflicts of interest among panel members; panelists may be biased by their own publications, inherent treatment philosophy, and research interests or by industry affiliations. The IOM recently recognized this problem by establishing criteria for identifying high-quality CPGs.[3] This report emphasized the need for limitation and full

Table 1
Definitions of levels of evidence for studies of therapy, prevention, etiology, and harm

Level		Study Type
1	a	Systematic reviews of randomized controlled trials
	b	Individual randomized controlled trials
	c	All or none studies
2	a	Systematic reviews of cohort studies
	b	Individual cohort studies
	c	Outcomes research, ecological studies
3	a	Systematic review of case control studies
	b	Individual case control studies
4		Case series
5		Expert opinion

Adapted from Oxford Centre for Evidence-Based Medicine Levels of Evidence Working Group. The Oxford 2011 levels of evidence. http://www.cebm.net/index.aspx?o=5653. Accessed August 5, 2012.

Table 2
NCCN categories guideline recommendations

Category	Level of Evidence	Level of Consensus
1	High	Uniform agreement
2A	Lower	Uniform agreement
2B	Lower	Minor disagreement
3	Any	Major disagreement

Adapted from Pfister DG, Ang KK, Brizel DM, et al. Head and neck cancers. J Natl Compr Canc Netw 2011;9(6):596–650.

disclosure of any conflicts of interest among panel members and transparency surrounding the development of CPGs.[3] Other investigators have suggested including unbiased methodologists in the expert panel, although their exact roles have yet to be defined.[9]

Another consideration when formulating CPGs is the target patient and physician populations; guidelines must take into account differences in the patient case mix and resources accessible by physicians, in addition to social and cultural factors.[10] Regional differences in CPGs for the same disease may reflect these variations.

Opponents of CPGs argue that they restrict physicians' autonomy in practicing medicine by dictating algorithms of care. In reality, CPGs are created to provide a framework and foundation on which individualized patient management can be constructed subject to several factors including the patient's performance status and personal desire. The NCCN explicitly states that physicians are "expected to use independent medical judgment in the context of individual clinical circumstances to determine a patient's care or treatment."[4]

Importance in Daily Practice

The recent emphasis on evidence-based medicine has resulted in a proliferation of clinical publications,[11] making it increasingly more difficult to keep up with the most current literature. Physicians are not only expected to read these studies but they are also expected to evaluate the strength of the evidence and the potential impact on clinical practice. In addition, the capability of otolaryngologists to understand and critique literature has yet to be determined.[12] CPGs serve the purpose of presenting physicians with practice recommendations based on the best available evidence and expert consensus; physicians can then individualize the care they deliver built on the framework offered by CPGs.

Role in Quality Assessment

The IOM has recommended developing a set of core quality measures to evaluate and monitor the quality of cancer care[1]; currently, quality metrics for the management of oral cavity and larynx cancers (but not oropharyngeal cancers) have been developed but are not yet validated. Since CPGs are built on the best available evidence, they can establish standards of care, designate quality indicators, and set priorities for quality improvement initiatives.[13]

Recently, Hessel and colleagues[14] established 4 main quality measures and 26 clinical end points based on institutional and NCCN guidelines, using these to evaluate the care delivered to patients with oral cavity cancers in a tertiary level of care department. The investigators reported an 88% or greater compliance with the 4 main quality metrics but more variable results for the clinical end points, thereby identifying areas of improvement.[14] Lewis and colleagues[15] used NCCN guidelines as a quality standard to evaluate the care received by patients with head and neck cancers referred to a tertiary care center with recurrent or persistent disease, finding that 43% of these patients had prereferral care that deviated from NCCN guidelines. In these instances, guidelines served to delineate specific metrics[14] and act as a quality standard[15]; being built on the best available evidence enables CPGs to have versatility in providing quality metrics.

Implications for Changing Policy

There has been recent emphasis on limiting the overuse of medical interventions with no proven benefit and the underuse of those with proven efficacy.[2] Because CPGs identify the most appropriate practices based on the best available evidence, they have a pivotal role in national quality initiatives and may potentially affect reimbursement policies.[12]

This role of CPGs has been demonstrated most clearly in the United Kingdom. In 1999, the National Institute for Health and Clinical Excellence (NICE) was established by the National Health Service (NHS) of England and Wales to develop CPGs, which are then published as general guidelines.[16] In addition, NICE makes recommendations to the NHS about reimbursement for medical interventions based on safety, clinical effectiveness, and cost, which are related to the CPGs they develop. This system is facilitated by the presence of universal health care; the United States, with its medley of private payers, has no such parallel agency.[17] The Centers for Medicare and Medicaid Services have begun pay-for-performance programs derived from evidence-based quality indicators and not from specific CPGs, although none currently apply to head and neck cancer care.

Pay-for-performance programs rely on specific performance indicators; there are no such standardized metrics for head and neck surgery, although this may soon change. Weber and colleagues[18] identified head and neck surgical performance measures based on those in the general surgery literature that include length of stay, perioperative wound infections, mortality, return to the operating room within 7 days of index surgery, and readmission within 30 days of discharge. An intradepartmental review of more than 2500 cases demonstrated that individual surgeon, patient comorbidities, and procedure acuity significantly affected the prevalence of negative performance indicators.[18] Although these metrics have yet to be standardized, such indicators may be tied to future performance incentives. Limited evidence, the flexibility inherent to CPGs, and identifying who would receive the incentive currently hinder the use of CPGs for this purpose, but may be overcome if incentives are prorated based on the priority of the measure and guideline goals are made more explicit.[19]

ESSENTIAL POINTS FOR THERAPEUTIC STANDARDS

Therapeutic standards in oncology are traditionally focused on obtaining the best clinical outcomes; namely, achieving the best survival with the fewest recurrences. For head and neck cancer, these standards must also account for functional outcomes related to swallowing, voice, and adequacy of the airway that are affected by both the patient's tumor and the sequelae of treatment.[20] Therefore, the goals of head and neck cancer management are to maximize locoregional control, survival, and functional outcomes. Because of the additional consideration of functional preservation, multidisciplinary treatment planning must also include such ancillary services as dentistry and prosthodontics, and speech language and pathology.

Current CPGs uphold these tenets to maximize clinical and functional outcomes. NCCN recommendations for oral cavity cancer management are primarily surgical with adjuvant therapy as indicated,[4] in part due to advances in reconstruction optimizing functional rehabilitation.[21] Laryngeal cancer was also largely treated with surgery and adjuvant radiation disease until the Veterans Affairs Laryngeal Cancer Study Group reported comparable survival outcomes with organ preservation in patients treated with induction chemotherapy and definitive radiation,[22] and RTOG 91–11 identified concurrent chemoradiation as providing the highest rates of organ preservation while maintaining oncologic outcomes.[23] Following these publications demonstrating the feasibility and efficacy of nonsurgical larynx preservation, there was increased interest in and use of chemoradiation for the treatment of advanced oropharyngeal cancer,[24,25] because open approaches for resecting large oropharyngeal cancers engender significant functional impairment. Recently, transoral approaches to the oropharynx have enabled comparable oncologic outcomes while minimizing functional morbidity; these include open approaches,[26] transoral laser microsurgery,[27] and transoral robotic surgery.[28,29]

Also impacting the management of oropharyngeal cancer is the increasing incidence of human papilloma (HPV)-associated cancers. Patients with this subset of oropharyngeal malignancies have significantly better overall and progression-free survival than their HPV-negative counterparts.[30] Consideration is currently being given to potential de-intensification of treatment of patients with HPV-positive oropharyngeal cancer; suggested strategies include surgery with adjuvant therapy dependent on histopathologic findings, the use of less toxic targeted agents, and lower radiation doses.[31] Clinical trials are needed to evaluate this properly; as should be standard for any head and neck cancer treatment, management should be based on the best available evidence and ad hoc treatment should be avoided.

MULTIDISCIPLINARY TREATMENT PLANNING

As early as 1937, Surgeon General Thomas Parran urged multidisciplinary cancer care.[32] Tumor boards have existed in the United States for at least 50 years, although their role has shifted significantly from an educational activity[33] to a working conference for multidisciplinary treatment planning. More recently, tumor boards have begun to represent quality assurance in cancer care.

The benefits of multidisciplinary treatment planning have yet to be fully realized. Majority of the existing literature extols the positive impact of multidisciplinary conferences, including improved coordination of care, survival, patient satisfaction, clinical trial recruitment, appropriate tumor staging, and even cost.[34] In the otolaryngology literature, only the impact of a tumor board on whether a diagnosis, tumor stage, or treatment plan was changed has been reported, with changes occurring 27% of the time.[35]

The impact of multidisciplinary treatment planning on NCCN guideline compliance has not yet been widely studied. Freeman and colleagues[36,37] reported that after instituting a thoracic malignancy conference, rates of patients undergoing a complete staging evaluation, multidisciplinary assessment before treatment initiation, and receiving treatment recommendations compliant with NCCN guidelines significantly increased for both esophageal and lung cancers. In addition, the time from diagnosis to treatment significantly decreased for both cohorts of patients.[36,37] Establishing a prostate multidisciplinary clinic was associated with a significant increase in NCCN guideline-adherent care for patients with prostate cancers, with a significant increase in the breadth of treatment options offered to patients.[38] However, a study reporting significantly more appropriate treatment received by patients with lung cancer presented at multidisciplinary team meetings noted no effect on overall survival[39]; further study is needed to determine the effect of improved guideline compliance on clinical outcomes. Possibly their most significant impact is serving as a forum for communication and coordination of care, critically important for the cancer patient.

There is evidence that not all multidisciplinary treatment planning conferences are created equal. Lamb and colleagues[40] performed a systematic review of studies evaluating the effectiveness of these conferences, reporting a failure to reach a treatment decision in up to 52% of cases, with recommended treatment not implemented in up to 16%. They concluded that team and social factors affect management decisions, and recommended that leadership and team skills training be included to help standardize the efficacy of these conferences.[40] Taylor and colleagues[41] evaluated the quality of multidisciplinary conferences by identifying specific metrics, such as the effectiveness of the meeting chair (whether or not discussions remained focused and an explicit treatment plan articulated for each patient) and clinical presentations (structured vs unprepared). Based on their criteria, they reported great variability in quality among multidisciplinary teams.[41]

Despite these differences among teams, obtaining multidisciplinary input in formulating treatment plans represents a quality improvement. A survey of multidisciplinary teams across tumor types found fairly consensual viewpoints regarding the positive effect of multidisciplinary planning on patient-centered clinical decision making.[42] Although further study is needed on the impact of multidisciplinary treatment planning on clinical outcomes and more work may be needed to standardize the effectiveness of tumor boards, implementation of these conferences has great potential for quality improvement in cancer care.

REGIONALIZATION OF CARE

Twenty-five years ago, Dr John Lore issued a plea that head and neck cancer surgeries be performed by qualified surgeons and not by "dabblers" lacking a high-volume case mix, ancillary resources, and continuing education in head and neck surgical oncology.[43] In 1999, the IOM advocated regionalization of cancer care by recommending that cancer patients undergoing procedures associated with high mortality rates should receive treatment at high-volume institutions.[1] Studies have shown that mortality rates from complex surgeries are lower when performed at high-volume centers[44,45] or by high-volume surgeons.[46] These relationships have not been widely explored for head and neck cancer. Kim and colleagues[47] used clinical registry data to report an increase in the number of neck dissections performed nationally and noted a trend toward regionalization.[48] Also using registry data, Gourin and colleagues[49] found a trend toward regionalization for oropharyngeal cancer surgery over a 20-year period; high-volume hospital care was associated with shorter hospital stays,[49] although survival was not examined.

Although examining outcomes of cancer surgeries in relation to hospital and surgeon volume is important, examining outcomes for a disease entity is perhaps more comprehensive. Chen and colleagues[50,51] reported significantly improved survival for patients with early-stage and advanced-stage laryngeal cancers when treated at high-volume facilities, independent of treatment modality. They also noted that most patients with advanced-stage laryngeal cancer were treated at high-volume centers, indicating that regionalization had occurred.[51]

In Weber's 2007 address as president of the American Head and Neck Society, he highlighted several strategies to improve the quality of head and neck cancer care, urging regionalization and discouraging "dabbling."[52] Studies have indicated that even without formal policy changes, regionalization of head and neck cancer care has been occurring; however, efforts to encourage and incentivize regionalization should be adopted to maximize the quality of care delivered to patients with head and neck cancers.

SUMMARY

In establishing criteria for improving the quality of cancer care, the IOM emphasized the development of CPGs, multidisciplinary treatment planning, and regionalization of care.[1] CPGs, developed by expert multidisciplinary panels and based on the best available evidence, provide a framework for physicians to optimize the cancer care they provide. CPGs may also establish quality standards and affect health policy. Multidisciplinary treatment planning and increasing regionalization of care improve the quality of head and neck cancer care, which should aim to maximize survival, provide locoregional control, and preserve function.

REFERENCES

1. Spinks T, Albright HW, Feeley TW, et al. Ensuring quality cancer care: a follow-up review of the Institute of Medicine's 10 recommendations for improving the quality of cancer care in America. Cancer 2012;118(10):2571–82.
2. Institute of Medicine. Crossing the quality chasm: a new health system for the 21st century. Washington, DC: National Academies Press; 2001.
3. Institute of Medicine. Clinical practice guidelines we can trust. Washington, DC: National Academies Press; 2011.
4. Pfister DG, Ang KK, Brizel DM, et al. Head and neck cancers. J Natl Compr Canc Netw 2011;9(6):596–650.
5. Scottish Intercollegiate Guidelines Network. Diagnosis and clinical management of head and neck cancer: a national clinical guideline. 2006. Available at: http://www.sign.ac.uk/pdf/sign90.pdf. Accessed July 30, 2012.
6. Machtay M, Rosenthal DI, Hershock D, et al. Organ preservation therapy using induction plus concurrent chemoradiation for advanced resectable oropharyngeal carcinoma: a University of Pennsylvania phase II trial. J Clin Oncol 2002; 20(19):3964–71.
7. Bonner JA, Harari PM, Giralt J, et al. Radiotherapy plus cetuximab for squamous-cell carcinoma of the head and neck. N Engl J Med 2006;354(6): 567–78.
8. Lorch JH, Goloubeva O, Haddad RI, et al. Induction chemotherapy with cisplatin and fluorouracil alone or in combination with docetaxel in locally advanced squamous-cell cancer of the head and neck: long-term results of the TAX 324 randomised phase 3 trial. Lancet Oncol 2011;12(2):153–9.
9. Akl EA, Karl R, Guyatt GH. Methodologists and context experts disagreed regarding managing conflicts of interest of clinical practice guidelines panels. J Clin Epidemiol 2012;65(7):734–9.
10. Haggard M. The relationship between evidence and guidelines. Otolaryngol Head Neck Surg 2007;137(Suppl 4):S72–7.
11. Wasserman JM, Wynn R, Bash TS, et al. Levels of evidence in otolaryngology journals. Otolaryngol Head Neck Surg 2006;134(5):717–23.
12. Shin JJ, Randolph GW, Rauch SD. Evidence-based medicine in otolaryngology, part 1: the multiple faces of evidence-based medicine. Otolaryngol Head Neck Surg 2010;142(5):637–46.

13. Browman GP, Brouwers M. The role of guidelines in quality improvement for cancer surgery. J Surg Oncol 2009;99(8):467–9.
14. Hessel AC, Moreno MA, Hanna EY, et al. Compliance with quality assurance measures in patients treated for early oral tongue cancer. Cancer 2010; 116(14):3408–16.
15. Lewis CM, Hessel AC, Roberts DB, et al. Prereferral head and neck cancer treatment: compliance with National Comprehensive Cancer Network treatment guidelines. Arch Otolaryngol Head Neck Surg 2010;136(12):1205–11.
16. Dent TH, Sadler M. From guidance to practice: why NICE is not enough. BMJ 2002;324(7341):842–5.
17. Clancy CM, Cronin K. Evidence-based decision making: global evidence, local decisions. Health Aff 2005;24(1):151–62.
18. Weber RS, Lewis CM, Eastman SD, et al. Quality and performance indicators in an academic department of head and neck surgery. Arch Otolaryngol Head Neck Surg 2010;136(12):1212–8.
19. Garber AM. Evidence-based guidelines as a foundation for performance incentives. Health Aff 2005;24(1):174–9.
20. Hutcheson KA, Lewin JS. Functional outcomes after chemoradiotherapy of laryngeal and pharyngeal cancers. Curr Oncol Rep 2012;14(2):158–65.
21. Genden EM, Ferlito A, Silver CE, et al. Contemporary management of cancer of the oral cavity. Eur Arch Otorhinolaryngol 2010;267(7):1001–17.
22. Induction chemotherapy plus radiation compared with surgery plus radiation in patients with advanced laryngeal cancer. The Department of Veterans Affairs Laryngeal Cancer Study Group. N Engl J Med 1991;324(24):1685–90.
23. Forastiere AA, Goepfert H, Maor M, et al. Concurrent chemotherapy and radiotherapy for organ preservation in advanced laryngeal cancer. N Engl J Med 2003;349(22):2091–8.
24. Zhen W, Karnell LH, Hoffman HT, et al. The National Cancer Data Base report on squamous cell carcinoma of the base of tongue. Head Neck 2004;26(8):660–74.
25. Chen AY, Schrag N, Hao Y, et al. Changes in treatment of advanced oropharyngeal cancer, 1985-2001. Laryngoscope 2007;117(1):16–21.
26. Holsinger FC, McWhorter AJ, Menard M, et al. Transoral lateral oropharyngectomy for squamous cell carcinoma of the tonsillar region: I. Technique, complications, and functional results. Arch Otolaryngol Head Neck Surg 2005;131(7): 583–91.
27. Pradier O, Christiansen H, Schmidberger H, et al. Adjuvant radiotherapy after transoral laser microsurgery for advanced squamous carcinoma of the head and neck. Int J Radiat Oncol Biol Phys 2005;63(5):1368–77.
28. Leonhardt FD, Quon H, Abrahao M, et al. Transoral robotic surgery for oropharyngeal carcinoma and its impact on patient-reported quality of life and function. Head Neck 2012;34(2):146–54.
29. de Almeida JR, Genden EM. Robotic surgery for oropharynx cancer: promise, challenges, and future directions. Curr Oncol Rep 2012;14(2):148–57.
30. Ang KK, Harris J, Wheeler R, et al. Human papillomavirus and survival of patients with oropharyngeal cancer. N Engl J Med 2010;363(1):24–35.
31. Sturgis EM, Ang KK. The epidemic of HPV-associated oropharyngeal cancer is here: is it time to change our treatment paradigms? J Natl Compr Canc Netw 2011;9(6):665–73.
32. Clark RL, Williams AC. Regionalization: a program for mobilization of cancer teams. Bull Am Coll Surg 1963;48:29–30.
33. Berman HL. The tumor board: is it worth saving? Mil Med 1975;140(8):529–31.

34. Patkar V, Acosta D, Davidson T, et al. Cancer multidisciplinary team meetings: evidence, challenges, and the role of clinical decision support technology. Int J Breast Cancer 2011;2011:831605.
35. Wheless SA, McKinney KA, Zanation AM. A prospective study of the clinical impact of a multidisciplinary head and neck tumor board. Otolaryngol Head Neck Surg 2010;143(5):650–4.
36. Freeman RK, Van Woerkom JM, Vyverberg A, et al. The effect of a multidisciplinary thoracic malignancy conference on the treatment of patients with esophageal cancer. Ann Thorac Surg 2011;92(4):1239–42 [discussion: 1243].
37. Freeman RK, Van Woerkom JM, Vyverberg A, et al. The effect of a multidisciplinary thoracic malignancy conference on the treatment of patients with lung cancer. Eur J Cardiothorac Surg 2010;38(1):1–5.
38. Korman H, Lanni T Jr, Shah C, et al. Impact of a prostate multidisciplinary clinic program on patient treatment decisions and on adherence to NCCN guidelines: the William Beaumont Hospital experience. Am J Clin Oncol 2013;36(2):121–5.
39. Boxer MM, Vinod SK, Shafiq J, et al. Do multidisciplinary team meetings make a difference in the management of lung cancer? Cancer 2011;117(22):5112–20.
40. Lamb BW, Brown KF, Nagpal K, et al. Quality of care management decisions by multidisciplinary cancer teams: a systematic review. Ann Surg Oncol 2011; 18(8):2116–25.
41. Taylor C, Atkins L, Richardson A, et al. Measuring the quality of MDT working: an observational approach. BMC Cancer 2012;12(1):202.
42. Lamb BW, Sevdalis N, Taylor C, et al. Multidisciplinary team working across different tumour types: analysis of a national survey. Ann Oncol 2012;23(5): 1293–300.
43. Lore JM Jr. Dabbling in head and neck oncology (a plea for added qualifications). Arch Otolaryngol Head Neck Surg 1987;113(11):1165–8.
44. Begg CB, Cramer LD, Hoskins WJ, et al. Impact of hospital volume on operative mortality for major cancer surgery. JAMA 1998;280(20):1747–51.
45. Birkmeyer JD, Siewers AE, Finlayson EV, et al. Hospital volume and surgical mortality in the United States. N Engl J Med 2002;346(15):1128–37.
46. Birkmeyer JD, Stukel TA, Siewers AE, et al. Surgeon volume and operative mortality in the United States. N Engl J Med 2003;349(22):2117–27.
47. Kim EY, Eisele DW, Goldberg AN, et al. Neck dissections in the United States from 2000 to 2006: volume, indications, and regionalization. Head Neck 2011; 33(6):768–73.
48. Gourin CG, Frick KD. National trends in oropharyngeal cancer surgery and the effect of surgeon and hospital volume on short-term outcomes and cost of care. Laryngoscope 2012;122(3):543–51.
49. Gourin CG, Forastiere AA, Sanguineti G, et al. Volume-based trends in surgical care of patients with oropharyngeal cancer. Laryngoscope 2011;121(4):738–45.
50. Chen AY, Pavluck A, Halpern M, et al. Impact of treating facilities' volume on survival for early-stage laryngeal cancer. Head Neck 2009;31(9):1137–43.
51. Chen AY, Fedewa S, Pavluck A, et al. Improved survival is associated with treatment at high-volume teaching facilities for patients with advanced stage laryngeal cancer. Cancer 2010;116(20):4744–52.
52. Weber RS. Improving the quality of head and neck cancer care. Arch Otolaryngol Head Neck Surg 2007;133(12):1188–92.

Survivorship—Competing Mortalities, Morbidities, and Second Malignancies

Pablo H. Montero-Miranda, MD, Ian Ganly, MD, PhD*

KEYWORDS

• Head and neck cancer • Competing mortalities • Survival analysis • Comorbidities

KEY POINTS

- The mortality from head and neck squamous cell cancer has declined over the past 30 years.
- There are many competing risk factors that contribute to death in cancer patients.
- Competing risk factors include the effects of age, gender, race, comorbidities, diet, quality of life (QOL), human papillomavirus (HPV) infection, and second primaries.
- The presence of these competing risk factors affect the survival outcome of patients with head and neck cancer.
- Traditional survival analysis using Kaplan-Meier statistics may not be appropriate in patients with multiple competing risk factors and may overestimate disease-specific survival (DSS) figures.
- Statistical models, which include competing risk factors in the survival analysis model, need to be developed.
- These statistical models should be incorporated into the design and analysis of future randomized controlled trials (RCTs) in head and neck cancer management.

Mortality of head and neck cancer has declined in the United States over the past 20 years.[1,2] This improvement has been linked to the use of multimodality treatment of advanced disease. Despite this improvement, DSS remains low.[3–6]

Patients who survive head and neck cancer are exposed to morbidity and mortality secondary to the same factors as the general population. It is also clear, however, that factors related to their cancer and cancer treatment predispose them to increased risk of mortality.[7]

Disclosure Statement: Dr Montero and Dr Ganly have no conflicts of interest.
Head and Neck Service, Department of Surgery, Memorial Sloan Kettering Cancer Center, New York, NY, USA
* Corresponding author. Head and Neck Service, Memorial Sloan Kettering Cancer Center, 1275 York Avenue, New York, NY 10021.
E-mail address: ganlyi@mskcc.org

Otolaryngol Clin N Am 46 (2013) 681–710
http://dx.doi.org/10.1016/j.otc.2013.04.008 oto.theclinics.com
0030-6665/13/$ – see front matter

Improvements in head and neck cancer treatment, even among patients with advanced disease, have led to a scenario where an increasing proportion of patients die from causes other than the primary cancer. These other causes of death are called competing mortalities. The quantification of overall mortality (OM) may not be an adequate representation of the benefits of treatment. Instead, it may merely be a reflection of the baseline host factors (age, gender, comorbidity status, and so forth) of the patients receiving active treatment and/or the result of the emergence of treatment-related factors and new malignancies.

During the past 20 years, there have been important advances not only in head and neck cancer treatment but also in the way that survival and the factors that affect it are understood, especially the competing causes of death. Examples of such competing risks for mortality are listed in **Box 1**. The most important competing risks are death due to patient comorbidities, treatment-related complications, and death secondary to second malignancies. These conditions have been analyzed before in other types of cancers[8–10] and are receiving greater attention in head and neck cancer.

The existence of competing mortalities may preclude the observation of the event of interest, generating negative results instead of improvements in survival.[11] Competing mortalities are especially important in the context where survival is prolonged due to the use of better treatments; if they are present, getting positive will be more unlikely, generating bias toward the null hypothesis.[12] This review analyzes these factors, how they affect survival, and how they can be integrated into survival analysis.

TRADITIONAL COMPETING MORTALITIES IN HEAD AND NECK CANCER

Effect of Age

Long life expectancy has resulted in more elderly patients with cancer.[13] It has been reported that by 2030, 70% of all cancers will be diagnosed in older adults. This will result in a major public health problem in the future.[14] Elderly patients are likely to have serious comorbidities that can affect treatment decisions. Not all elderly patients will have serious coexistent disease, however, and some elders are healthy people. Unfortunately, older patients are often undertreated because of their age and not because of the presence of chronic diseases.[15] This has been reported before and seems especially true in head and neck cancer patients.[16–18]

In head and neck cancer patients, increasing age has been associated with poor survival.[19,20] When severe comorbidities are not present, however, age is not

Box 1
Competing mortality factors

Age

Gender

Race

Marital (partner) status

Comorbidities

Behavior lifestyles

BMI

QOL

Second primaries

HPV infection

necessarily an independent predictor of poor survival.[21] In a matched-pair analysis, Pytynia and colleagues[22] have shown there was no difference in OS, DSS, or recurrence-free survival (RFS) rates between patients younger than 40 years and older than 40 years when adjusted by comorbidity status.

Age does not necessarily mean poor outcome.[23] There is no evidence that advanced age alone is a contraindication for radical surgery. There are reports that surgery can be safely performed in older head and neck cancer patients.[24,25] This is also true for advanced reconstructive surgery; there is no evidence that there is a significant increased incidence of flap lost or mortality in the elderly.[26] Multiple reports have shown that radiotherapy alone is effective and well tolerated among older patients in good health condition.[27–31] In patients treated with chemoradiotherapy, however, age has been associated with reduced chemotherapy compliance.[32] Unfortunately, an increased incidence of noncancer death has been reported in older patients submitted to chemoradiation regimes, probably secondary to acute and late toxicities.[23] Adequate evaluation, effective management of toxicities, and tailored treatment regimes should help reduce this problem.[27]

In a population-based analysis of RCTs undertaken by Mell and colleagues,[33] competing mortality risk was significantly associated with increasing age and increasing comorbidity in a multivariable model. Older patients with comorbidities were more likely to die of noncancer causes. The investigators suggested that these patients should receive a tailored treatment based on their high risk and that they should be excluded from high-risk therapies evaluated in RCT.[33]

Older patients are at risk of receiving substandard treatment based on a doctor's bias related to age.[34] In addition, families or patients themselves may refuse standard treatment just because of age. This decision is usually based on QOL concerns. There is prospective evidence, however, that QOL in patients treated for head and neck cancer does not differ significantly 1 year after treatment between patients older than 70 and patients younger than 60.[35]

The effect of age on overall survival (OS) is probably clouded because of the presence of comorbidities. Although it has been reported that older patients have a lower OS, this could be a consequence of comorbidities or substandard treatment.[17] Bhattacharyya,[36] in a analysis of 2508 patients with larynx, tongue, and tonsil cancer extracted from the Surveillance Epidemiology and End Results (SEER) database, have shown that when survival was adjusted by cancer-related factors and standard treatment, no significant difference was found between patients older and younger than 70. Substandard treatment is a significant poor prognostic factor in older patients.[18] Therefore, head and neck cancer treatment in elderly patients should be based on comprehensive assessment of preexistent medical conditions and patient choice, not just on chronologic age.[18,21,37] How elderly patients can be appropriately included in RCT to test new therapies, avoiding the bias related to age, is a question to be resolved.

Effect of Gender, Partner Status, and Sociocultural Factors

Female gender has been identified as a competing risk of mortality in a recent analysis of predictors of OS.[33,38] Information about the effect of gender on survival and prognosis is contradictory. Previous reports by the RTOG in head and neck cancer suggested a worse survival in men, especially if they were single.[39] Some population-based studies have also suggested a poorer survival time in men.[40,41] A more recent analysis by the RTOG on the impact of partner status reported that the presence of a partner improves outcomes: partnered women and men have a better OS than unpartnered women and men.[42] The same analysis showed the protective effect of female gender, partnered and unpartnered, on survival and locoregional control.

Differences in prognosis between genders have also been linked to the presence of HPV. HPV infection seems to be more frequent among men than women (10.1% vs 3.6%).[43] Saba and colleagues,[44] in a SEER database analysis from 1977 to 2006, reported a higher incidence of oropharyngeal cancer among men, likely related to the higher incidence of HPV infection among them. They failed to find a difference in survival between men and women in the whole period.[44] In a similar SEER analysis, however, Brown and colleagues[45] compared survival differences between gender and race between 1977–1991 and 1992–2006. In this analysis, they found better survival rates among white women compared with white and black men in the first period but an improved survival among white men over the other groups in the second period.

In other head and neck cancer sites outside of the oropharynx, the effect of gender on survival is more difficult to assess. A recent matched-pair analysis of patients, with tumors from different localizations in the head and neck, treated in a single institution with the same multidisciplinary approach failed to show any difference in OS, RFS, and DSS after stratification by gender and adjusted by other variables.[46]

The poor prognosis in single men in some of the previous reports cited could have different explanations. This could be due to a lack of partner and family support, emotional problems, or lack of medical insurance, which are more common among single men.[42] Also, gender and marital status have been related to other protective factors, such as high educational level and high socioeconomic status (SES). Lower educational level and lower SES have been shown to be important detrimental prognostic factors in head and neck oncology.[47–49] Chen and colleagues[50] have reported less mortality for patients with oral cavity and pharyngeal cancer among patients with at least 12 years of education. Similar results have been found in groups of patients treated in RTOG protocols, with significantly better OS and locoregional control in patients with college or technical education.[51] Poor overall health and lack of support systems probably explains most of the differences in survival among these groups.

Gender differences on survival could be related to social-cultural rather than biologic factors. Theses aspects and the emergent influence of gender differences in HPV infection need further investigation and could be important objectives of public health policies.

Effect of Race

The incidence of head and neck cancer in the African American population is greater than that in the white population in the United States. In addition, outcomes are also poorer in African American patients with head and neck cancer.[41,52,53] These differences are independent of comorbidities, clinical characteristics, and treatment modality.[41] It has been suggested that outcome differences between patients of different races are related to social factors rather than biologic differences.[54] These social factors include SES, educational level, lower income, lack of health insurance, and late diagnosis.[55,56]

It has also been suggested that there are differences in the distribution of sites affected and the stage at diagnosis between different races.[57] For example, in oral cavity cancer, it has been reported that black patients are more likely to present with advanced disease, even when socioeconomic and insurance status are adjusted for.[58] Larynx cancer is more frequent among black patients than white, although it is not necessarily diagnosed at a more-advanced stage. Advanced oropharyngeal cancer also occurs more frequently in black patients than white patients.[59] These differences have been linked to preference in tobacco use among black people, with more use of mentholated cigarettes. In addition, African Americans are less likely to stop smoking than whites.[60,61]

Although the incidence and stage are higher in black patients, this does not necessarily mean that black patients have poorer outcome. Arbes and colleagues[47] and Ragin and colleagues[58] analyzed 2 series of oral cancer patients and failed to show a decrease in OS among African American patients compared with white patients when other demographic characteristics were adjusted for. Chen and colleagues,[59] in a matched-pair analysis, showed no significant differences between cases and controls in RFS, DSS, or OS among black patients and white patients. Bach and colleagues,[62] in a multisite meta-analysis, were not able to find a difference in survival among races in head and neck cancer. In contrast, however, some investigators have noticed differences in DSS, with poor DSS in black patients.[58,63,64] In general, it is thought that the differences in survival among races are due to demographic factors rather than biologic factors.[54]

An exception to this concept may be in HPV-related head and neck cancer. Settle and colleagues,[65] in a retrospective and prospective analysis of head and neck cancer patients treated in a single institution, showed that the decrease in OS among African American patients was explained mainly by a worse OS of oropharynx cancer patients. HPV-positive white patients were 9-fold more frequent than HPV-positive black patients in that analysis. Other recent analyses have shown poorer survival rates for African American patients compared with white patients in tonsil and base of tongue cancers. HPV would have a major role in this survival difference.[44,45] These findings raise the question about the importance of some racial factors in HPV infection and how this could affect prognosis, especially in oropharynx carcinoma. Further analyses of biologic factors that could explain these differences are needed.

Effect of Comorbidities and Lifestyle Behavior

Comorbidities become more common with increasing age and reduce life expectancy.[66] The prevalence of comorbidities among head and neck cancer patients is high (**Table 1**). The most frequent are cardiovascular (30%–40%) and respiratory (10%–13%) and are almost 2-fold more frequent than in the general population.[67,68] The proportion of head and neck cancer patients with moderate to severe comorbidities has been reported to be approximately 21% and is just exceeded by the incidence among lung cancer and colorectal cancer patients, 40% and 25%, respectively.[69]

Comorbidities affect treatment decision making and prognosis.[70–72] For patients with head and neck cancer, the prognostic effect of comorbidities have been widely studied and demonstrated.

Comorbidity assessment

There are different instruments to assess the comorbidity status of cancer patients. Most of these instruments are adapted from other chronic conditions and some of them have been specifically designed for head and neck cancer patients (**Table 2**).[72–76] The most commonly used are the Kaplan-Feinstein, adult comorbidity evaluation (ACE) 27, Charlson index, and Washington University Head and Neck Comorbidity Index (WUHNCI). These instruments capture comorbidity information in a retrospective or prospective way. This information can be used for survival prediction, QOL evaluation, or functional outcome.[77]

Effect of comorbidities on the prognosis of head and neck cancer patients

Patients with severe comorbidities and older age are less likely to undergo aggressive treatments (discussed previously).[21,70] Patients with comorbidities are more likely to

Table 1
Prevalence of comorbidity in patients with head and neck cancer

Author	Country	Patients (N)	Site	Index Used	Comorbidity Prevalence (%)	Prevalence of Moderate/Severe Comorbidity (%)
Singh et al,[97] 1998	US	70	Head and neck (<45 yo)	ACE 27	—	30
de Cassia Braga Ribeiro et al,[175] 2003	Brazil	110	Oral cavity	CI	53.6	8.2
Paleri et al,[176] 2003	UK	182	Larynx	ACE 27	64.5	55.1
Ribeiro et al,[177] 2000	US	530	Oral cavity, oropharynx	CI	39.1	—
Piccirillo et al,[72] 2004	US	1086	ACE 27	ACE 27	53.9	24.1
Borggreven et al,[178] 2005	Netherlands	100	Head and neck	ACE 27	83	57
Alho et al,[179] 2007	Finland	221	Head and neck	CI	48.4	48.4
Castro et al,[180] 2007	Brazil	90	Larynx	ACE 27	88.9	16.7
				CI	65.6	18.9
Sanabria et al,[181] 2007	Brazil	310	Head and neck (>70 yo)	ACE 27	75	29.4
Datema et al,[79] 2010	Netherlands	1282	Head and neck	ACE 27	36.4	19

Abbreviations: ACE 27, adult comorbidity evaluation 27; CI, charlson index.

From Paleri V, Wight RG, Silver CE, et al. Comorbidity in head and neck cancer: a critical appraisal and recommendations for practice. Oral Oncol 2010;46(10):712–9; with permission.

Table 2
Characteristics of the most frequently used comorbidities indexes in head and neck cancer

Index Name	Year	Developed For	Number of System Evaluated	Number of Comorbidity Ailment	Severity Scale of	Also Includes
Kaplan-Feinstein index[66]	1974	General medical (diabetes mellitus)	6	12	Grade 0 to 3	Malignancies Alcoholism Psychocomotor impairment
Charlson index[73]	1986	Breast cancer	9	19	Severity weighted by 1–6 score. Grade from 0 to 3 according to the sum of weights.	Malignancies AIDS
ACE 27[69]	2000	Head and neck cancer	8	27	Grades 1 to 3. Score is defined according to the highest ranked single ailment	Alcohol abuse Illicit drugs Body weight
Washington University Head and Neck Comorbidity Index[74]	2003	Head and neck cancer	4	7	Severity weighted by 1–4 scale. Score from 0 to 15 according to the sum of weights	Malignancies

receive palliative therapy rather than curative treatment.[67,71] It has been recommended that older patients without comorbidities be treated the same as younger patients but with close geriatric observation and more-supportive treatment.[70]

The effect of comorbidities on the prognosis of head and neck cancer patients has been widely reported as an independent predictor on outcome (**Table 3**). This risk of death, estimated by Piccirillo and colleagues[67,72] for patients with moderate to severe comorbidities, was 2 to 3 times more compared with patients without comorbidities, adjusting for other patient and tumor characteristics. Reid and colleagues,[78] in a large series of patients from the SEER and Medicare databases, reported an increased relative hazard for patients with Charlson index scores 1 and 2 or more, of 1.3 and 1.8, respectively. This seems extremely important in short-term mortality (less than 6 month). In a review by Datema and colleagues[79] of the Netherlands cancer registries, 5.8% of patients treated died in the first 6 months, and this mortality rate was mainly explained by chronic comorbidities. In 2 analyses of patients with larynx cancer, it has been reported that the 5-year OS for patients with comorbidities was 15% compared with the 5-year OS of 54% to 74% for patients without comorbidities.[80,81] In oral cavity cancer, similar reports have shown a 10% 5-year survival among patients with severe comorbidities versus 49% in patients without comorbidities.[82] In oropharynx cancer, the same phenomena has been observed, with prognosis reported as 18% versus 40% for patients with and without comorbidities, respectively.[83]

Alcohol and tobacco use effect on head and neck cancer

The burden of disease in head and neck cancer patients is highly determined by lifestyles; approximately 25% of head and neck cancer patients could be classified as alcoholic (using the Michigan Alcoholism Screening Test protocol) and more than 80% of patients as ever-smokers.[84–86] The effect of tobacco and alcohol use on OS in these patients has been previously reported.[87,88] Hall and colleagues[89] estimated 18% of deaths were not related to cancer but were related to other diseases associated with tobacco use after a matched-pair analysis with healthy controls. Duffy has shown that smoking status was the strongest predictor of poor OS, with a hazard ratio of 2 for former smokers and 2.4 for current smokers.[88] Among alcohol users, after controlling for smoking, there is an increased risk of death that has been estimated as 2-fold for patients with alcoholism and 2.76-fold for patients with systemic alcohol-related disease compared with nonalcohol users.[84] Patients with severe alcoholism are at high risk of dying from cardiovascular disease, pulmonary disease, and other alcohol-related conditions.[84]

The effect of alcohol and smoking is also associated with local and regional control of head and neck cancer. In an analysis by Fortin and colleagues,[86] the local control rate among a series of head and neck cancer patients treated with radiotherapy was

Table 3
Increased risk of mortality with higher comorbidity burden

Authors	Patients Number	Index Used	HR (95% CI) for Overall Survival
Reid et al,[78] 2001	9386	CI	Score 1: 1.33 (1.21–1.47) Score ≥2: 1.83 (1.64–2.05)
Piccirillo et al,[72] 2004	1086	ACE 27	Moderate: 1.92 (1.50–2.48) Severe: 2.48 (1.77–3.47)
Datema et al,[79] 2010	1282	ACE 27	Moderate 1.38 Severe 2.23

Modified from Paleri V, Wight RG, Silver CE, et al. Comorbidity in head and neck cancer: a critical appraisal and recommendations for practice. Oral Oncol 2010;46(10):712–9; with permission.

significantly better for never-smokers than for active smokers (5-year local control 75% vs 67%) and for never-drinkers than active drinkers. There was no significant effect for tobacco and alcohol with regional and distant failure. Regardless of the effect on locoregional control, the information available about the effect of tobacco or alcohol use on DSS is less clear and contradictory and is mainly based on small studies.[90–93]

Complications with comorbidities

Patients with severe comorbidities also have a higher incidence of complications and mortality secondary to cancer treatment.[94,95] The most frequent complications are cardiovascular (12%) and respiratory (11%).[96] Complications tend to be more severe in patients with high-risk diseases, even among younger patients.[97]

After treatment of head and neck cancer, the incidence of new comorbidities remains high for the first 6 to 12 months. After this time, the incidence of cardiovascular disease and diabetes returns to overall population rates but not for chronic respiratory disease, anemia, or depression.[68] This is probably a multifactorial phenomenon influenced by the short-term and long-term effects of treatment and the burden of alcohol and tobacco use in most of these patients. On a separate issue, the risk of other malignant diseases remains elevated among these patients after 12 months of treatment, especially in the groups of patients treated with chemotherapy (discussed later).

Effect of Body Mass Index and Diet

A low body mass index (BMI) has been associated with increased risk of head and neck cancer, especially among drinkers and smokers.[98] Rather than being an independent risk factor, however, low BMI is more likely a marker of poor chronic nutritional status secondary to tobacco and alcohol use.[99,100] Malnutrition and weight loss have been associated with poor prognosis in head and neck cancer, but this seems a consequence of tobacco/alcohol use or an effect of cancer and cancer-treatment rather than an independent predictor.[88,101,102] A better BMI could potentially improve treatment results from oncologic as well as QOL perspectives. For example, patients with BMI greater than 25 who undergo chemoradiation therapy are shown to have better swallowing function.[103]

Two large population studies have found different results. Mell and colleagues[33] reported that lower BMI is an independent risk factor of treatment-related mortality in a competing risk analysis. A similar finding appeared when recurrence and second malignancies were analyzed, showing a high incidence of lower BMI among patients with cancer-related events. Gaudet and colleagues,[104] in a large prospective analysis, reported that smoking patients with BMI greater than 24.9 have a 28% higher risk of dying of head and neck cancer than smoking patients with BMI greater than 25. This result was not observed, however, among nonsmokers.

Despite these observations, when OS has been measured, low BMI has not been independently associated with poor survival in the few cases studies that have addressed this question.[105]

Other pretreatment healthy behaviors have been reported to influence survival. High intakes of poultry, vegetables, and vitamin C were observed to improve survival in head and neck cancer patients.[92] These protective effects were not observed among patients with high intake of animal proteins or high fat intake.[92] A prospective analysis carried out by Sandoval and colleagues[106] suggested that high intake of vegetables before and after diagnosis of oral cancer may reduce the risk of recurrence, overall mortality, and cancer mortality in oral cancer patients. The number of patients is small, however, and failed to show significance in a multivariate analysis. In a recent analysis by Duffy and colleagues,[88] fruit and vegetable intake failed to predict survival in head and neck cancer patients after adjustment for tobacco and alcohol use or tumor characteristics.

The effect of dietary factors has also been analyzed with respect to the incidence of new primaries of the upper aerodigestive tract. It has been suggested that some dietary factors (like low citrus fruit intake) could contribute with alcohol and smoking to increase the risk of second primary cancers among patients with head and neck cancers.[107,108]

Effect of Quality of Life

Health-related QOL has been increasingly measured in head and neck cancer patients in the context of prospective trials. The scales used to measure QOL give important information about the impact of disease and treatment on patients. It also allows analyzing any association between QOL and survival outcomes.[109] In a recent review of the literature, published between 1982 and 2008, Montazeri[110] reported that 4 of the 8 studies analyzing the association between QOL and survival of head and neck cancer patients failed to demonstrate any survival effect. It has been proposed that there is not a strong relationship between QOL and survival. Some specific factors, however, could be influencing long-term survival, such as poor satisfaction, eating/speech problems, and presence of pain 1 year after treatment.[111,112] These factors could potentially help detect patients at high risk of poor survival.[112]

Effect of Second Primary Malignancies

Head and neck cancer patients have a high risk of morbidity and mortality because of second primary malignancies. This is a problem for patients with early stage head and neck cancer because these patients often survive for a long time. Second primaries are also important for survivors of aggressive multimodality therapy for advanced disease. Second primary tumors of the upper aerodigestive tract are common among head and neck patients due to the chronic DNA damage within the squamous epithelium from carcinogenic exposure.[113] The carcinogenic effect of tobacco and alcohol is multistep and synergistic. It also predisposes patients to multiple precancerous and cancerous lesions in the aerodigestive tract, upper esophagus, and lungs. Consequently, some types of secondary tumors are more frequent than in the general population and are a source of mortality that competes with the primary index tumor. Second primary tumors are the most important cause of death among head and neck cancer survivors.[114,115]

The actuarial rate of second primary tumors of the aerodigestive tract has been reported to be between 9% and 14%.[116,117] Leon and colleagues[118] established that the annual incidence of second cancers among head and neck cancer patients is 3.8%. This increases to 5.1% in patients with a third tumor and to 7.8% in patients with a fourth tumor. The head and neck is the most common site of second malignancies (30%–50%), followed by the lung (34%). Most of these cancers are squamous cell carcinomas (86%).[117,118] Haughey and colleagues,[116] in a meta-analysis of second cancers, described a prevalence of 14.2% in 40,287 patients with head and neck cancer. Most of the second cancers are metachronous, as was described by Liao et al. The site with highest prevalence of second cancers is the oral cavity, and approximately 50% of aerodigestive tract second primaries were detected by 2 years from index tumor presentation.[116] They are not uncommon, however, even after 5 years. For this reason, lifetime follow-up is recommended, with close endoscopic surveillance recommended during the first 2 years after the index tumor.

Previous reports have shown that second malignancies are generally detected earlier or at least in a less-advanced stage than the index cancer, probably due to more-intense surveillance.[119,120] Despite this, patients with second malignancies have a lesser survival than patients with primary malignancies.[119,120]

Survival with second primaries or successive tumors

Second primaries or successive tumors have been reported to adversely affect the survival of head and neck cancer patients.[116,117,119] Leon and colleagues[118] described a 10% decrease in 5-year OS with each new second malignancy, regardless if they were treated or not. The effect on survival of the second primary is influenced by the location of the new tumor.[121,122] Second primary cancers arising in the esophagus and lungs are significantly associated with a poorer prognosis than second primary tumors arising in the head and neck region.[122,123] It has been hypothesized that this poor prognosis could be secondary to the effect of previous treatment (eg, radiotherapy) or more-aggressive biologic behavior.[120]

Jones[117] described some factors that were more common among patients with second primary tumors:

- Younger age (second primary tumors more likely in men younger than 60 years)
- Laryngeal and oral cavity index tumor sites
- Small primary tumors
- Absence of neck metastases at the time of index tumor diagnosis

Lin and colleagues[124] reported that tobacco and alcohol use was associated with a 5-fold and 2-fold increased risk of second primary tumors, respectively. Radiotherapy to the index tumor was not associated with an increased risk of developing a second tumor. Patients with a second primary can be treated successfully with surgery or nonsurgical treatment. Patients treated aggressively have a better survival than patients without treatment.[119] The proportion of patients who are considered candidates for radical surgery decreases, however, with successive primaries.[118]

The effect of previous radiotherapy on survival after a new primary is unclear. Dolan and colleagues,[125] in a series of 358 patients with second primaries, reported that metachronous cancers are significantly associated with poor survival when the cancer arises within previously irradiated tissue. Other investigators have reported, however, no significant differences for previously irradiated patients.[117,126]

Site of second primary tumors

The increasing risk of second primaries is not restricted to the aerodigestive tract. Morris and colleagues,[115] in a recent analysis of the SEER database, described an incidence of 22.6% of second primary malignancies if all other sites are included (colorectal, bladder, kidney, skin, and cervix). They estimated the incidence of observed to expect ratio of second primary cancer is 2.2 compared with the general population. Most of the excess is explained by second primaries arising in the upper aerodigestive tract, followed by colorectal cancer and bladder, both of which are linked to tobacco use (**Fig. 1**). The risk of other common cancers, such as breast and prostate cancer, was not elevated over the general population.

Morris and colleagues[127] have demonstrated the risk of second primary malignancies differs significantly by the subsite of index head and neck cancer. The higher observed-to-expected second-cancer ratio was for hypopharynx (3.5×), followed by oropharynx (3.0×), oral cavity (2.8×) and larynx (1.9×). Hypopharynx and larynx are most commonly associated with second primaries in the lung. Oropharynx and oral cavity are most commonly associated with second primaries in the head and neck.

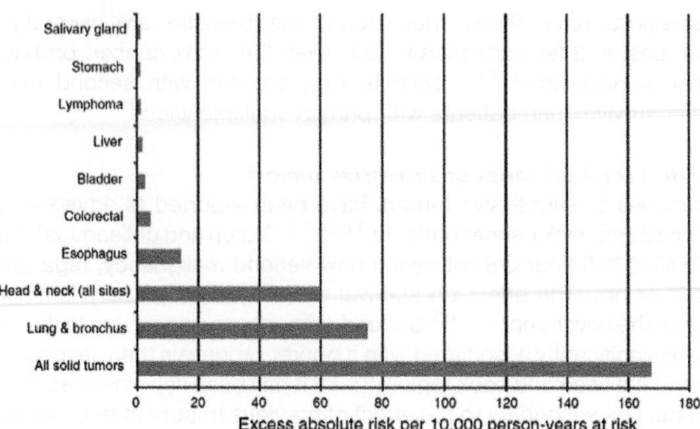

Fig. 1. Sites of second primaries (sites of SPM at meaningfully elevated risk after an index HNSCC, ranked by excess absolute risk per 10,000 person-years at risk). (*From* Morris LG, Sikora AG, Hayes RB, et al. Anatomic sites at elevated risk of second primary cancer after an index head and neck cancer. Cancer Causes Control 2011;22(5):671–9; with permission.)

Morris and colleagues[127] described a significant decrease in the incidence of second primaries among patients with oropharyngeal cancer in the past 10 years. This phenomenon could be linked to the etiologic shift in oropharyngeal carcinoma from a tobacco and alcohol–related cancer to an HPV-related carcinoma.[128] Further analyses are needed, but there are some reports suggesting a decreased risk of second primaries among HPV-positive oropharyngeal carcinoma.[129,130] An increasing incidence of anogenital cancer after an oral cavity/pharyngeal cancer, and vice versa, has been reported linking sexual behavior in the development of this disease.[131]

Mortality risk factors with second primaries

In an analysis of how second primaries act as competing risk factors for mortality, Rose and colleagues[38] identified increasing age, African American race, unmarried status, higher SES, advantage stage, nonsurgical treatment, and hypopharyngeal/oral cavity sites as independent risk factors of death among patients with second primaries.

The lack of effective preventative measures of second primary malignancies in survivors of head and neck cancer emphasizes the importance of tobacco and alcohol cessation among these patients and also the increasing importance of safe sexual behavior practice.

EFFECT OF HPV INFECTION ON OUTCOMES AND SECOND MALIGNANCIES

Squamous cell carcinomas of the head and neck are increasingly understood as having different biologic behaviors that may be linked to etiologic factors. A shift in the epidemiology of head and neck cancer has been consistently reported during the past 30 years, especially affecting oropharyngeal cancer. In 1983, Syrjanen and colleagues[132] described the presence of cellular changes secondary to HPV infection in oral squamous cell carcinomas. After this, HPV was identified in different sites of the head and neck, although with different prevalence. The oropharynx appeared as the most important site for this infection. The emergence of HPV as an etiologic factor in head and neck cancer has been systematically reviewed in the literature since then. It is now known that HPV-related oropharyngeal carcinomas are a unique subtype of head and neck carcinomas, demonstrating that HPV-related squamous cell carcinoma is a different entity from the classic alcohol and tobacco–induced SCC with a distinct clinical and prognostic profile.[133]

HPV and Oropharynx Carcinoma Outcome

The incidence of oropharynx carcinoma has risen during the past 30 years, with other sites showing either a stable or decreased incidence.[134,135] This phenomenon has been called an "epidemic" and is attributed to changes in the etiologic factors of oropharyngeal carcinomas with a decreased use of tobacco/alcohol and changes in sexual behavioral patterns emerging over the past several decades.[128,136] Oropharynx is the most likely site to be HPV positive in head and neck, and this accounts for this increasing incidence of head and neck cancers in this site (**Fig. 2**).

The available literature of retrospective series and prospective studies strongly suggests that HPV-positive oropharyngeal cancers have a better prognosis (**Table 4**):

- Mellin and colleagues[137] showed, in a group of patients treated for tonsil cancer, a significant improvement in DSS among patients with HPV-related tonsillar carcinoma.
- Lindel and colleagues[138] carried out a retrospective analysis of outcome after curative radiotherapy for tonsillar carcinoma and observed a lower risk of local failure for HPV-positive patients in a multivariate analysis adjusted by T stage and alcohol consumption. This analysis failed, however, to show a significant effect on OS and DSS. The investigators of this study attributed the benefit to local control as a favorable increase in sensitivity to radiotherapy.[138]

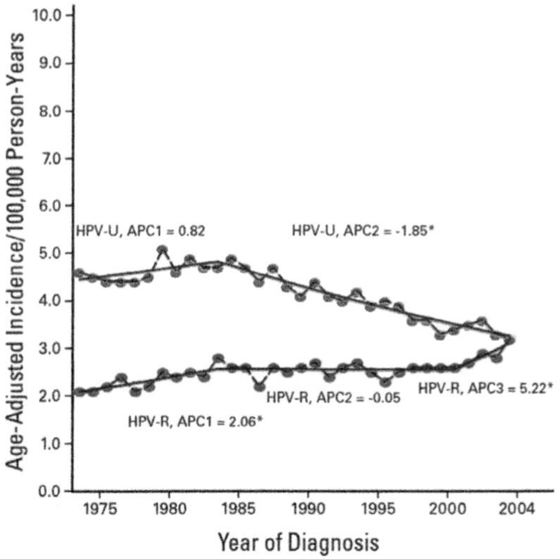

Fig. 2. Decreasing incidence of HPV-unrelated carcinomas of head and neck: age-adjusted incidence by calendar year of diagnosis for HPV-related sites (including base of tongue, lingual tonsil, tonsil, oropharynx, and Waldeyer ring) and HPV-unrelated sites (including other and unspecified parts of tongue excluding base of tongue, gum, floor of mouth, palate, other parts of mouth). The annual percentage change (APC) in incidence is shown for HPV-related (HPV-R) and HPV-unrelated (HPV-U) oral squamous cell carcinomas. An asterisk for the APC value denotes statistical significance at $P<.05$. (*From* Chaturvedi AK, Engels EA, Anderson WF, et al. Incidence trends for human papillomavirus-related and -unrelated oral squamous cell carcinomas in the United States. J Clin Oncol 2008;26(4):612–9; with permission.)

Table 4
Retrospective case series demonstrating effects of HPV status on survival

Author	Patients Number	Assays	Outcome HPV Positive vs HPV Negative: Endpoint	HR or OR (95% CI)	*P* Value
Mellin et al,[137] 2000	60	PCR	Risk of relapse	0.24	.025
Gillison et al,[182] 2000	253	PCR and ISH	DSS	0.41 (0.20–0.88)	.020
Schwartz et al,[155] 2001	254	PCR	OS	0.34 (0.14–0.83)	—
Lindel et al,[138] 2001	99	PCR	Local failure	0.31 (0.09–0.99)	.048
Weinberger et al,[183] 2004	120	p16	OS	0.42 (0.20–0.90)	.021

Data from Ang KK, Sturgis EM. Human papillomavirus as a marker of the natural history and response to therapy of head and neck squamous cell carcinoma. Semin Radiat Oncol 2012;22(2):128–42.

- Another analysis from Li and colleagues[139] in tonsil cancer patients showed an improvement in survival for those patients with HPV-related disease, even when adjusted for age, gender, tumor characteristics, and treatment.

Review of clinical trials of locally advanced oropharyngeal cancer show similar trends in survival (**Table 5**). The first prospective analysis by Kumar and colleagues[140] (University of Chicago Medical Center study 9921) showed a better OS and DSS among HPV-positive tumor patients. In 2008, a prospective analysis by Fakhry and colleagues[141] (Eastern Cooperative Oncology Group study 2399) demonstrated a 61% reduction in risk of death and 62% lower risk of progression for patients with HPV-positive oropharyngeal carcinoma than for HPV-negative patients. Patients with HPV-positive status showed a significantly better response rate to chemoradiation than HPV-negative patients (84% vs 57%, respectively).

Ang and colleagues,[130] in a post hoc analysis of the results of Radiation Therapy Oncology Group (RTOG) 0129, demonstrated that HPV status was an independent predictor of survival. HPV-positive patients with stage III and IV oropharyngeal carcinoma had a significantly better OS than non-HPV patients (3-year OS of 82.4% vs 57.1% for HPV-negative cancer). They developed a risk model for death from oropharyngeal squamous cell carcinoma on the basis of HPV status, pack-years of tobacco

Table 5
Clinical trials analyzing on the effect of HPV status on survival

Author	Patients Number	Assays	Outcome HPV Positive vs HPV Negative: Endpoint	HR or OR (95% CI)	*P* Value
Fakhry et al,[141] 2008	96	ISH and p16	Tumor progression	0.27 (0.10–0.75)	.01
Ang et al,[130] 2010	323	ISH and p16	OS	0.42 (0.27–0.66)	<.001
			Progression-free survival	0.49 (0.33–0.74)	<.001
Rischin et al,[142] 2010	185	p16	OS	0.36 (0.17–0.74)	.004
			Failure-free survival	0.39 (0.20–0.74)	<.001
Posner et al,[143] 2011	111	PCR (E6-E7)	OS	0.20 (0.10–0.38)	<.0001
Lassen et al,[184] 2011	794	p16	OS	0.62 (0.49–0.78)	<.001
			DSS	0.58 (0.41–0.81)	.001

Data from Ang KK, Sturgis EM. Human papillomavirus as a marker of the natural history and response to therapy of head and neck squamous cell carcinoma. Semin Radiat Oncol 2012;22(2):128–42.

smoking, tumor stage, and nodal stage, that showed that the risk of death significantly increased with each additional pack-year of tobacco smoking.

The TROG 02.02 phase III trial on 172 oropharynx cancer patients (59% of them were HPV positive), also reported a better OS (91% vs 74%) and RFS for HPV-positive patients (87% vs 72%) than HPV-negative patients, although they failed to show a significant improvement in the time to failure.[142] A subset analysis of oropharyngeal cancer patients in the TAX 324 phase III trial, where 50% of the evaluable patients were HPV positive, showed a significantly improved survival for HPV-positive patients (82%) versus 35% for HPV-negative patients at 5 years.[143]

The synergistic effect of HPV infection and tobacco use was also addressed by Ang and colleagues[130] in their analysis of RTOG 0129. The found a deleterious effect of smoking history and HPV-positivity on survival of oropharyngeal cancer patients: 82% (169 out of 206) of HPV-positive patients were ever-smokers versus 58% among HPV-negative patients. Smoking was an independent predictor of survival in both groups, and the magnitude of this effect increased with the pack per year history. Using HPV status, smoking history, lymph node categories, and T status, they could stratify patients into 3 different risk groups. Although most of the patients with HPV-positive tumors fall into the low-risk category (3-year survival: 94%), patients with HPV-positive tumors but with smoking history more than 10 pack-years were in an intermediate risk of survival (3-year survival: 67%). Maxwell and colleagues[144] compared the DSS and the risk of recurrence among HPV-positive oropharyngeal carcinomas based on tobacco use. They found a significant increase in risk of recurrence for HPV-positive tobacco users than never-users (hazard ratio [HR] 5.2), but tobacco status did not affect DSS or OS. HPV-positive patients, however, have a significantly better OS and DSS than HPV-negative patients.

The protective effect of HPV status on survival in oropharyngeal cancer is widely demonstrated based mainly in post hoc analysis of RCTs and case series. Changes in treatment scheme or, at least, less-aggressive treatments for HPV-positive oropharyngeal carcinomas could be expected in the future. These changes should be based, however, in trials specifically designed to address the most effective treatment of HPV-positive and HPV-negative patients.[145]

HPV and Oral Cavity Cancer Outcomes

In contrast to oropharyngeal carcinoma, a decrease in the incidence of oral cavity cancer has been reported in the past 30 years.[146] A possible explanation is the reduction in the prevalence of smoking and alcohol use in the general population during the last 40 years.[147] It is also possible to hypothesize an etiologic shift in oral cavity cancer to an HPV-related disease, similar to that for oropharynx cancer. Reports on the relationship between HPV and oral cancer pathogenesis, however, are conflicting:

- Some investigators have dismissed a link between oral cavity cancer and HPV infection, based on the very low prevalence rates reported in some studies.[148–150]
- In contrast, other investigators have reported that the infection of oral cavity cancer cells by HPV could be as high as oropharynx, approximately 60% or 70%.[151,152]

Problems in the detection methods used in oral cavity could lead to these differences. The relationship between oral cavity cancer and HPV infection is therefore not a closed case, and further research is necessary to elucidate its role.

Chaturvedi and colleagues[153,154] explored the potential difference in survival for HPV-unrelated sites of oral cavity versus HPV-related sites in oropharynx, using

SEER database registries from 1973 to 2004. Apparently, the improvement in survival in the past 30 years has affected mainly the oropharynx. They found significantly greater survival rates for HPV-related sites (oropharynx) than for HPV-unrelated sites (oral cavity) during the period 1993 to 2004, for all stages in patients treated with radiation therapy. When survival rates were analyzed across calendar periods, the improvement was more pronounced for HPV-related sites. Similar results have been reported in other analysis of national cancer registers from Sweden and Norway.

There are few cases series that address the effect of HPV status in oral cavity cancer prognosis as a different entity from oropharynx. Schwartz and colleagues[155] reported from a series of 254 patients with oral squamous cell carcinoma (15% HPV positive), an improvement in OS and DSS for HPV-positive patients after adjustment for patient and tumor characteristics. This analysis included, however, a few patients with oropharynx cancer that could have affected the final results. An analysis by Zhao and colleagues,[156] limited to oral cavity sites, reported an independent prognostic effect on the OS after adjustment for histologic grade, TNM stage, and tobacco use. HPV-positive status was significantly correlated with better OS in this series. Recently, Duray and colleagues,[157] in a series of oral cavity cancer patients, showed a high incidence of HPV-related cancers (44%, using PCR detection); however, in this series, HPV-positive patients had a significant increased risk of recurrence than HPV-negative patients and worse DSS.

An attempt to make a subsite analysis of oral cavity cancer has inconclusive information. Harris and colleagues[158] compared the overexpression of HPV p16 (INK4a) using *in situ* hybridization (ISH) and polymerase chain reaction (PCR) in oral tongue cancer. They found that p16 (INK4a) was more sensitive. When it is overexpressed, it is associated with an improved DSS. An analysis restricted to floor of mouth by Simonato and colleagues,[159] however, failed to demonstrate any survival benefit for HPV-positive patients (17.2% of the cohort).

A meta-analysis by Ragin and Taioli,[160] based in 23 outcome studies of patients with head and neck cancer in relation to HPV infection, published up to 2007, failed to demonstrate any survival benefit for HPV-positive or HPV-negative patients in sites of head and neck other than the oropharynx.

Although the presence of HPV infection among oral cavity cancer patients could be underestimated, the impact of HPV infection on survival of oral cancer is less clear than in patients with HPV-associated oropharyngeal cancers.

HPV and Second Primaries

As discussed previously, second primary tumors are an important problem in head and neck cancer patients. The emerging effect of HPV on second primary incidence is a developing issue and it is currently being intensively studied. In a recent analysis of second primaries developing after treatment of an index head and neck cancer, Morris and colleagues[128] described a significant and dramatic decrease in the incidence of second malignancies among survivors of oropharyngeal cancer, especially during the first decade of the twenty-first century. They reported a decline in the risk ranging from 1.2% to 7.8% annually since 1991. Before 1990, the oropharynx represented the site of head and neck index tumor second most often associated with the development of second primaries in the head and neck; after 1991, second primaries in patients treated for oropharyngeal occur less frequently than patients treated for squamous cell cancers arising other head and neck sites. This phenomenon can be explained in terms of the etiologic shift in oropharyngeal carcinoma from a tobacco and alcohol-related cancer to an HPV-related carcinoma. Further analyses are needed, but other reports have also suggested a decreased risk of second primaries among HPV-positive oropharyngeal carcinoma survivors.[129,130]

Outside the classic sites of second primaries, an increasing incidence of anogenital cancers after oral cavity/pharyngeal cancers, and vice versa, has been reported, further linking sexual behavior related to transmission of HPV that can cause infection that contributes to the development of HPV-associated cancers.[131] Similarly, patients with cervical cancer history seem to be at increased risk of developing second primary malignancies in the oropharynx and anogenital region but not in the oral cavity.[161,162]

Another topic of interest is whether or not HPV infection can cause the development of multiple primaries in the oropharynx or beyond it, in a similar way that the field of cancerization theory explains multifocal disease. An initial case report has been published describing the presence of multiple HPV-positive primaries in oropharynx and nasopharynx.[163]

HPV detection in lung lesions has been recently mentioned in the differential diagnosis of lung cancer versus head and neck cancer metastasis.[164,165]

The progress in the understanding of HPV-related biology should offer increasing knowledge of the development of multifocal disease and metachronic tumors and eventually preventive measures to control the increased risk that patients are subject to.

FUTURE SURVIVORSHIPS ISSUES IN HEAD AND NECK CANCER

Over the past 30 years, the methods by which cancer results are reported have improved since the first effort to standardize information about survival by the World Health Organization.[166,167] A better understanding of how host variables and host lifestyles, as well as tumor intrinsic characteristics, affect survival has led to significant changes in the way we understand survivorship, how patients are accrued in RCTs and how results are interpreted.

Head and neck cancer mortality has declined in the past 20 years.[2] The explanation for this is not clear but may be based on improvements on therapies, decline of tobacco use, and emergence of new etiologic factors, such as HPV, leading to a different survival profile. During the past 10 years, better multimodality therapies have shown important improvements in survival of head and neck cancer patients, especially in those with advanced-stage disease. The patients who survive head and neck cancer live longer and are subject to cancer relapse but are also exposed to the evolution of their other chronic diseases, the long-term toxic effects of the treatment received, and the risk of second primaries. How these new factors or competing risks of mortality are interpreted in survival analysis is an important survivorship issue.

In most cancer studies, the time to an event of interest is the main outcome measured.[168] This is usually known as survival time. This time could represent the time from diagnosis to death of any cause (OS), the time to recurrence of cancer (RFS), or the time to death of cancer (DSS). More-specific survival data should be useful in specific situations, such as local recurrence or distant metastasis (eg, local or distant RFS, respectively). Some patients have the event of interest; others do not have the event during the time of observation or are lost to follow-up (censored). The methods of analyzing survival and recurrence data are well known, comprising Kaplan-Meier curves, log rank tests, hazard ratios, and Cox proportional hazard function.

Competing Risk in Follow Up

There is a possibility that some patients are exposed to a different event, which prevents continued monitoring of the follow-up. If follow-up stops because a patient has experienced a different defined event, the problem may be viewed as a competing risk. Competing risk refers to the existence of different causes of failure that can affect the probability of experiencing the event of interest.[169] These could be a different event (death of other causes, death of other cancers, and so forth) or a repetitive event (multiple recurrences). In this situation, the Kaplan-Meier method could be inappropriate, and more-advanced methods should be used, such as the mixture model or cumulative incidence method. Mixture models, or cure models, specifically allow modeling different types of event. Cumulative metrics use the sum of event specific probabilities (ie, each patient is entered as many times as events suffered and is censored on the time of next event).[170]

Selection of Endpoint in Cancer Epidemiology

OS or OM represents the endpoint of choice in cancer epidemiology. To directly quantify the effect of treatment on cancer, however, the DSS or cancer-specific mortality is more important. Both are frequently used in clinical reports as endpoints, both can be easily calculated using actuarial methods, and both can precisely estimate the event of interest. Unfortunately, neither of these metrics escapes from competing risk events.

OS is widely used because it is clinically important, it is an unambiguous character, and the event information can be obtained easily from government agencies.[171] It requires, however, longer follow-up time, and subsequently there is more risk of loss of patients during follow-up, which make studies more expensive, and which, therefore, may delay dissemination of effective therapies.

Disease-Specific Survival

DSS can be measured instead of OS. It is a more precise metric that reports cancer-specific death, allowing for a better comparison of the efficacy of treatments. Although its use has some drawbacks (the event of interest is more difficult to assess), it is more subjective (the problem of bias of cause of death), and full records are not always available. In DSS, a death unrelated to index cancer is censored at the time of death. Then, a death from other causes is considered a success. This masks the effectiveness of cancer treatment considering patients who die of other diseases as being cured. Therefore, the use of DSS in a population of patients with a high risk of competing causes of mortality could falsely inflate the DSS.[172]

Mell and colleagues,[33] in a recent analysis of competing risk of mortality in head and neck cancer patients, illustrated this point. They have shown that, in a group of patients with homogeneous oncologic characteristics and similar DSS, it is possible to recognize subgroups of patients with markedly different OS based on their competitive risk of death. They identified risk based on the age, comorbidity conditions, BMI, gender, and distance traveled to get treatment. This analysis allowed them to classify patients into low or high risk of death secondary to noncancer causes. Those patients who are high risk follow the competing disease pathway, leading to noncancer mortality (**Fig. 3**). They have shown how much the risk of competitive causes of death affects the OS calculation. Theoretically, in a scenario of high risk of competing causes of death, the OS and the DSS could not reflect the improvements in treatment just due to the high prevalence of noncancer causes of death. Rose and colleagues,[38] using the SEER database, identified that the presence of competing risk factors could influence the sample size necessary to achieve an 80% power in RCTs. Using competing risk methods versus standard sample size estimation, this group reported an increase in the sample size of 42% was necessary to achieve an 80% power among high-risk patients. This illustrates how the lack of a correct competing risk analysis can affecti the design of an RCT.

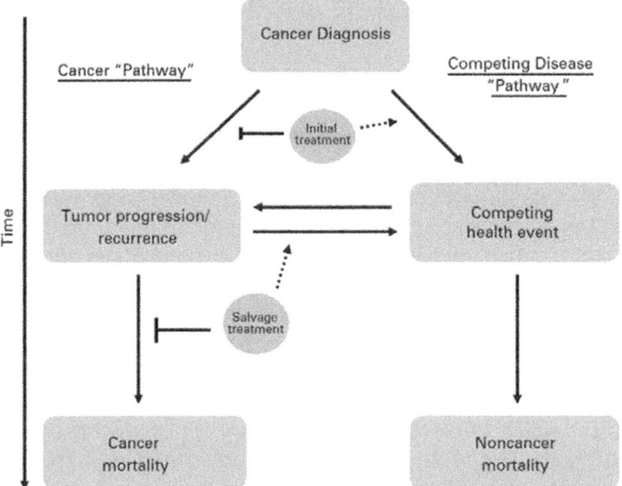

Fig. 3. Noncancer pathway of mortality (schematic representation of clinical event pathways in patients with competing risks). (*From* Mell LK, Dignam JJ, Salama JK, et al. Predictors of competing mortality in advanced head and neck cancer. J Clin Oncol 2010;28(1):15–20; with permission.)

Clinical Decision Making

Once the increasing importance of competing risk factors of mortality in cancer survival estimation is understood, it is important to analyze how this information could be useful in clinical decision making. It is possible to recognize different levels of importance. The first level is the individual decision making: how these factors affect the treatment and prognosis of a unique patient. The second level is a population level: how these factors could affect the design and interpretation of RCTs that determine how the individual patients are treated.

Nomograms could offer the best available answer to the first question. Nomograms have appeared in the past 10 years as an accurate prognostic tool for individual patients. Although the terms, *nomogram* and *prediction model*, are used indistinctively, a nomogram is the simple graphic representation or calculation device that is based on a statistical prediction model. This is a numeric probability of the occurrence of a clinical event based on a logistic or progression hazard analysis (Cox regression) of significant prognostic variables that assign a score to each of them.[173] The nomogram, constructed using not only tumor characteristics but also host and treatment-related characteristics, could predict the probability of an event based on the sum of scores obtained from the different variables analyzed. These are presented in a user-friendly form through a graphic or computerized interface, incorporating many of the variables analyzed in this review as predictors of competing risk of mortality. Nomograms have been widely tested in other types of cancers, but their use in head and neck cancer has been limited.[174]

The competing risk of mortality factors could be incorporated in the selection of new therapies through RCT in different ways, such as setting the target population, taking into account the distribution and risk stratification of competing cause of death, and using competing-risk methods in the determination of sample size.[38] Also, it has been suggested that the use of multiple primary cause-specific endpoints, instead of composite endpoints, like OS or DSS, in a setting of high risk of competing risk mortalities should be done incorporating competing risk of mortality as events in the subsequent analysis.[11]

SUMMARY

The existence of adverse factors that affect survival of patients with head and neck cancer, distinct from those related to the cancer itself, is well known. Age, chronic comorbidities, lifestyle behaviors, risk of second primaries, and, more recently, HPV infection affect the risk of morbidity and mortality among head and neck cancer survivors. These factors are especially important in a scenario of patients who live longer because of better treatment, even in advanced-stage disease. Besides these factors, the effect of new therapies that increase survival can also put patients at an increased risk of adverse outcome due to severe treatment-related morbidity.

The use of classic metrics, such as OS, to measure outcomes could fail to recognize that head and neck cancer survivors are exposed to an increased risk of death because of other causes different from their primary cancer. Incorporating competing mortalities into the analysis of outcome endpoints could lead to a better understanding of the different factors that influence and determine survival in head and neck cancer patients. These factors will have increasing importance in the design, analysis, and implementation of RCTs of future therapies.

REFERENCES

1. Pulte D, Brenner H. Changes in survival in head and neck cancers in the late 20th and early 21st century: a period analysis. Oncologist 2010;15(9):994–1001.
2. National Cancer Institute, USA. A Snap Shot in Head and Neck Cancers. Available at: http://www.cancer.gov/aboutnci/servingpeople/snapshots/head-neck.pdf. Accessed March 10, 2012.
3. Adelstein DJ, Saxton JP, Rybicki LA, et al. Multiagent concurrent chemoradiotherapy for locoregionally advanced squamous cell head and neck cancer: mature results from a single institution. J Clin Oncol 2006;24(7):1064–71.
4. Bernier J, Domenge C, Ozsahin M, et al. Postoperative irradiation with or without concomitant chemotherapy for locally advanced head and neck cancer. N Engl J Med 2004;350(19):1945–52.
5. Bonner JA, Harari PM, Giralt J, et al. Radiotherapy plus cetuximab for locoregionally advanced head and neck cancer: 5-year survival data from a phase 3 randomised trial, and relation between cetuximab-induced rash and survival. Lancet Oncol 2010;11(1):21–8.
6. Cooper JS, Pajak TF, Forastiere AA, et al. Postoperative concurrent radiotherapy and chemotherapy for high-risk squamous-cell carcinoma of the head and neck. N Engl J Med 2004;350(19):1937–44.
7. Argiris A, Brockstein BE, Haraf DJ, et al. Competing causes of death and second primary tumors in patients with locoregionally advanced head and neck cancer treated with chemoradiotherapy. Clin Cancer Res 2004;10(6):1956–62.
8. Fish EB, Chapman JA, Link MA. Competing causes of death for primary breast cancer. Ann Surg Oncol 1998;5(4):368–75.
9. Ng AK, Bernardo MP, Weller E, et al. Long-term survival and competing causes of death in patients with early-stage Hodgkin's disease treated at age 50 or younger. J Clin Oncol 2002;20(8):2101–8.
10. Huddart RA, Norman A, Shahidi M, et al. Cardiovascular disease as a long-term complication of treatment for testicular cancer. J Clin Oncol 2003;21(8):1513–23.

11. Mell LK, Jeong JH. Pitfalls of using composite primary end points in the presence of competing risks. J Clin Oncol 2010;28(28):4297–9.
12. Manola JB, Gray RJ. When bad things happen to good studies. J Clin Oncol 2011;29(26):3497–9.
13. Howlader N, Noone A, Krapcho M, et al, editors. SEER Cancer Statistics Review, 1975-2008. Bethesda (MD): National Cancer Institute. Available at: http://seer.cancer.gov/csr/1975_2010/. Based on November 2010 SEER data submission, posted to the SEER web site 2011. Accesed December 30, 2011.
14. Smith BD, Smith GL, Hurria A, et al. Future of cancer incidence in the United States: burdens upon an aging, changing nation. J Clin Oncol 2009;27(17):2758–65.
15. Samet J, Hunt WC, Key C, et al. Choice of cancer therapy varies with age of patient. JAMA 1986;255(24):3385–90.
16. Derks W, de Leeuw JR, Hordijk GJ, et al. Reasons for non-standard treatment in elderly patients with advanced head and neck cancer. Eur Arch Otorhinolaryngol 2005;262(1):21–6.
17. Sanabria A, Carvalho AL, Vartanian JG, et al. Factors that influence treatment decision in older patients with resectable head and neck cancer. Laryngoscope 2007;117(5):835–40.
18. van der Schroeff MP, Derks W, Hordijk GJ, et al. The effect of age on survival and quality of life in elderly head and neck cancer patients: a long-term prospective study. Eur Arch Otorhinolaryngol 2007;264(4):415–22.
19. Jones AS, Beasley N, Houghton D, et al. The effects of age on survival and other parameters in squamous cell carcinoma of the oral cavity, pharynx and larynx. Clin Otolaryngol Allied Sci 1998;23(1):51–6.
20. Sarini J, Fournier C, Lefebvre JL, et al. Head and neck squamous cell carcinoma in elderly patients: a long-term retrospective review of 273 cases. Arch Otolaryngol Head Neck Surg 2001;127(9):1089–92.
21. Bernardi D, Barzan L, Franchin G, et al. Treatment of head and neck cancer in elderly patients: state of the art and guidelines. Crit Rev Oncol Hematol 2005;53(1):71–80.
22. Pytynia KB, Grant JR, Etzel CJ, et al. Matched analysis of survival in patients with squamous cell carcinoma of the head and neck diagnosed before and after 40 years of age. Arch Otolaryngol Head Neck Surg 2004;130(7):869–73.
23. Grenman R, Chevalier D, Gregoire V, et al. Treatment of head and neck cancer in the elderly: European Consensus (panel 6) at the EUFOS Congress in Vienna 2007. Eur Arch Otorhinolaryngol 2010;267(10):1619–21.
24. Clayman GL, Eicher SA, Sicard MW, et al. Surgical outcomes in head and neck cancer patients 80 years of age and older. Head Neck 1998;20(3):216–23.
25. Derks W, De Leeuw JR, Hordijk GJ, et al. Elderly patients with head and neck cancer: short-term effects of surgical treatment on quality of life. Clin Otolaryngol Allied Sci 2003;28(5):399–405.
26. Kesting MR, Holzle F, Wolff KD, et al. Use of microvascular flap technique in older adults with head and neck cancer: a persisting dilemma in reconstructive surgery? J Am Geriatr Soc 2011;59(3):398–405.
27. Syrigos KN, Karachalios D, Karapanagiotou EM, et al. Head and neck cancer in the elderly: an overview on the treatment modalities. Cancer Treat Rev 2009;35(3):237–45.
28. Pignon T, Horiot JC, Van den Bogaert W, et al. No age limit for radical radiotherapy in head and neck tumours. Eur J Cancer 1996;32A(12):2075–81.

29. Metges JP, Eschwege F, de Crevoisier R, et al. Radiotherapy in head and neck cancer in the elderly: a challenge. Crit Rev Oncol Hematol 2000;34(3): 195–203.
30. Schofield CP, Sykes AJ, Slevin NJ, et al. Radiotherapy for head and neck cancer in elderly patients. Radiother Oncol 2003;69(1):37–42.
31. Huang SH, O'Sullivan B, Waldron J, et al. Patterns of care in elderly head-and-neck cancer radiation oncology patients: a single-center cohort study. Int J Radiat Oncol Biol Phys 2011;79(1):46–51.
32. Kubicek GJ, Kimler BF, Wang F, et al. Chemotherapy in head and neck cancer: clinical predictors of tolerance and outcomes. Am J Clin Oncol 2011;34(4): 380–4.
33. Mell LK, Dignam JJ, Salama JK, et al. Predictors of competing mortality in advanced head and neck cancer. J Clin Oncol 2010;28(1):15–20.
34. Lalami Y, de Castro G Jr, Bernard-Marty C, et al. Management of head and neck cancer in elderly patients. Drugs Aging 2009;26(7):571–83.
35. Derks W, de Leeuw RJ, Hordijk GJ, et al. Quality of life in elderly patients with head and neck cancer one year after diagnosis. Head Neck 2004;26(12): 1045–52.
36. Bhattacharyya N. A matched survival analysis for squamous cell carcinoma of the head and neck in the elderly. Laryngoscope 2003;113(2):368–72.
37. Genden EM, Rinaldo A, Shaha AR, et al. Treatment considerations for head and neck cancer in the elderly. J Laryngol Otol 2005;119(3):169–74.
38. Rose BS, Jeong JH, Nath SK, et al. Population-based study of competing mortality in head and neck cancer. J Clin Oncol 2011;29(26):3503–9.
39. Konski AA, Pajak TF, Movsas B, et al. Disadvantage of men living alone participating in Radiation Therapy Oncology Group head and neck trials. J Clin Oncol 2006;24(25):4177–83.
40. Goldberg HI, Lockwood SA, Wyatt SW, et al. Trends and differentials in mortality from cancers of the oral cavity and pharynx in the United States, 1973-1987. Cancer 1994;74(2):565–72.
41. Molina MA, Cheung MC, Perez EA, et al. African American and poor patients have a dramatically worse prognosis for head and neck cancer: an examination of 20,915 patients. Cancer 2008;113(10):2797–806.
42. Dilling TJ, Bae K, Paulus R, et al. Impact of gender, partner status, and race on locoregional failure and overall survival in head and neck cancer patients in three radiation therapy oncology group trials. Int J Radiat Oncol Biol Phys 2011;81(3):e101–9.
43. Gillison ML, Broutian T, Pickard RK, et al. Prevalence of oral HPV infection in the United States, 2009-2010. JAMA 2012;307(7):693–703.
44. Saba NF, Goodman M, Ward K, et al. Gender and ethnic disparities in incidence and survival of squamous cell carcinoma of the oral tongue, base of tongue, and tonsils: a surveillance, epidemiology and end results program-based analysis. Oncology 2011;81(1):12–20.
45. Brown LM, Check DP, Devesa SS. Oropharyngeal cancer incidence trends: diminishing racial disparities. Cancer Causes Control 2011;22(5):753–63.
46. Roberts JC, Li G, Reitzel LR, et al. No evidence of sex-related survival disparities among head and neck cancer patients receiving similar multidisciplinary care: a matched-pair analysis. Clin Cancer Res 2010;16(20):5019–27.
47. Arbes SJ Jr, Olshan AF, Caplan DJ, et al. Factors contributing to the poorer survival of black Americans diagnosed with oral cancer (United States). Cancer Causes Control 1999;10(6):513–23.

48. Paterson IC, John G, Adams Jones D. Effect of deprivation on survival of patients with head and neck cancer: a study of 20,131 cases. Clin Oncol (R Coll Radiol) 2002;14(6):455–8.
49. Macfarlane GJ, Sharp L, Porter S, et al. Trends in survival from cancers of the oral cavity and pharynx in Scotland: a clue as to why the disease is becoming more common? Br J Cancer 1996;73(6):805–8.
50. Chen AY, DeSantis C, Jemal A. US mortality rates for oral cavity and pharyngeal cancer by educational attainment. Arch Otolaryngol Head Neck Surg 2011; 137(11):1094–9.
51. Konski A, Berkey BA, Kian Ang K, et al. Effect of education level on outcome of patients treated on Radiation Therapy Oncology Group Protocol 90-03. Cancer 2003;98(7):1497–503.
52. Gourin CG, Podolsky RH. Racial disparities in patients with head and neck squamous cell carcinoma. Laryngoscope 2006;116(7):1093–106.
53. Goodwin WJ, Thomas GR, Parker DF, et al. Unequal burden of head and neck cancer in the United States. Head Neck 2008;30(3):358–71.
54. Worsham MJ, Divine G, Kittles RA. Race as a social construct in head and neck cancer outcomes. Otolaryngol Head Neck Surg 2011;144(3):381–9.
55. Conway DI, Petticrew M, Marlborough H, et al. Socioeconomic inequalities and oral cancer risk: a systematic review and meta-analysis of case-control studies. Int J Cancer 2008;122(12):2811–9.
56. Shiboski CH, Schmidt BL, Jordan RC. Racial disparity in stage at diagnosis and survival among adults with oral cancer in the US. Community Dent Oral Epidemiol 2007;35(3):233–40.
57. Nichols AC, Bhattacharyya N. Racial differences in stage and survival in head and neck squamous cell carcinoma. Laryngoscope 2007;117(5):770–5.
58. Ragin CC, Langevin SM, Marzouk M, et al. Determinants of head and neck cancer survival by race. Head Neck 2011;33(8):1092–8.
59. Chen LM, Li G, Reitzel LR, et al. Matched-pair analysis of race or ethnicity in outcomes of head and neck cancer patients receiving similar multidisciplinary care. Cancer Prev Res (Phila) 2009;2(9):782–91.
60. Gandhi KK, Foulds J, Steinberg MB, et al. Lower quit rates among African American and Latino menthol cigarette smokers at a tobacco treatment clinic. Int J Clin Pract 2009;63(3):360–7.
61. Kabat GC, Morabia A, Wynder EL. Comparison of smoking habits of blacks and whites in a case-control study. Am J Public Health 1991;81(11):1483–6.
62. Bach PB, Schrag D, Brawley OW, et al. Survival of blacks and whites after a cancer diagnosis. JAMA 2002;287(16):2106–13.
63. Murdock JM, Gluckman JL. African-American and white head and neck carcinoma patients in a university medical center setting. Are treatments provided and are outcomes similar or disparate? Cancer 2001;91(Suppl 1):279–83.
64. Settle K, Taylor R, Wolf J, et al. Race impacts outcome in stage III/IV squamous cell carcinomas of the head and neck after concurrent chemoradiation therapy. Cancer 2009;115(8):1744–52.
65. Settle K, Posner MR, Schumaker LM, et al. Racial survival disparity in head and neck cancer results from low prevalence of human papillomavirus infection in black oropharyngeal cancer patients. Cancer Prev Res (Phila) 2009;2(9): 776–81.
66. Kaplan MH, Feinstein AR. The importance of classifying initial co-morbidity in evaluating the outcome of diabetes mellitus. J Chronic Dis 1974;27(7–8): 387–404.

67. Piccirillo JF, Vlahiotis A. Comorbidity in patients with cancer of the head and neck: prevalence and impact on treatment and prognosis. Curr Oncol Rep 2006;8(2):123–9.
68. Landis SH, El-Hariry IA, van Herk-Sukel MP, et al. Prevalence and incidence of acute and chronic comorbidity in patients with squamous cell carcinoma of the head and neck. Head Neck 2012;34(2):238–44.
69. Piccirillo JF. Importance of comorbidity in head and neck cancer. Laryngoscope 2000;110(4):593–602.
70. Derks W, de Leeuw RJ, Hordijk GJ. Elderly patients with head and neck cancer: the influence of comorbidity on choice of therapy, complication rate, and survival. Curr Opin Otolaryngol Head Neck Surg 2005;13(2):92–6.
71. Piccirillo JF, Costas I. The impact of comorbidity on outcomes. ORL J Otorhinolaryngol Relat Spec 2004;66(4):180–5.
72. Piccirillo JF, Tierney RM, Costas I, et al. Prognostic importance of comorbidity in a hospital-based cancer registry. JAMA 2004;291(20):2441–7.
73. Charlson ME, Pompei P, Ales KL, et al. A new method of classifying prognostic comorbidity in longitudinal studies: development and validation. J Chronic Dis 1987;40(5):373–83.
74. Piccirillo JF, Lacy PD, Basu A, et al. Development of a new head and neck cancer-specific comorbidity index. Arch Otolaryngol Head Neck Surg 2002; 128(10):1172–9.
75. Reid BC, Alberg AJ, Klassen AC, et al. A comparison of three comorbidity indexes in a head and neck cancer population. Oral Oncol 2002;38(2):187–94.
76. Piccirillo JF, Costas I, Claybour P, et al. The measurement of comorbidity by cancer registries. J Registry Manag 2003;30:8–14.
77. Paleri V, Wight RG, Silver CE, et al. Comorbidity in head and neck cancer: a critical appraisal and recommendations for practice. Oral Oncol 2010;46(10): 712–9.
78. Reid BC, Alberg AJ, Klassen AC, et al. Comorbidity and survival of elderly head and neck carcinoma patients. Cancer 2001;92(8):2109–16.
79. Datema FR, Ferrier MB, van der Schroeff MP, et al. Impact of comorbidity on short-term mortality and overall survival of head and neck cancer patients. Head Neck 2010;32(6):728–36.
80. Feinstein AR, Schimpff CR, Andrews JF Jr, et al. Cancer of the larynx: a new staging system and a re-appraisal of prognosis and treatment. J Chronic Dis 1977;30(5):277–305.
81. Lacy PD, Piccirillo JF. Development of a new staging system for patients with recurrent laryngeal squamous cell carcinoma. Cancer 1998;83(5):910–7.
82. Pugliano FA, Piccirillo JF, Zequeira MR, et al. Clinical-severity staging system for oral cavity cancer: five-year survival rates. Otolaryngol Head Neck Surg 1999; 120(1):38–45.
83. Pugliano FA, Piccirillo JF, Zequeira MR, et al. Clinical-severity staging system for oropharyngeal cancer: five-year survival rates. Arch Otolaryngol Head Neck Surg 1997;123(10):1118–24.
84. Deleyiannis FW, Thomas DB, Vaughan TL, et al. Alcoholism: independent predictor of survival in patients with head and neck cancer. J Natl Cancer Inst 1996;88(8):542–9.
85. Franceschi S, Talamini R, Barra S, et al. Smoking and drinking in relation to cancers of the oral cavity, pharynx, larynx, and esophagus in northern Italy. Cancer Res 1990;50(20):6502–7.

86. Fortin A, Wang CS, Vigneault E. Influence of smoking and alcohol drinking behaviors on treatment outcomes of patients with squamous cell carcinomas of the head and neck. Int J Radiat Oncol Biol Phys 2009;74(4):1062–9.
87. Farshadpour F, Kranenborg H, Calkoen EV, et al. Survival analysis of head and neck squamous cell carcinoma: influence of smoking and drinking. Head Neck 2011;33(6):817–23.
88. Duffy SA, Ronis DL, McLean S, et al. Pretreatment health behaviors predict survival among patients with head and neck squamous cell carcinoma. J Clin Oncol 2009;27(12):1969–75.
89. Hall SF, Groome PA, Rothwell D. The impact of comorbidity on the survival of patients with squamous cell carcinoma of the head and neck. Head Neck 2000; 22(4):317–22.
90. Pytynia KB, Grant JR, Etzel CJ, et al. Matched-pair analysis of survival of never smokers and ever smokers with squamous cell carcinoma of the head and neck. J Clin Oncol 2004;22(19):3981–8.
91. Koch WM, Lango M, Sewell D, et al. Head and neck cancer in nonsmokers: a distinct clinical and molecular entity. Laryngoscope 1999;109(10):1544–51.
92. Dikshit RP, Boffetta P, Bouchardy C, et al. Lifestyle habits as prognostic factors in survival of laryngeal and hypopharyngeal cancer: a multicentric European study. Int J Cancer 2005;117(6):992–5.
93. Schantz SP, Byers RM, Goepfert H, et al. the implication of tobacco use in the young-adult with head and neck-cancer. Cancer 1988;62(7):1374–80.
94. Ferrier MB, Spuesens EB, Le Cessie S, et al. Comorbidity as a major risk factor for mortality and complications in head and neck surgery. Arch Otolaryngol Head Neck Surg 2005;131(1):27–32.
95. Pelczar BT, Weed HG, Schuller DE, et al. Identifying High-Risk Patients before Head and Neck Oncologic Surgery. Arch Otolaryngol 1993;119(8):861–4.
96. Buitelaar DR, Balm AJ, Antonini N, et al. Cardiovascular and respiratory complications after major head and neck surgery. Head Neck 2006;28(7):595–602.
97. Singh B, Bhaya M, Zimbler M, et al. Impact of comorbidity on outcome of young patients with head and neck squamous cell carcinoma. Head Neck 1998;20(1): 1–7.
98. Gaudet MM, Olshan AF, Chuang SC, et al. Body mass index and risk of head and neck cancer in a pooled analysis of case-control studies in the International Head and Neck Cancer Epidemiology (INHANCE) Consortium. Int J Epidemiol 2010;39(4):1091–102.
99. Nieto A, Sanchez MJ, Martinez C, et al. Lifetime body mass index and risk of oral cavity and oropharyngeal cancer by smoking and drinking habits. Br J Cancer 2003;89(9):1667–71.
100. Franceschi S, Dal Maso L, Levi F, et al. Leanness as early marker of cancer of the oral cavity and pharynx. Ann Oncol 2001;12(3):331–6.
101. Couch M, Lai V, Cannon T, et al. Cancer cachexia syndrome in head and neck cancer patients: part I. Diagnosis, impact on quality of life and survival, and treatment. Head Neck 2007;29(4):401–11.
102. Kubrak C, Olson K, Jha N, et al. Nutrition impact symptoms: key determinants of reduced dietary intake, weight loss, and reduced functional capacity of patients with head and neck cancer before treatment. Head Neck 2010;32(3):290–300.
103. McRackan TR, Watkins JM, Herrin AE, et al. Effect of body mass index on chemoradiation outcomes in head and neck cancer. Laryngoscope 2008;118(7): 1180–5.

104. Gaudet MM, Patel AV, Sun J, et al. Prospective studies of body mass index with head and neck cancer incidence and mortality. Cancer Epidemiol Biomarkers Prev 2012;21(3):497–503.
105. Doerr TD, Marks SC, Shamsa FH, et al. Effects of zinc and nutritional status on clinical outcomes in head and neck cancer. Nutrition 1998;14(6):489–95.
106. Sandoval M, Font R, Manos M, et al. The role of vegetable and fruit consumption and other habits on survival following the diagnosis of oral cancer: a prospective study in Spain. Int J Oral Maxillofac Surg 2009;38(1):31–9.
107. Day GL, Shore RE, Blot WJ, et al. Dietary factors and second primary cancers: a follow-up of oral and pharyngeal cancer patients. Nutr Cancer 1994;21(3):223–32.
108. Dikshit RP, Boffetta P, Bouchardy C, et al. Risk factors for the development of second primary tumors among men after laryngeal and hypopharyngeal carcinoma. Cancer 2005;103(11):2326–33.
109. Urba S, Gatz J, Shen W, et al. Quality of life scores as prognostic factors of overall survival in advanced head and neck cancer: analysis of a phase III randomized trial of pemetrexed plus cisplatin versus cisplatin monotherapy. Oral Oncol 2012;48(8):723–9.
110. Montazeri A. Quality of life data as prognostic indicators of survival in cancer patients: an overview of the literature from 1982 to 2008. Health Qual Life Outcomes 2009;7:102.
111. Mehanna HM, De Boer MF, Morton RP. The association of psycho-social factors and survival in head and neck cancer. Clin Otolaryngol 2008;33(2):83–9.
112. Karvonen-Gutierrez CA, Ronis DL, Fowler KE, et al. Quality of life scores predict survival among patients with head and neck cancer. J Clin Oncol 2008;26(16):2754–60.
113. Slaughter DP, Southwick HW, Smejkal W. Field cancerization in oral stratified squamous epithelium; clinical implications of multicentric origin. Cancer 1953;6(5):963–8.
114. Vikram B. Changing patterns of failure in advanced head and neck cancer. Arch Otolaryngol 1984;110(9):564–5.
115. Morris LG, Sikora AG, Hayes RB, et al. Anatomic sites at elevated risk of second primary cancer after an index head and neck cancer. Cancer Causes Control 2011;22(5):671–9.
116. Haughey BH, Gates GA, Arfken CL, et al. Meta-analysis of second malignant tumors in head and neck cancer: the case for an endoscopic screening protocol. Ann Otol Rhinol Laryngol 1992;101(2 Pt 1):105–12.
117. Jones AS, Morar P, Phillips DE, et al. Second primary tumors in patients with head and neck squamous cell carcinoma. Cancer 1995;75(6):1343–53.
118. Leon X, Martinez V, Lopez M, et al. Second, third, and fourth head and neck tumors. A progressive decrease in survival. Head Neck 2012;34(12):1716–9.
119. Liao CT, Kang CJ, Chang JT, et al. Survival of second and multiple primary tumors in patients with oral cavity squamous cell carcinoma in the betel quid chewing area. Oral Oncol 2007;43(8):811–9.
120. Robinson E, Neugut AI, Murray T, et al. A comparison of the clinical characteristics of first and second primary head and neck cancers. A population-based study. Cancer 1991;68(1):189–92.
121. Erkal HS, Mendenhall WM, Amdur RJ, et al. Synchronous and metachronous squamous cell carcinomas of the head and neck mucosal sites. J Clin Oncol 2001;19(5):1358–62.
122. Schwartz LH, Ozsahin M, Zhang GN, et al. Synchronous and metachronous head and neck carcinomas. Cancer 1994;74(7):1933–8.

123. McDonald S, Haie C, Rubin P, et al. Second malignant tumors in patients with laryngeal carcinoma: diagnosis, treatment, and prevention. Int J Radiat Oncol Biol Phys 1989;17(3):457–65.
124. Lin K, Patel SG, Chu PY, et al. Second primary malignancy of the aerodigestive tract in patients treated for cancer of the oral cavity and larynx. Head Neck 2005;27(12):1042–8.
125. Dolan R, Vaughan C, Fuleihan N. Metachronous cancer: prognostic factors including prior irradiation. Otolaryngol Head Neck Surg 1998;119(6):619–23.
126. Farhadieh RD, Otahal P, Rees CG, et al. Radiotherapy is not associated with an increased rate of Second Primary Tumours in Oral Squamous Carcinoma: a study of 370 patients. Oral Oncol 2009;45(11):941–5.
127. Morris LG, Sikora AG, Patel SG, et al. Second primary cancers after an index head and neck cancer: subsite-specific trends in the era of human papillomavirus-associated oropharyngeal cancer. J Clin Oncol 2011;29(6):739–46.
128. Sturgis EM, Ang KK. The epidemic of HPV-associated oropharyngeal cancer is here: is it time to change our treatment paradigms? J Natl Compr Canc Netw 2011;9(6):665–73.
129. Licitra L, Perrone F, Bossi P, et al. High-risk human papillomavirus affects prognosis in patients with surgically treated oropharyngeal squamous cell carcinoma. J Clin Oncol 2006;24(36):5630–6.
130. Ang KK, Harris J, Wheeler R, et al. Human papillomavirus and survival of patients with oropharyngeal cancer. N Engl J Med 2010;363(1):24–35.
131. Sikora AG, Morris LG, Sturgis EM. Bidirectional association of anogenital and oral cavity/pharyngeal carcinomas in men. Arch Otolaryngol Head Neck Surg 2009;135(4):402–5.
132. Syrjanen K, Syrjanen S, Lamberg M, et al. Morphological and immunohistochemical evidence suggesting human papillomavirus (HPV) involvement in oral squamous cell carcinogenesis. International journal of oral surgery 1983; 12(6):418–24.
133. Gillison ML. Human papillomavirus-associated head and neck cancer is a distinct epidemiologic, clinical, and molecular entity. Semin Oncol 2004;31(6): 744–54.
134. Frisch M, Hjalgrim H, Jaeger AB, et al. Changing patterns of tonsillar squamous cell carcinoma in the United States. Cancer Causes Control 2000;11(6):489–95.
135. Shiboski CH, Schmidt BL, Jordan RC. Tongue and tonsil carcinoma: increasing trends in the U.S. population ages 20-44 years. Cancer 2005;103(9):1843–9.
136. Gillison ML, D'Souza G, Westra W, et al. Distinct risk factor profiles for human papillomavirus type 16-positive and human papillomavirus type 16-negative head and neck cancers. J Natl Cancer Inst 2008;100(6):407–20.
137. Mellin H, Friesland S, Lewensohn R, et al. Human papillomavirus (HPV) DNA in tonsillar cancer: clinical correlates, risk of relapse, and survival. Int J Cancer 2000;89(3):300–4.
138. Lindel K, Beer KT, Laissue J, et al. Human papillomavirus positive squamous cell carcinoma of the oropharynx: a radiosensitive subgroup of head and neck carcinoma. Cancer 2001;92(4):805–13.
139. Li W, Thompson CH, O'Brien CJ, et al. Human papillomavirus positivity predicts favourable outcome for squamous carcinoma of the tonsil. Int J Cancer 2003; 106(4):553–8.
140. Kumar B, Cordell KG, Lee JS, et al. EGFR, p16, HPV Titer, Bcl-xL and p53, sex, and smoking as indicators of response to therapy and survival in oropharyngeal cancer. J Clin Oncol 2008;26(19):3128–37.

141. Fakhry C, Westra WH, Li S, et al. Improved survival of patients with human papillomavirus-positive head and neck squamous cell carcinoma in a prospective clinical trial. J Natl Cancer Inst 2008;100(4):261–9.
142. Rischin D, Young RJ, Fisher R, et al. Prognostic significance of p16INK4A and human papillomavirus in patients with oropharyngeal cancer treated on TROG 02.02 phase III trial. J Clin Oncol 2010;28(27):4142–8.
143. Posner MR, Lorch JH, Goloubeva O, et al. Survival and human papillomavirus in oropharynx cancer in TAX 324: a subset analysis from an international phase III trial. Ann Oncol 2011;22(5):1071–7.
144. Maxwell JH, Kumar B, Feng FY, et al. Tobacco use in human papillomavirus-positive advanced oropharynx cancer patients related to increased risk of distant metastases and tumor recurrence. Clinical cancer research : an official journal of the American Association for Cancer Research 2010;16(4):1226–35.
145. Mehanna H, Olaleye O, Licitra L. Oropharyngeal cancer—is it time to change management according to human papilloma virus status? Curr Opin Otolaryngol Head Neck Surg 2012;20(2):120–4.
146. Chaturvedi AK, Engels EA, Anderson WF, et al. Incidence trends for human papillomavirus-related and -unrelated oral squamous cell carcinomas in the United States. J Clin Oncol 2008;26(4):612–9.
147. Sturgis EM, Cinciripini PM. Trends in head and neck cancer incidence in relation to smoking prevalence: an emerging epidemic of human papillomavirus-associated cancers? Cancer 2007;110(7):1429–35.
148. Herrero R, Castellsague X, Pawlita M, et al. Human papillomavirus and oral cancer: the International Agency for Research on Cancer multicenter study. J Natl Cancer Inst 2003;95(23):1772–83.
149. Applebaum KM, Furniss CS, Zeka A, et al. Lack of association of alcohol and tobacco with HPV16-associated head and neck cancer. J Natl Cancer Inst 2007;99(23):1801–10.
150. Sugiyama M, Bhawal UK, Kawamura M, et al. Human papillomavirus-16 in oral squamous cell carcinoma: clinical correlates and 5-year survival. Br J Oral Maxillofac Surg 2007;45(2):116–22.
151. Kulkarni SS, Vastrad PP, Kulkarni BB, et al. Prevalence and distribution of high risk human papillomavirus (HPV) Types 16 and 18 in Carcinoma of cervix, saliva of patients with oral squamous cell carcinoma and in the general population in Karnataka, India. Asian Pac J Cancer Prev 2011;12(3):645–8.
152. da Silva CE, da Silva ID, Cerri A, et al. Prevalence of human papillomavirus in squamous cell carcinoma of the tongue. Oral Surg Oral Med Oral Pathol Oral Radiol Endod 2007;104(4):497–500.
153. Hammarstedt L, Lu Y, Marklund L, et al. Differential survival trends for patients with tonsillar, base of tongue and tongue cancer in Sweden. Oral Oncol 2011;47(7):636–41.
154. Nygard M, Aagnes B, Bray F, et al. Population-based evidence of increased survival in human papillomavirus-related head and neck cancer. Eur J Cancer 2012;48(9):1341–6.
155. Schwartz SR, Yueh B, McDougall JK, et al. Human papillomavirus infection and survival in oral squamous cell cancer: a population-based study. Otolaryngol Head Neck Surg 2001;125(1):1–9.
156. Zhao D, Xu QG, Chen XM, et al. Human papillomavirus as an independent predictor in oral squamous cell cancer. Int J Oral Sci 2009;1(3):119–25.

157. Duray A, Descamps G, Decaestecker C, et al. Human papillomavirus DNA strongly correlates with a poorer prognosis in oral cavity carcinoma. Laryngoscope 2012.
158. Harris SL, Thorne LB, Seaman WT, et al. Association of p16(INK4a) overexpression with improved outcomes in young patients with squamous cell cancers of the oral tongue. Head Neck 2011;33(11):1622–7.
159. Simonato LE, Garcia JF, Sundefeld ML, et al. Detection of HPV in mouth floor squamous cell carcinoma and its correlation with clinicopathologic variables, risk factors and survival. Journal of oral pathology & medicine : official publication of the International Association of Oral Pathologists and the American Academy of Oral Pathology 2008;37(10):593–8.
160. Ragin CC, Taioli E. Survival of squamous cell carcinoma of the head and neck in relation to human papillomavirus infection: review and meta-analysis. Int J Cancer 2007;121(8):1813–20.
161. Rose Ragin CC, Taioli E. Second primary head and neck tumor risk in patients with cervical cancer–SEER data analysis. Head Neck 2008;30(1):58–66.
162. Spitz MR, Sider JG, Schantz SP, et al. Association between malignancies of the upper aerodigestive tract and uterine cervix. Head Neck 1992;14(5):347–51.
163. McGovern SL, Williams MD, Weber RS, et al. Three synchronous HPV-associated squamous cell carcinomas of Waldeyer's ring: case report and comparison with Slaughter's model of field cancerization. Head Neck 2010;32(8):1118–24.
164. Bishop JA, Ogawa T, Chang X, et al. HPV analysis in distinguishing second primary tumors from lung metastases in patients with head and neck squamous cell carcinoma. Am J Surg Pathol 2012;36(1):142–8.
165. Umudum H, Rezanko T, Dag F, et al. Human papillomavirus genome detection by in situ hybridization in fine-needle aspirates of metastatic lesions from head and neck squamous cell carcinomas. Cancer 2005;105(3):171–7.
166. Miller AB, Hoogstraten B, Staquet M, et al. Reporting results of cancer treatment. Cancer 1981;47(1):207–14.
167. Eisenhauer EA, Therasse P, Bogaerts J, et al. New response evaluation criteria in solid tumours: revised RECIST guideline (version 1.1). Eur J Cancer 2009; 45(2):228–47.
168. Clark TG, Bradburn MJ, Love SB, et al. Survival analysis part I: basic concepts and first analyses. Br J Cancer 2003;89(2):232–8.
169. Satagopan JM, Ben-Porat L, Berwick M, et al. A note on competing risks in survival data analysis. Br J Cancer 2004;91(7):1229–35.
170. Clark TG, Bradburn MJ, Love SB, et al. Survival analysis part IV: further concepts and methods in survival analysis. Br J Cancer 2003;89(5):781–6.
171. Abrams J. Disease-free survival versus overall survival as a primary end point for adjuvant colon cancer studies: a commentary. J Clin Oncol 2005;23(34): 8564–5.
172. Machtay M, Glatstein E. Just another statistic. Oncologist 1998;3(3):III–IIV.
173. Iasonos A, Schrag D, Raj GV, et al. How to build and interpret a nomogram for cancer prognosis. J Clin Oncol 2008;26(8):1364–70.
174. Kattan MW. Nomograms are superior to staging and risk grouping systems for identifying high-risk patients: preoperative application in prostate cancer. Curr Opin Urol 2003;13(2):111–6.
175. de Cassia Braga Ribeiro K, Kowalski LP, Latorre Mdo R. Perioperative complications, comorbidities, and survival in oral or oropharyngeal cancer. Arch Otolaryngol Head Neck Surg 2003;129(2):219–28.

176. Paleri V, Wight RG, Davies GR. Impact of comorbidity on the outcome of laryngeal squamous cancer. Head Neck 2003;25(12):1019–26.
177. Ribeiro KC, Kowalski LP, Latorre MR. Impact of comorbidity, symptoms, and patients' characteristics on the prognosis of oral carcinomas. Arch Otolaryngol Head Neck Surg 2000;126(9):1079–85.
178. Borggreven PA, Kuik DJ, Langendijk JA, et al. Severe comorbidity negatively influences prognosis in patients with oral and oropharyngeal cancer after surgical treatment with microvascular reconstruction. Oral Oncol 2005;41(4):358–64.
179. Alho OP, Hannula K, Luokkala A, et al. Differential prognostic impact of comorbidity in head and neck cancer. Head Neck 2007;29(10):913–8.
180. Castro MA, Dedivitis RA, Ribeiro KC. Comorbidity measurement in patients with laryngeal squamous cell carcinoma. ORL J Otorhinolaryngol Relat Spec 2007;69(3):146–52.
181. Sanabria A, Carvalho AL, Vartanian JG, et al. Comorbidity is a prognostic factor in elderly patients with head and neck cancer. Ann Surg Oncol 2007;14(4):1449–57.
182. Gillison ML, Koch WM, Capone RB, et al. Evidence for a causal association between human papillomavirus and a subset of head and neck cancers. J Natl Cancer Inst 2000;92(9):709–20.
183. Weinberger PM, Yu Z, Haffty BG, et al. Prognostic significance of p16 protein levels in oropharyngeal squamous cell cancer. Clin Cancer Res 2004;10(17):5684–91.
184. Lassen P, Eriksen JG, Krogdahl A, et al. The influence of HPV-associated p16-expression on accelerated fractionated radiotherapy in head and neck cancer: evaluation of the randomised DAHANCA 6&7 trial. Radiother Oncol 2011;100(1):49–55.

Erratum

CORRECTION: In the June 2013 issue of Otolaryngologic Clinics of North America, in the article by Dr Malcolm Taw, Dr Chau Nguyen, and Dr Marilene Wang on Complementary and Integrative Treatments for Rhinosinusitis, a sentence in the summary section was intended to state: 'For example, Palmer[41] elegantly describes this transition whereby "generations of doctors and scientists were taught to envision bacteria as single cells that float or swim through some fluid... in fact, rhinologists continue to foster this view"; however, biofilms are not just single cells, but are structurally and metabolically heterogeneous multicellular communities.'[153]

This statement was misprinted as '... however, structured community of cells enclosed in a matrix of polysaccharides, nucleic acids, and proteins.'

Otolaryngol Clin N Am 46 (2013) 711
http://dx.doi.org/10.1016/j.otc.2013.07.002
0030-6665/13/$ – see front matter Published by Elsevier Inc.

Index

Note: Page numbers of article titles are in **boldface** type.

A

Age, effect of, on survivorship in cancers of head and neck, 682–683
Alcohol, and tobacco interaction, 508–509
  and tobacco use, effect on survivorship in cancers of head and neck, 688–689
  tobacco as risk factor independent of, 508
Anemia, inherited aplastic, Fanconi anemia as, 568

C

Cancer care, multidisciplinary treatment planning in, 675–676
  regionalization of, 676–677
  therapeutic standards for, 674
Cetuximab, concurrent with accelerated radiation therapy, in cancers of head and neck, 648–649
Chemoradiation, concurrent, versus induction chemotherapy, in cancer of head and neck, 652
  concurrent with radiation therapy, in squamous cell carcinomas of head and neck, 646–647
  in cancers of head and neck, 631
  in locally advanced oropharynngeal cancer, 646
  in resectable or unresectable cancers of head and neck, 646–647
Chemotherapy, in Fanconi anemia, 573
  induction, in cancer of head and neck, 649–652
    versus concurrent chemoradiation trial results, in cancer of head and neck, 652
    with taxane-containing regimens, in cancer of head and neck, 650–652
Cisplatin, high-dose, and concurrent radiation therapy, in cancers of head and neck, 647
Clinical practice guidelines, considerations for, 672–674
  definition of, 672
  for changing policy, 674
  importance of daily practice, 673
  role in quality assessment, 673–674

D

DNA in tumor tissue, human papillomavirus and, 512–513

E

Epidermal growth factor receptor, and squamous cell carcinoma of head and neck, 589–590
  inhibition of, radiation therapy and, 631–632

Otolaryngol Clin N Am 46 (2013) 713–718
http://dx.doi.org/10.1016/S0030-6665(13)00093-5 oto.theclinics.com

F

Fanconi anemia, and human papillomavirus, 570
as inherited aplastic anemia, 568
association with head and neck squamous cell carcinoma, 569–570
chemotherapy in, 573
clinical diagnosis of, 569
clinical outcomes/complications/concerns in, 573–574
genes implicated in, 568–569
graft-versus-host disease in, 574
hematopoietic stem cell transplantation and, 574
otolaryngologists awareness of, **567–577**
prognosis in, genotype as predictor of, 573
radiation therapy in, 572–573
risk for cancers in, 568
solid tumors in, 569
therapeutic options in, 570–573
Fluorodeoxyglucose positron emission tomography/computed tomography, for evaluation of squamous cell carcinoma of oral cavity, 608–609

G

Graft-versus-host disease, in Fanconi anemia, 574

H

Head and neck, cancers of, accelerated radiation therapy and hyperfractionation in, 647
adjuvant concurrent chemoradiation therapy in, 652–653
and human papillomavirus, limitations of studies on, 511
chemoprevention of, 580
chemoradiation in, 631
clinical decision making in, 699–700
disease-specific survival in, 698
high-dose cisplatin concurrent with radiation therapy in, 647
incidence of, 579
induction chemotherapy in, 649–652
versus concurrent chemoradiation trial results, 652
with taxane-containing regimens, 650–652
resectable or unresectable, chemoradiation in, 646–647
standardizing treatment of, **671–679**
survivorship in, competing mortalities, morbidities, and second malignancies and, **681–710**
effect of age on, 682–683
effect of alcohol and tobacco use on, 688–689
effect of body mass index and diet on, 689–690
effect of comorbodities and lifestyle behavior on, 685–689
effect of gender, partner status, and sociocultural factors on, 683–684
effect of quality of life on, 690
effect of race on, 684–685
effect of second primary malignancies on, 690–692
future issues in, 697–700
with concurrent cetuximab in, 648–449

squamous cell carcinoma of, altered gene expression profiles in, 557–559
altered genes in, 547–552
associated with Fanconi anemia, 569–570
causes of, 545
comparative genomic hybridization in, 552–555
cyclooxygenase inhibitors and, 588
effect of human papillomavirus infection on outcomes in, 692–697
epidermal growth factor receptor and, 589–590
epigenetic alterations in, 555–557
genetic alterations in, 546–555
genomics studies in, future goals for, 560–561
green tea polyphenols and, 588
implications for therapy in, 559–560
next-generation sequencing and, 546–547
oncogenes and, 549–552
P53-targeted agents and, 589
progression of, 546
promoter methylation in, 555–557
radiation therapy and concurrent chemoradiation in, 646–647
systemic treatment before, during, and after definitive treatment, **645–656**
thiazolidinediones and, 589
tumor suppressor genes and, 547–549
"Vogelgram" for, 580
Human papillomavirus, and cancers of head and neck, limitations of studies on, 511
and carcinogenesis, 523
and Fanconi anemia, 570
and oropharyngeal cancer, epidemiologic studies linking, 522–523
as cause of oropharyngeal cancer, 511
basics of, 522–523
Human papillomavirus-associated cancer epidemic, emergence of, 510–516
Human papillomavirus infection, and outcome of cancer of oral cavity, 695–696
effect on incidence of second primaries, 676–697
effect on outcome of oropharyngeal carcinoma, 693–695
effect on outcomes of squamous cell carcinoma of head and neck, 692–697
Human papillomavirus-positive and HPV-nagative cancers, exposures and biology associated with, 514
survival in, genomic differences and, 529
Human papillomavirus vaccination, 516–517
Hyperfractionation, and accelerated radiation therapy, in cancers of head and neck, 647

L

Laser microsurgery, transoral, in oropharyngeal cancers, 618–619, 623
Leukoplakia, oral, natural history and treatment of, 582–584
Lifestyle behavior, effect of, on survivorship in cancers of head and neck, 685–689
Lymph nodes, cervical, primary metastases to, radiation therapy for, 633

O

Oncogenes, and squamous cell carcinoma of head and neck, 549–552
Oral cavity, cancers of, and oropharyngeal cancer, survivors of, functional assessment and rehabilitation of, **657–670**

Oral (*continued*)
variation in burden, by country, 509–510
and pharyngeal cancers, tobacco as risk factor for, 508
functional outcomes of, 658–659
outcome in, human papillomavirus infection and, 695–696
posttreatment rehabilitation in, 663–665
pretreatment functional assessment in, 660–661
treatment of, preventing/reducing functional problems following, 662–663, 664
carcinomas of, and oropharyngeal carcinomas, epidemiology of, **507–520**
future burdens of, 517
squamous cell carcinomas of, and oropharyngeal squamous cll carcinoma, genomics of, **545–566**
and squamous cell carcinoma of oropharynx, evaluation and staging of, **599–613**
diagnosis and evaluation of, 600
direct transoral surgery in, 616
early stage, neck dissection in, 617
evaluation and staging of, novel approaches in, 607–609
FDG-PET/CT for, evaluation of, 608–609
genetic polymorphisms and, 585–586
incidence of, 615
loss of heterozygocity and, 585
mandibulotomy/mandiblectomy approach to, 616
molecular epidemiology of, 585–586
pharyngotomy approach to, 617
primary, secondary, and tertiary prevention for, 581–582
prognostic staging for, 602–603
screening for, 581
sentinel lymph node biopsy in, 607–608, 617–618
surgical interventions in, **615–628**
Oral premalignancy, **579–597**
chemoprevention of, 586
retinoids and, 586–588
Oropharyngeal cancers, and cancer of oral cavity, survivors of, functional assessment and rehabilitation of, **657–670**
variation in burden, by country, 509–510
biology of, and response to therapy, impact of human papillomavirus on, **521–543**
early T-category, radiation therapy for, 632
epidemiologic studies linking human papillomavirus to, 511–512
functional outcomes of, 659–660
human papillomavirus-associated, epidemic of, 514, 515
human papillomavirus-driven, survival for, 514–516
locally advanced, chemoradiation in, 646
surgical innovations in, 618–623
transoral laser microsurgery in, 618–619, 623
transoral robotic surgery in, 619
Oropharyngeal carcinoma, and oral cavity carcinomas, epidemiology of, **507–520**
future burdens of, 517
intensity-modulated proton therapy for, 636, 637, 638–639, 640–641
intensity-modulated radiation therapy for, 633–639
outcome of, effect of human papillomavirus infection on, 693–695

Oropharyngeal squamous cell carcinoma, and squamous cell carcinoma of oral cavity, evaluation and staging of, **599–613**
diagnosis and evaluation of, 601–602
direct transoral surgery in, 616
human papillomavirus-positive, clinical implications of, 523–525
clinical presentation of, 524
de-escalation of treatment, 523
and patient selection for, 535–539
induction chemotherapy in, 532
novel targeted therapies in, 533–535
prevention of, 524–525
status determination, 525
surgical alterations in, 533
survival benefit in, mechanisms of, 528–529
survival disparity in, 528
survival in, 525–528
treatment implications for, 529–532
treatment regimens in, 525–528
incidence of, 615
mandibulotomy/mandiblectomy approach to, 616
neck dissection and sentinel lymph node biopsy in, 617–618
pharyngotomy approach to, 617
prognostic staging for, 602, 603–606, 608
HPV status, 604
smoking status, 604–605, 606
survival stratification, 605
TNM staging, 603–604
surgical interventions in, **615–628**
Oropharyngeal tumors, fractionation radiation therapy in, 630–631
management of, advances in radiation oncology for, **629–643**

P

Pharyngeal cancers, and cancers of oral cavity, tobacco as risk factor for, 508
Proton therapy, intensity-modulated, for oropharyngeal carcinoma, 636, 637, 638–639, 640–641

R

Radiation oncology, advances in, for management of oropharyngeal tumors, **629–643**
Radiation therapy, accelerated, and hyperfraction, in cancers of head and neck, 647
concurrent with high-dose cisplatin, in cancers of head and neck, 647
epidermal growth factor receptor inhibition and, 631–632
for early T-category oropharyngeal cancer, 632
for primary metastases to cervical lymph nodes, 633
fractionation, in oropharyngeal tumors, 630–631
in Fanconi anemia, 572–573
intensity-modulated, for oropharyngeal carcinoma, 633–639
unilateral, for tonsillar carcinoma, 633, 634
with concurrent cetuximab, in cancers of head and neck, 648–649

Radiation (*continued*)
with concurrent chemoradiation, in squamous cell carcinomas of head and neck, 646–647
Retinoids, and oral premalignancy, 586–588
Robotic surgery, transoral, development of, 619–620
functional results of, 620, 621, 660
in oropharyngeal cancers, 619
oncologic results of, 620–623

S

Sentinel lymph node biopsy, in squamous cell carcinomas of oral cavity, 607–608, 617–618
Stem cell transplantation, hematopoietic, Fanconi anemia and, 574

T

Taxane-containing regimens, with induction chemotherapy, in cancer of head and neck, 650–652
Thiazolidinediones, and squamous cell carcinoma of head and neck, 589
Tobacco, and alcohol interaction, 508–509
and alcohol use, effect on survivorship in cancers of head and neck, 688–689
as risk factor for oral cavity and pharyngeal cancers, 508
as risk factor independent of alcohol, 508
Tobacco epidemic, evolution of, 507–510
variation by country, 509
Tonsillar carcinoma, unilateral radiation therapy for, 633, 634
Tumor suppressor genes, and squamous cell carcinoma of head and neck, 547–549

Printed and bound by CPI Group (UK) Ltd, Croydon, CR0 4YY
03/10/2024
01040478-0002